HEALTH PLANNING
Qualitative Aspects and Quantitative Techniques

THE JOHNS HOPKINS MONOGRAPHS IN INTERNATIONAL HEALTH

Health Manpower in a Developing Economy:
Taiwan, A Case Study in Planning
>by Timothy D. Baker and Mark Perlman (1967)

The Health Center Doctor in India
>by Harbans S. Takulia, Carl E. Taylor, S. Prakash Sangal, and Joseph D. Alter (1967)

Health Manpower Planning in Turkey:
An International Research Case Study
>by Carl E. Taylor, Rahmi Dirican, and Kurt W. Dueschle (1968)

Health and Disease in Four Peruvian Villages:
Contrasts in Epidemiology
>by Alfred A. Buck, Tom T. Sasaki, and Robert I. Anderson (1968)

Health Manpower in Peru:
A Case Study in Planning
>by Thomas L. Hall (1969)

Health and Disease in Chad:
Epidemiology, Culture, and Environment in Five Villages
>by Alfred A. Buck, Robert I. Anderson, Tom T. Sasaki, and Kazuyoshi Kawata (1970)

Health and Disease in Rural Afghanistan
>by Alfred A. Buck, Robert I. Anderson, Kazuyoshi Kawata, I. Willard Abrahams, Ronald A. Ward, and Tom T. Sasaki (1972)

Health Planning: Qualitative
Aspects and Quantitative Techniques
>edited by William A. Reinke assisted by Kathleen N. Williams (1972)

HEALTH PLANNING
Qualitative Aspects and Quantitative Techniques

Edited by William A. Reinke

Assisted by Kathleen N. Williams

The Johns Hopkins University
School of Hygiene and Public Health
Department of International Health
Baltimore, Maryland
1972

Support for the preparation of this volume was provided by the United States
Agency for International Development. Information and conclusions in the book
do not necessarily reflect the position of the Agency or the United States
Government. The United States Government retains an irrevocable right to
reproduce this publication in whole or in part.

Composed and Printed by the Waverly Press, Inc.
Baltimore, Maryland 21202

Table of Contents

Preface

While dedicated effort continues to enlarge the body of medical knowledge, a growing number of voices are being raised to express concern that the existing knowledge be used effectively to make quality health care generally available. In the health field, the gap between what is scientifically and technologically possible and what is actually being accomplished is very disturbing—all the more so when health care is proclaimed to be a right instead of a privilege and when those who need the services take the proclamation seriously, for the economic and social cost of an imperfect and inefficient fulfillment of that right is tremendous.

As a result, we are witnessing accelerated interest in the application of modern management methods to health services, systematic appraisal of health care systems and their components, and rational planning to allocate scarce health resources efficiently according to accepted priorities.

As the need for planning becomes more generally appreciated, troublesome questions are raised concerning the nature of this planning. On the one hand, the growing body of available quantitative techniques suggests that planning can and should be a straightforward, systematic assessment of the benefits and costs (monetary and otherwise) associated with alternative approaches. On the other hand, in recognition of the political, social, and cultural realities of a given planning environment we are forced to admit that many policies, priorities, and courses of action are the result of subjective considerations that defy tidy methodological packaging. To the question of whether health planning is art or science, we can answer only that it contains ingredients of both; hopefully, with the passage of time, it will contain more of the latter and less of the former.

Comprehensive health planning is broad in scope, not only with respect to the services covered, but also in terms of the variables to be considered and the methods to be employed. As a minimum the planner must cope with demographic and epidemiologic variables, with human, physical, and financial resources, and with the disciplines of economics, sociology, political science, statistics, and operations research. The literature in any one of these fields is voluminous, and to keep abreast of developments in all of them is impossible. Moreover, most of the literature is not addressed specifically to the matter of health planning. The resulting need for a concise, integrated, multidisciplinary digest of planning methodology seems obvious.

This need has become particularly obvious in the course of our experience at Johns Hopkins University with an educational program in comprehensive health planning. A large proportion of the participants in this program are practical administrators without recent formal training in the various disciplines in question. Yet we take care not to spend excessive time in remedial teaching. Our program is built around small group workshops in which the students actually participate in the planning process. Under such circumstances, they come to recognize the extent to which planning can be methodical and to apply the methods at their command. Thus, a digest of health planning concepts and methods is essential for the participants in order that they may get to the practice of planning quickly, but knowledgeably. Hopefully, this volume will serve the same purpose for others engaged in planning at various levels.

The material covered herein is extensive, although obviously not exhaustive. For this reason, we make extensive use of associated reading lists. Annotated primary readings are cited for each of the topical areas with the aim of guiding the reader to the minimum body of information required for a reasonably comprehensive understanding of the subject in question. For the reader interested in broader and deeper insights, secondary reading lists are provided, as well as a listing of bibliographies on various aspects of health planning.

The book is divided into four parts. Part I provides an introduction and places the planning process in some perspective. Part II emphasizes the various aspects of information gathering which form the health planning base. Part III deals with specific methods of analyzing and synthesizing the component sets of information. Since the first three parts are especially relevant to planning for personal health care services, Part IV considers the special features of mental health, environmental health, and population planning.

A volume such as this requires a number of authors with individual areas of expertise but with a common background of experience and competence in the teaching and practice of health planning. Those who have contributed herein meet these qualifications and we are grateful indeed for their generous support in the writing. They in turn are each indebted for the counsel of others too numerous to mention. Four individuals must be given special recognition, however, for their long-standing guidance and support of health planning in general and this volume in particular: Drs. Carl E. Taylor, Timothy D. Baker, Ernest L. Stebbins, and John C. Hume.

William A. Reinke
Editor

Baltimore
January, 1972

List of Contributors

Unless otherwise noted, the contributors to this volume listed below are members of the faculty of The Johns Hopkins University School of Hygiene and Public Health

Timothy D. Baker, M.D., M.P.H. Assistant Dean and Professor of International Health and Public Health Administration

Philip D. Bonnet, M.D. Professor of Medical Care and Hospitals

Margaret Bright, Ph.D. Professor of Epidemiology and Behavioral Sciences

Thomas L. Hall, M.D., Dr.P.H. Deputy Director, Carolina Population Center, University of North Carolina, Chapel Hill, North Carolina

M. Alfred Haynes, M.D., M.P.H. Professor and Chairman, Department of Community Medicine, Charles R. Drew Postgraduate Medical School, Los Angeles, California

Cornelius W. Krusé, Dr.P.H. Professor and Chairman, Department of Environmental Health

Paul V. Lemkau, M.D. Professor and Chairman, Department of Mental Hygiene

Wallace Mandell, Ph.D., M.P.H. Professor of Mental Hygiene

Vicente Navarro, M.D., Dr.P.H. Associate Professor of Medical Care and Hospitals and International Health

William A. Reinke, Ph.D. Professor of International Health, Public Health Administration, Biostatistics, and Medical Care and Hospitals

A. Peter Ruderman, Ph.D. Lecturer in International Health; Professor of Health Administration, University of Toronto School of Hygiene, Toronto, Canada

Ernest L. Stebbins, M.D., M.P.H. Dean Emeritus and Professor of Public Health Administration and International Health

Carl E. Taylor, M.D., Dr.P.H. Professor and Chairman, Department of International Health

Kathleen N. Williams, M.A. Research Assistant, Department of International Health

I

Planning in Perspective

History and Background of Health Planning in the United States

ERNEST L. STEBBINS and KATHLEEN N. WILLIAMS

HEALTH PLANNING THROUGH VOLUNTARY EFFORTS

In the United States, efforts at health planning until quite recently were either decentralized to state or local governments or initiated by private or nongovernmental agencies. Most frequently these planning efforts were disease-oriented, i.e., categorical approaches directed toward specific health problems. Consider, for example, the work of the National Tuberculosis Association, which was established at the beginning of the twentieth century. A nationwide network of voluntary health workers under the guidance of a central organization dramatized the problem of tuberculosis in the nation and stimulated the development of programs in state or local governmental agencies for prevention and treatment of that disease.

This pattern of health planning and program development has been followed by a number of voluntary agencies, such as the American Cancer Society, American Public Health Association, National Foundation for Infantile Paralysis, and a host of others. An effort was made to coordinate the activities of these voluntary health agencies and to achieve some degree of comprehensive planning by the creation of the National Health Council, which provided a means of communication among these various organizations and afforded limited coordination of their activities.

The first serious effort at health manpower planning was a study of medical education in the United States and Canada conducted by Abraham Flexner, which clearly focused attention upon the need for adequately trained physicians and revealed the sad state of medical education at the time (1). This report had a major influence on the establishment of standards of medical education and the improvement of physician training and education in the United States.

The economic crisis and the Great Depression of the late 1920's and early 1930's focused attention upon the rising costs of medical care and the inequities of the distribution of health and medical services in the nation. In its 1933 report, the Committee on the Cost of Medical Care dramatized the serious

3

deficiencies in the existing system of personal health services (2). This study clearly demonstrated the inability of a large proportion of the population to obtain high-quality medical care because of the rising cost of these services. Recommendations of the Committee included proposals for prepayment systems for medical care needs, and they undoubtedly were at least partially responsible for the introduction of proposed legislation for compulsory health insurance (the Wagner Bill, introduced in the late 1930's) and the health provisions of the Social Security Act of 1935.

During this same period, a joint committee of the American Public Health Association and the National Health Council, chaired by Dr. Haven Emerson, carried out a study of the provision of full-time local health services in the nation. The findings and recommendations of this committee were not released for publication until the end of World War II, at which time the report, which came to be known as the Emerson Report, was published (3). Because of the conservatism of the committee, recommendations were limited to the then-accepted traditional public health services—environmental sanitation, communicable disease control, maternal and child heath, vital statistics, and public health laboratory services. This report set minimal standards for full-time, local health services, based upon the very limited scope of activity then generally accepted, and made the grievous error of stating these minimal standards in terms of number of health personnel per population unit and per capita expenditure. In the rapidly expanding field of public health, these minimum standards were inadequate almost before they were promulgated.

During this same period, the New York Academy of Medicine undertook an ambitious study of the problems of provision of personal health and medical services under the theme of "Medicine in the Changing Order." This project, guided by a distinguished committee of physicians and staffed by a highly-qualified, multidisciplinary group of experts, analyzed and further defined the problems of provision of quality medical care to the total population. Because of the highly controversial issues then being debated, however, no startling new proposals came out of this learned dissertation (10 volumes), and the report had little impact on health planning in the nation (4).

Aging of the population, with its associated increase in chronic illness, was recognized as a major and expanding problem of medical care during the 1950's. Under the auspices of the American Medical Association, the American Hospital Association, and the American Public Health Association, a Commission on Chronic Illness was established to carry out a detailed study of the extent and nature of chronic illness in the nation. Although sponsored by three professional organizations, the Commission was unique in that it included a broad representation of consumer groups including organized labor, industry, commercial insurance interests, and the general public. An exhaustive five-year study led to a voluminous report which contributed greatly to existing knowledge about the problem of caring for the chronically ill (5).

Unfortunately, conflicting interests and minority opinions expressed by commission members weakened the impact of recommendations and hampered implementation of proposed plans.

National Commision on Community Health Services

The most recent, largely voluntarily supported, national effort at comprehensive health planning was the National Commission on Community Health Services. This Commission was created under the sponsorship of the American Public Health Association and the National Health Council and was financed by both private foundations and the United States Public Health Service and the Vocational Rehabilitation Administration. It carried out a four-year study of community health needs and existing services with the stated purpose of developing a blueprint for a system of preventive and curative medical services and environmental health protection for the next decade. The Commission consisted of a mixture of health professionals and representatives of organized labor, industry, and the community at large. Its work was carried out through three major projects: a National Task Forces project, a Community Action Studies project, and a Communications project.

The *Task Forces* project consisted of six groups dealing with environmental health, comprehensive personal health services, health manpower, health care facilities, financing of health services and facilities, and organization of community health services. Each task force was made up of approximately 15 recognized leaders in its particular field of study, who were charged with studying the problem and making recommendations for the development and improvement of health services for the next decade. The task forces were given a high degree of autonomy, and their recommendations, while obviously influencing the Commission's report, were published unmodified and unedited as individual task force reports (6-11).

The *Community Action Studies* project guided the development of detailed studies in 21 communities throughout the United States (12). The communities selected for self-study, while not strictly a cross-section of the country, did include different geographical regions and areas of differing population density and differing socioeconomic conditions. Each community established a broadly representative advisory group responsible for the study and for the subsequent findings and recommendations in important problem areas. The findings of the Task Forces project and the Community Action Studies project formed the basis for the deliberations of the National Commission and the development of its recommendations.

The *Communications* project was an effort to test public reaction to the findings of the various task forces and the community studies. Nearly a year before the conclusion of the Commission's report, four regional conferences were held, in San Francisco, Chicago, Atlanta, and Philadelphia. Each of these conferences was attended by approximately 300 representatives of all segments of the population, including labor, industry, professionals, and community leaders, in approximately equal proportions.

The report of the Commission was published in early 1966 (13). Its recommendations and those of the six task forces dealt with almost every phase of community health services. Many of its recommendations have already been implemented through legislation or administrative action. Its most significant recommendations were that community health services need greater federal participation and that comprehensive health planning must take place on a continuing basis. The Commission assumed that high-quality personal health services and a healthy environment were civic rights and that government at all levels, together with nongovernmental agencies and private citizens, had a responsibility to provide, within the limits of their resources, superior community health services.

The Commission recognized that existing political boundaries and local autonomy represent major obstacles to comprehensive health planning and the development of excellent community health services. The Commission also enunciated the concept of the "problem shed" and the need for a mechanism for dealing with health problems by a combination of political subdivisions representing the "community of solution." It recognized that the "community of solution" might differ from one health problem to another and recommended regional or areawide planning bodies corresponding to the problem areas. In the provision of personal health services, the Commission recommended a "single system," eventually combining into one system of medical service all of the many and fragmented programs of both the public and private sector.

HEALTH PLANNING IN THE NATIONAL GOVERNMENT
Presidential Commissions

Health Needs of the Nation

In 1951, the President of the United States appointed a Commission on the Health Needs of the Nation, which was broadly representative of the health professions and also of consumers, particularly organized labor and industry. The Commission gathered detailed information concerning available health services, facilities, and manpower and their adequacy to meet health needs, and assembled panels of experts to explore health needs and the extent to which these needs were being met. It also held open hearings to determine consumer opinion as to the adequacy of existing programs and services. The Commission compiled a voluminous report, known as the Magnuson Report, which contained previously unavailable information clearly identifying deficiencies in existing systems (14). The report also provided important recommendations for the correction of the deficiencies with major federal participation in financing more adequate services and facilities; however, as it was published shortly before a change in administration, it had little impact on the new administration or the Congress.

Heart Disease, Cancer, and Stroke

In February of 1963, President Kennedy appointed a Commission on Heart Disease, Cancer, and Stroke "to recommend steps to reduce the incidence of these diseases through new knowledge and more complete utilization of the medical knowledge we already have." The Commission was made up of approximately 30 prominent citizens, predominantly specialists in one of the three specified diseases. It gathered much information concerning the extent of the problems and the existence of services and facilities to care for individuals suffering from heart disease, cancer, and stroke. This information was obtained from approximately 50 professional organizations in the health field and from several hundred individuals, again primarily specialists in one of these three diseases.

In a surprisingly short time (about seven months), the Commission published a two-volume report with some major recommendations and certain legislative proposals, some of which were not directly related to the specific charge of the Commission (15). Among the important recommendations was the establishment of a nationwide network of Regional Medical Programs, based in medical schools or medical centers and related to satellite centers in community hospitals and through them to practicing physicians, which would provide exemplary care for victims of heart disease, cancer, and stroke, or "related diseases." With almost unprecedented speed, the recommendations were enacted into law (as the Heart Disease, Cancer, and Stroke Amendments of 1965), and the Regional Medical Programs were authorized.

Significant Legislation

Hill-Burton Act

In 1946, Congress enacted the Hospital Survey and Construction Act (Hill-Burton Act, P.L. 79-725) to provide federal aid to states for hospital facilities. An important condition of this legislation was that each state create a Hospital Planning Council, charged with the responsibility for assessing the need for new hospital construction (according to a prescribed formula of hospital beds per population unit). Each state's planning council was required to submit a plan detailing the appropriate priorities for meeting these needs. Annual revision of the plans was mandatory.

Amendments to the Act in 1954 broadened the scope of the program to include nursing homes, rehabilitation facilities, chronic disease facilities, and diagnostic or treatment centers. The most far-reaching revisions to the basic law came in 1964 with the passage of the Hospital and Medical Facilities Amendments (Hill-Harris Act, P.L. 88-443), which established a new grant program setting aside funds exclusively for modernization or replacement of both public and nonprofit private hospitals and other facilities. This resulted in a sharp increase in the percentage of projects for additions, alterations, and replacements, and shifted the emphasis from rural to urban hospital needs.

To reflect the changes required under the terms of the Hill-Harris amendments, three new state plan procedures were adopted. First, minimim and uniform national standards for assessing the physical condition of hospitals were put into effect. Second, bed capacity was now to be measured on the basis of newly-established square footage minimums. Third, a new formula for assessing bed need was developed, incorporating previous utilization data, projected population estimates, and a desirable occupancy factor. Since 1962, planning, rather than construction *per se*, has been stressed, as funds became available for regional planning of hospital and other health facilities through Hill-Burton channels.

Since its inception, Hill-Burton program planning has provided over 10,000 projects in 50 states and territories. Federal funds obligated to these projects came to more than $3.7 billion, or roughly one-third their total cost ($12 billion). By 1969, almost 470,000 in-patient beds had been provided in approved projects, almost 75 percent of them in general hospitals. In addition, out-patient facilities in approved projects (exclusive of those connected with general hospitals) totaled more than 2,700, of which nearly 50 percent were public health centers (16).

The Hospital Planning Councils created through this legislation have been among the more active planning institutions in the health field in the United States over the past quarter century. The Hill-Burton program has introduced systematic statewide planning, established minimum standards, and improved the quality of health care in rural America. It has also been criticized for focusing too narrowly on hospital construction alone and for failing to encourage or initiate more sophisticated plans for the organization and distribution of health care services (17). New amendments to the Public Health Service Act in the mid-1960's have attempted to compensate for these deficiencies, with mixed results.

Regional Medical Programs

Legislative action growing out of the work of the President's Commission on Heart Disease, Cancer, and Stroke resulted in 1965 in a significant amendment (P.L. 89-239) to the Public Health Service Act. Regionalization was the basic tenet of this new program, and "cooperative regional arrangements" were to be organized from *existing* medical centers, clinical research centers, and hospitals (18). Unlike other major health legislation, the regions envisaged by the Regional Medical Programs Act were not necessarily to be considered coterminous with state boundaries, and in fact only one-half of the 56 regions are statewide. The remainder are divided between areawide and multistate regions.

The initial scope of this program covered only heart disease, cancer, stroke, and related diseases. A subsequent amendment in 1970 (P.L. 91-515) greatly expanded the program by specifically including kidney diseases and all other major diseases and conditions (19). Although the basic format of RMP remains categorical, a shift in emphasis to diversified health delivery systems has taken place, especially with respect to the recent development of Health Maintenance Organizations (HMO's) (20). This same amendment also extended the program to include prevention and rehabilitation in addition to diagnosis and treatment.

Local participation, especially of health care providers, in planning is a second basic feature of the Regional Medical Program. This emphasis on local representation and areawide planning signified an important departure from past health legislation, as it attempted to elicit workable plans and projects from sources outside the usual official state or federal agencies. To this end, Regional Advisory Councils have been created in all 56 regions, charged with the responsibility for evaluating the over-all health care needs within each region. These advisory groups are obliged to include provider representatives from state and local health departments, medical schools in the region, teaching hospitals, practicing physicians, and other general public organizations, and are required to assess and approve all project applications before they are submitted to the 20-member National Advisory Council, which has the ultimate responsibility of recommending approval or disapproval of funding.

A third feature of the RMP is the dual nature of the funding mechanism—namely, a planning phase and an operational phase. The first fiscal year of the RMP saw planning grants approved for only seven programs. By 1971, however, planning grants for all 56 regions had been awarded, covering 100 percent of the United States population. Once regions had been awarded planning grants, they were able to apply for funds to cover operating expenses of all projects in their jurisdiction. By 1971, 55 regions were operational, and the one remaining was expected to be so within the next year. The bulk of the operational projects initially was devoted to continuing education and training but the functional emphasis has shifted to organization and delivery for patient services and improvement of manpower productivity and distribution. Such projects have been primarily for either heart disease or some combination of all diseases covered by the legislation, although support for programs in cancer and kidney diseases has grown. The emphasis on planning has not been downgraded, however. Continued planning and evaluation are considered integral parts of RMP, and as a result all projects are granted monies to carry out further planning activities.

Although these features—regionalization, local participation, and funding for both planning and operations—are considered notable manifestations of progress in federal health planning legislation, some drawbacks to the Regional Medical Programs have become increasingly troublesome as the program moves into its seventh year. Many projects have been criticized as being too fragmented and insufficiently incorporated into an over-all regional plan, thereby casting doubt on the wisdom of such decentralization of planning efforts. Also, substantial surpluses of funds in the early years of the program, resulting from unspent appropriations, led to Congressional questioning of new budgetary requests for RMP (and, by extension, of other health programs as well). For example, funds authorized in the first four fiscal years of the program totaled $405 million ($50 million in 1966, $90 million in 1967, $200 million in 1968, and $65 million in 1969), but the 55 regions had received only $145 million in both planning and operational grants (19). This underspending played a part in decreased funding for RMP just at the point when the program might have developed significant, large-scale projects in health care services and planning which could have served as models for the entire country.

Finally, the emphasis on the direct federal-regional relationship means that RMP projects have not easily been incorporated into or dovetailed with already existing federal or state programs (or vice versa), leading to both duplications and gaps in health care delivery, health manpower education and training, and research. One contribution that the Comprehensive Health Planning amendment to the Public Health Service Act may make to health planning in the United States—which the Regional Medical Programs are not in a position to make—is to function as a means for the various federal, state, and regional programs to be brought together in a more coordinated health care system.

Comprehensive Health Planning Act

The purpose of the Comprehensive Health Planning Act (P.L. 89-749) of 1966, as stated in the preamble to the act, was to promote comprehensive planning for health services, manpower, and facilities at every level of government, primarily through a strengthening of leadership and capacities of state health agencies (21). This legislation (known widely as the Partnership for Health Act) and its 1967 amendments (P.L. 90-174) authorized the disbursement of federal funds through five separate mechanisms:

(a) formula grants to a single state agency for planning (with amounts to be determined on the basis of state population and per capita income);

(b) project grants for the development of regional or local health plans and coordination of existing and planned health services, manpower, and facilities;

(c) project grants for training and education in health planning;

(d) formula grants to state health and mental health authorities for public health services (again based on population and per capita income); and

(e) project grants for health services development.

The project grants in all cases may be awarded only to those programs drawn up in accordance with plans developed by the State Health Planning Agency, in order to assure coordination of state and local planning efforts. In contrast to the original Regional Medical Programs, however, the project grants are not restricted to specific (disease) categorical programs, in order to encourage the more flexible use of funds and promote a *general* strengthening of state and local health services (17).

The Partnership for Health law calls for each state to establish a single adminstrative agency, known as the "a" agency, for all CHP activities within its borders, to appoint an advisory State Health Planning Council, and to develop an over-all state plan which encompasses the state and local activities to be funded. CHP "b" agencies include public or private organizations at the local or areawide (often multicounty) level which undertake both comprehensive planning and specific projects for their particular regions. As of 1971, approximately 160 grants had been approved for areawide health planning under the auspices of Section 314(b) of the law. The state "a" agency is not responsible for detailed planning, but rather is expected to review, coordinate, and supervise efforts undertaken by community, areawide, and other state planning groups (i.e., the "b" agencies) and to encourage cooperation among all private and public agencies and organizations concerned with health services, manpower, and facilities. The "a" agencies are charged with the ultimate responsibility for approval of areawide planning and the final authority for approval or disapproval rests with the "a" agency insofar as "b" agency program development is concerned. Despite this concentration of responsibility at the state level, there is a specific emphasis in the CHP program on improving health planning and health services at the community level, in that the state is required to provide satisfactory assurance to the federal government that funds will be used to strengthen services and agencies in the various political subdivisions.

Project grants to CHP "c" agencies, which now number about 23 university-based training programs, are intended to improve health planning skills among health professionals, other professional and lay groups, and consumers. Specifically, these training programs seek to provide the manpower and planning expertise needed on the staffs of the "a" and "b" agencies. Funds for these educational programs are granted directly to the sponsoring agencies. This particular section of the CHP Act has not received as much attention or money as have the programs of the "a" and "b" agencies and, in fact, runs some risk of being cut off completely as funds are diverted to newer projects such as Health Maintenance Organizations (HMO's).

One striking component of the CHP legislation is its concern with consumer participation. A majority of the membership of the State Planning Council must be composed of consumer representatives broadly reflecting public and private interests and all geographic and socioeconomic groups. In addition, widespread and active consumer participation in the development and operation of projects supported by CHP funds is called for, including programs for the training of consumers for their role in comprehensive health planning.

To balance the consumer viewpoint in CHP agencies, representatives from Regional Medical Programs are required on both CHP "a" and "b" agency councils. Since all CHP statewide agencies include at least part of one RMP, cooperation is fostered between the two programs through interlocking board and committee memberships; through joint studies, data banks, and other complementary activities; and through cooperative channels for review of RMP grant proposals by CHP agencies (20).

Planning under CHP auspices has tended to focus on facilities and/or manpower. With regard to the former, "a" and "b" agencies have developed standards and guidelines to be used in planning new facilities or renovating or relocating existing facilities. A number of states have established a review system, so that proposals for new facilities (or changes in present facilities) can be evaluated in terms of local needs and over-all community health plans. Bilateral or multilateral agreements among health facilities and institutions are specifically approved as a means of providing efficient and economical services. To monitor and control the development of health facilities, some states (e.g., New York and California) have granted a franchising authority to allow or disallow applications for building or expanding hospitals, opening new clinics, and so forth. Other states (e.g., Maryland) utilize the licensure authority within the "a" agency to control the nature and development of new health facilities. This is done by means of the "certification of need" program, which specifies that all newly proposed hospitals and nonprofit related institutions must conform to areawide plans before the institutions can be licensed to operate. Both "a" and "b" agencies are to help the facilities in determining whether the proposed location and/or services will contribute positively to meeting the needs of the population in the area in question (22, 23).

Section 314 (e) of the Partnership for Health Act has been used in the past year or so to promote the idea of Health Maintenance Organizations (HMO's) until such time as legislation directly pertaining to the concept may be passed. The objectives of HMO's have been summarized as follows: (1) to provide alternatives to the present fee for service, private practice health system in the United States; (2) to promote greater efficiency and better quality control within the system; (3) to improve the distribution of health services in both rural and urban areas, and among the poor, the medically indigent, and the more affluent; (4) to bring about some control on spiraling costs; and (5) to provide incentives for health maintenance rather than purely curative medicine (24).

The concept of HMO's has been fostered in part by the success of some longstanding pioneer prepaid group health organizations, such as Kaiser-Permanente and the Health Insurance Plan of New York, but HMO's have several basic features which distinguish them from previous types of health organizations. First, it is an *organized system,* including both facilities and manpower, which takes on the responsibility for providing directly or otherwise assuring the availability of a range of health services (not just ensuring payment for such services if the patient can secure them). Second, these health services shall encompass a *comprehensive set of maintenance and treatment activities,* including primary and emergency care, acute and chronic in-patient care, and rehabilitation, which has been agreed upon between the providers and consumers. The third feature is an *enrolled population,* i.e., individuals or groups who voluntarily elect to join the HMO through a formal contractual arrangement for a stated time period. The contract also specifies that the enrollee will use the HMO as his main source of health care. The fourth element is the basic *financial plan* through which prenegotiated and fixed payments are made in advance on a periodic basis (specified in the contract) on behalf of the individual or family enrolled in the HMO. Implicit in this arrangement is an incentive to the HMO to keep its clients healthy and to treat illness early, in order to keep costs down by minimizing the use of relatively expensive procedures and other costly resources (25). Finally, a *managing organization* will serve to assure fiscal, legal, public, and professional accountability. This management organization may be any of a variety of groups, including insurance companies, medical groups or societies, hospitals, or consumer groups (26).

Federal legislation on HMO's has been proposed through several channels, including both direct Congressional proposals and options under Medicare or under the still-to-be-considered National Health Insurance Standards Act. Some $23 million has been requested for the first fiscal year to underwrite the initial developmental costs of about 100 HMO's. An additional $22 million has been asked for to cover the operating costs of HMO's located in medically underserved areas (24). The target by the mid-1970's is some 1,700 HMO's serving possibly one-fifth of the United States population; by the end of the decade, the goal is a sufficient number of HMO's to cover 90 percent of the population (26).

Health Manpower Planning

Planning for health manpower by official governmental agencies and by professional groups, foundations, and other unofficial agencies in the United States dates back at least to the Flexner Report of 1910 (1). Health manpower planning, like other health planning in the United States, has rarely been comprehensive in nature. It has usually dealt with one profession at a time and has not had close linkages among plan recommendations, implementation, and evaluation. Early planning efforts include the Lee-Jones study (27), a part of the Commission on Medical Care of the early 1930's.

During World War II health manpower, like all manpower, assumed great importance as men were diverted from the civilian population to the armed forces overseas. Both the United States Public Health Service and the American Medical Association engaged in health manpower planning to help ensure civilian coverage (28-30).

Increasing public concern over the lack of physicians in the 1950's led the Surgeon General to appoint a special consultant group on medical education, chaired by Frank Bane with William Stewart as Chief of Study Staff. The report of this Commission (*Physicians for a Growing America,* or the Bane Report) recommended major increases in the number of physicians trained in the United States by increasing the size of classes and by creating new medical schools (31). (Plans for dental manpower were also briefly discussed.) Through the provision of larger amounts of federal funding, new schools were created and enrollment in many existing schools was expanded. In fact, implementation of the Commission's recommendations was so effective that in 1968 the Committee's goal of 330,000 physicians by 1975 was exceeded (32).

In 1966, problems of skyrocketing health costs and implementation of Medicare and Medicaid led President Johnson to establish the National Advisory Commission on Health Manpower to develop recommendations for action by government and private institutions for improving the availability and utilization of health manpower. This Commission prepared an extensive two-volume report on all types of health professionals, as well as covering the effect of health care systems on productivity (33). Although the report stressed efficiency, use of ancillary personnel, and quality of health professional training in health manpower planning, the stated shortage of 50,000 physicians was given the greatest attention by the news media and legislators.

Implementation of this report came first in the form of the Health Manpower Act of 1968 (P.L. 90-490), which covered both Health Professions Training (Title I) and Nurses Training (Title II). Federal funds were to be disbursed through construction grants, grants directly to health training institutions (partly on the basis of increased enrollment), special project grants, and student loans and scholarships. Titles III and IV extended appropriations for the Allied Health Professions Program and Health Research Facilities, respectively.

Another health manpower planning program during the 1960's was the Task Force on Health Manpower of the National Commission on Community Health Services (described earlier). The report of this Task Force, like that of the National Advisory Commission, covered all types of health manpower and stressed quality, education, recruitment, and the administration and organization of services as a basis for improvement of health manpower productivity (8).

The most recent efforts in health manpower planning in the United States have led to the Comprehensive Health Manpower Training Act of 1971 (P.L. 92-157). Implementation of this legislation provides direct support for the costs of education in the health professions, backed by an authorization of $2.8 billion extending through fiscal 1974.

Nursing concern for planning for personnel to meet the needs of society has a long history. The Bane Report had been antedated by the National League of Nursing report, *Nurses for a Growing Nation,* by two years (34). In the early 1960's, at the time the recommendations of the Bane Report were implemented, the Surgeon General formed a consulting group on nursing headed by Lucile Petry Leone which presented a plan outlining the needs and goals for nursing in the United States (35). Planning for nursing has been greatly aided by the work of the American Nurses' Association in their collection of data on nurse manpower (36).

Allied health professions were given a substantial boost with the passage of the Health Training Improvement Act of 1970 (P.L. 91-519), which authorized funds for construction of teaching facilities, grants to upgrade the quality of training (especially through special projects for experimentation, demonstration, and basic institutional improvement), scholarships and loans, and work study programs. One section calls for projects aimed at identifying potential allied health personnel who might otherwise be lost to the professions due to financial, educational, or cultural needs and assisting them to complete an appropriate training program. Returning veterans of the United States armed forces are specifically noted in this regard.

National planning efforts in health manpower in the United States have been supplemented by regional planning efforts, such as those by WICHE for the Western Region and for the Upper Midwest by a special health manpower study commission headed by Osler Peterson (37, 38). There have also been state studies such as those in Maryland by the State Planning Commission and the Council for Higher Education (39, 40). Most state or regional studies emphasize the difficulty of planning for health manpower at less than a national level, because of the uncertainties of interstate migration of health professionals.

In summary, there have been numerous planning efforts in health manpower in the United States. In general, early efforts were fragmentary and lacked direct links among planning, implementation, and evaluation. Despite this, over the long run educational institutions have responded to society's needs (as expressed in the various planning documents) by either improving the quality of professionals or increasing their quantity through expanded enrollment and new institutions.

References

1. Flexner, Abraham. *Medical Education in the United States and Canada.* New York: The Carnegie Foundation for the Advancement of Teaching, 1910.
2. Falk, I. S., Rorem, C. R., and Ring, M. D. *The Costs of Medical Care.* Chicago: University of Chicago Press, 1933.
3. Emerson, Haven. *Local Health Units for the Nation.* A Report for the American Public Health Association, Committee on Administrative Practice, Subcommittee on Local Health Units. New York: The Commonwealth Fund, 1945.
4. New York Academy of Medicine. *Medicine in the Changing Order.* New York: The Commonwealth Fund, 1947.
5. Commission on Chronic Illness. *Chronic Illness in the United States.* Volumes 1-4. Cambridge: Harvard University Press, 1956-1959.
6. National Commission on Community Health Services. *Changing Environmental Hazards: Challenges to Community Health.* Report of the

Task Force on Environmental Health. Washington, D.C.: Public Affairs Press, 1967.

7. National Commission on Community Health Services. *Comprehensive Health Care: A Challenge to American Communities*. Report of the Task Force on Comprehensive Personal Health Services. Washington, D.C.: Public Affairs Press, 1967.

8. National Commission on Community Health Services. *Health Manpower: Action to Meet Community Needs*. Report of the Task Force on Health Manpower. Washington, D.C.: Public Affairs Press, 1967.

9. National Commission on Community Health Services. *Health Care Facilities: The Community Bridge to Effective Health Services*. Report of the Task Force on Health Care Facilities. Washington, D.C.: Public Affairs Press, 1967.

10. National Commission on Community Health Services. *Financing Community Health Services and Facilities*. Report of the Task Force on Financing of Health Services. Washington, D.C.: Public Affairs Press, 1967.

11. National Commission on Community Health Services. *Health Administration and Organization in the Decade Ahead*. Report of the Task Force on Organization of Community Health Services. Washington, D.C.: Public Affairs Press, 1967.

12. National Commission on Community Health Services. *A Self-Study Guide for Community Action Planning*. Report of the Community Action Studies Project. New York: American Public Health Association, 1967.

13. National Commission on Community Health Services. *Health Is a Community Affair*. Cambridge: Harvard University Press, 1966.

14. U.S. President's Commission on the Health Needs of the Nation. *Building America's Health*. Volumes 1-5. Washington, D.C.: Government Printing Office, 1952-1953.

15. U.S. President's Commission on Heart Disease, Cancer, and Stroke. *A National Program to Conquer Heart Disease, Cancer, and Stroke*. Washington, D.C.: Government Printing Office, 1964.

16. Health Facilities Planning and Construction Service. *Hill-Burton Program Progress Report*. U.S.P.H.S. Publication No. 930-F-3. Silver Spring, Maryland: Department of Health, Education and Welfare, Health Services and Mental Health Administration, 1968.

17. Kane, D. A. "Comprehensive Health Planning: A Study in Creative Federalism." *American Journal of Public Health* 59:1706-1712, 1969.

18. Division of Regional Medical Programs. *Guidelines. Regional Medical Programs*. Revised. Washington, D.C.: Department of Health, Education and Welfare, Health Services and Mental Health Administration. May, 1968.

19. Division of Regional Medical Programs. "P.L. 91-515. Heart Disease, Cancer, Stroke, and Kidney Disease Amendments of 1970." *News, Information, Data* 4: No. 51S. Rockville, Maryland: Department of Health, Education and Welfare, Health Services and Mental Health Administration, November 20, 1970.

20. Regional Medical Programs Service. *Fact Book on Regional Medical Programs*. Rockville, Maryland: Department of Health, Education and Welfare, Health Services and Mental Health Administration, August, 1971.

21. Public Law 89-749. *Comprehensive Health Planning and Public Health*

Services Amendments of 1966. Section 2 (a) and (b). Washington, D.C.: Government Printing Office, 1966.

22. "Certification of Need Review Set for Health Facilities." *Maryland Comprehensive Health Planning Agency News* 1: No. 3, September, 1970.
23. "Certification of Need Program—Progress Report." *Maryland Comprehensive Health Planning Agency News—Information* 2: No. 3, April 20, 1971.
24. Myers, B. A. "Health Maintenance Organizations: Objectives and Issues." Paper presented at the Annual Conference of State Comprehensive Health Planning Agencies, Washington, D.C., April 7, 1971. Rockville, Maryland: Department of Health, Education and Welfare, Health Services and Mental Health Administration, n.d.
25. "HMOs—The Key Experimental Unit in Health Plans." *American Medical News*, pp. 10-11, June 7, 1971.
26. *Health Maintenance Organizations. The Concept and Structure.* Rockville, Maryland: Department of Health, Education and Welfare, Health Services and Mental Health Administration, n.d.
27. Lee, Roger I. and Jones, Lewis W. *The Fundamentals of Good Medical Care.* Chicago: University of Chicago Press, 1933.
28. Ciocco, A. and Altman, I. "Statistics on the Patient Load of Physicians in Private Practice." *Journal of the American Medical Association* 121:506-513, 1943.
29. Ciocco, A. and Altman, I. "The Patient Load of Physicians in Private Practice. A Comparative Statistical Study of Three Areas." *Public Health Reports* 58:1329-1351, 1943.
30. Dickinson, F. G. "Analysis of Questionnaire on Medical Care of Civilians during World War II." *Journal of the American Medical Association* 134:369-374, 1947.
31. Bane, G. *Physicians for a Growing America.* Report of the Surgeon General's Consultant Group on Medical Education. U.S.P.H.S. Publication No. 709. Washington, D.C.: Government Printing Office, 1959.
32. "The MD Shortage." Editorial. *AMA News*, August 30, 1971.
33. *Report of the National Advisory Commission on Health Manpower.* Volumes I and II. Washington, D.C.: Government Printing Office, 1967.
34. *Nurses for a Growing Nation.* New York: National League for Nursing, 1957.
35. Surgeon-General's Consultant Group on Nursing. *Toward Quality in Nursing. Needs and Goals.* Washington, D.C.: Government Printing Office, 1963.
36. *Facts about Nursing. A Statistical Summary.* New York: American Nurses' Association, 1969.
37. *The West's Manpower Needs.* Boulder, Colorado: Western Interstate Commission for Higher Education, 1960.
38. Health Manpower Study Commission. *Health Manpower for the Upper Midwest.* St. Paul, Minnesota: Hill Family Foundation, 1966.
39. *Medical Education and Research Needs in Maryland.* Baltimore: Committee on Medical Care, Maryland State Planning Commission, 1962.
40. Baker, T. D., Cassidy, J. E., Galkin, J. D., *et al. Projection of Maryland's Health Manpower Needs through the 1980's.* Baltimore: Maryland Council for Higher Education, 1968.

ADDITIONAL READINGS

Primary

Conant, Ralph W. *The Politics of Community Health*. Washington, D.C.: Public Affairs Press, 1968.
Case history approach to political factors in community health planning.
Kissick, W. L., editor. "Dimensions and Determinants of Health Policy." *Milbank Memorial Fund Quarterly* 46: No. 1, Part 2, January, 1968.
A series of broadly ranging papers presented as a symposium on health care delivery.
National Commission on Community Health Services. *Health Is a Community Affair*. Cambridge: Harvard University Press, 1966.
This document, developed from studies in depth of representative communities and from recommendations of community and health leaders across the nation, is the first group effort to deal with the entire range of problems in community health services.
National Commission on Community Health Services. *Action-Planning for Community Health Services*. Washington, D.C.: Public Affairs Press, 1967.
Detailed self-studies in a number of communities in the United States.
Roemer, M. I. *The Organization of Medical Care under Social Security*. Geneva: International Labour Office, 1969.
A study based on the experience of eight countries in the organization of medical care under social security. Subject sections deal with general background components of medical care, resource development and allocation, quality, costs, and coordination.
Roemer, R., Frink, J., and Kramer, C. "Environmental Health Services. Multiplicity of Jurisdictions and Comprehensive Environmental Management." *Milbank Memorial Fund Quarterly* 49:419-509, No. 4, Part 1, October, 1971.
A quite complete review of the problems of jurisdictions in environmental health services and the obstacles to comprehensive health planning.
Wilson, R. N. *Community Structure and Health Action. A Report on Process Analysis*. Washington, D.C.: Public Affairs Press, 1968.
A study of community structure and leadership, community process and decision-making, and the use of process analysis in obtaining perspectives on community and health.

Secondary

Cater, D. "Comprehensive Health Planning. I. Creative Federalism." *American Journal of Public Health* 58: 1022-1025, 1968.
Coggeshall, L. T. *Planning for Medical Progress through Education*. Evanston, Illinois: Association of American Medical Colleges, 1965.
Hilleboe, H. E. and Schaefer, M. "Administrative Requirements for Comprehensive Health Planning at the State Level." *American Journal of Public Health* 58: 1039-1046, 1968.
National Conference on Public Health Training. *Third Report to the Surgeon General*. Washington, D.C.: Government Printing Office, 1967.

Milt, Harry, editor. *Meeting the Crisis in Health Care Services in our Communities.* Report of the 1970 National Health Forum. New York: National Health Council, 1970.

Rogers, P. G. "Comprehensive Health Planning. IV. The Partnership for Health Programs." *American Journal of Public Health* 58:1036-1038, 1968.

Willard, W. R. "Comprehensive Health Planning. II. Diverse Factors in Regional Medical Planning." *American Journal of Public Health* 58:1026-1030, 1968.

Yarborough, R. W. "Alleviating Fragmented Systems of Health Care: The Regional Medical Programs." *Journal of Medical Education* 45:411-415, 1970.

2

Stages of the Planning Process

CARL E. TAYLOR

Planning has moved from an intuitive, spontaneous, and subjective projection of activity based on past experience to a much more deliberate, systematic, and objective process of mobilizing information and organizing resources. The process of planning needs first of all to be itself planned (1).

Experience in health planning has led to the identification of a series of systematic stages in the planning process (2). To a considerable extent these stages parallel the commonly accepted steps of the scientific method as applied to research. Planning explores the uncertainties of how the best use can be made of limited resources to meet priority needs. It has, therefore, much of the intellectual challenge of research.

Planning is a dynamic process; hence it is not in practice a single movement up a rigidly structured static stairway of steps. Rather it is an unending upward spiral of incremental efforts toward improvement. The purpose of the present categorization of the elements of the planning process is to provide a general framework or outline of what needs to be done to ensure a systematic approach.

In reality, many activities should be carried out concurrently, providing a mutually supportive flow back and forth between various stages of the process depending on local conditions and requirements. Such variations will lead at different times and places to great differences in the balance between the amount of planning input required for various steps of the process. Important determinants are the level of development of the country and such mundane questions as whether data are already available or must be laboriously gathered. The structure and function of the planning machinery must also be adjusted to local conditions. Flexibility is desirable, especially at the start, when adaptations are more necessary and more frequent.

FIRST STAGE—PLANNING THE PLANNING AND DEVELOPING PLANNING COMPETENCE

In any planning structure the policy-making body must represent the political power structure, the general public, and health professionals (3-7). The balance among these three groups is determined largely by the type of planning to be undertaken. In broad-gauge comprehensive planning it is particularly important to ensure that the health activities fit general public desires; hence the proportionate representation of consumers should be great. In many types of program planning and project planning, which should themselves fit in with a general comprehensive plan, the particular competence required is more technical in nature; thus, representation on the policy-making group can be weighted more toward the health professional.

The planning unit is the main executive arm of the planning commission and should have its core group composed of an appropriate balance of the types of health professionals most involved in relevant health activities. Because many judgments in planning are based on financial considerations, someone with a background in economics is needed. Similarly, competence in the social sciences and principles of administration is desirable.

In general, the planning unit should be closely associated with the administrative structure but not directly involved in administration. Its success is often determined by its ability to make itself useful to administrators. This may involve undertaking a variety of service tasks for the administrative or institutional units with which the planners work. Effective planning, however, requires the ability to move easily at all administrative and organizational levels and lines of communication. It is, therefore, important to keep from getting tied down with routine chores. While it is desirable to be as high as possible in the administrative hierarchy in order to gain as much authority as possible, it is also important to refrain from dissipating too much technical energy around conference tables of policy makers and committees which talk rather than act. Moreover, access to the most peripheral units in field work brings an important realism into planning.

Since planning is largely an educational enterprise, substantial effort must be devoted to teaching the planning methods to be used throughout the administrative structure. Once the members of the planning unit have themselves received the best training available, they should organize special training programs for those with whom they work. Some of the most effective planning organizations have devoted a great deal of energy to organizing short courses in planning which are attended by all levels of health personnel (8). In addition to teaching technical planning, data gathering skills, economic theory, and analytic methodology, such a systematic educational program can have a unique impact by developing enthusiasm and an esprit of cooperative action.

SECOND STAGE—STATEMENTS OF POLICY AND BROAD GOALS

Planning policies and goals must be politically determined (4, 6). The first lesson for the health planner to learn is that he must not impose his own personal predilections on the planning process. Instead, skill must be developed in gauging and mobilizing political opinions. Planning can itself be an excellent educational process in modifying public attitudes and especially in demonstrating major areas of deficiency which require attention. The process of getting consumer participation in United States regional programs provides an outstanding example of the quick education that the assumption of responsibility brings (9). In order to set the stage for effective implementation of the plan it is essential to make sure at the start that planning goals fit the policies of the political group responsible for implementation (10, 11).

One of the best educational maneuvers that a planning group can use in conditioning the political structure to which it is responsible is to require the policy-making group to go through the difficult exercise of explicitly stating plan aims. Too often goals are left so vague and general that they are little more than platitudes. By taking the time at the beginning to get policy makers to arrive at explicit statements, much time is saved later when the details of planning and implementation are being worked out. An important step at this stage is to distinguish clearly between long-term goals and short-range objectives. Both should be stated with clear recognition of time and priority implications.

Planners can profitably promote the idea among policy makers that planning is their best way of being leaders rather than followers of public opinion. To ensure that planning is dynamic rather than static, they must recognize its cyclic nature. After following the steps of the planning process through a plan period, the time comes when policy makers are back to the first step again and must revise the plan objectives on the basis of experience gained. Continuity must be maintained by constantly looking ahead to the next plan period.

THIRD STAGE–DATA GATHERING

If planning had no other reason to exist, it would not be hard to justify it on the basis of improvements made in the information systems within the health services (8, 12). Some planning groups serve primarily as statistical units, and just by making information available to appropriate decision makers they have a major planning impact. For instance, the National Health Council has for many years fulfilled a useful voluntary role in the United States by collecting and analyzing information (3, 13). The relative amount of time which a planning unit must devote to data gathering depends, of course, on the existing statistical organization. Where the sources of information are good, the planning unit needs only to adjust the data to particular planning objectives. Where data are deficient, the planning unit may have to set up their own surveys or other data gathering systems. Depending on local conditions they have the choice of organizing periodic surveys or establishing continuing reporting mechanisms for their own particular data within the general statistical organization of the health services.

A particular benefit of good planning is that it provides a basis for judgment in sharpening the selection of truly useful data. A well-known weakness of statistical organizations is that they collect so much junk. Tradition and habit, along with borrowed forms, maintain a flow of irrelevant and redundant numbers which make it difficult to sort out truly meaningful data. To start with, the burden of excessive form-filling may cause outright fabrication or at the best rushed estimation at the peripheral unit where the data start. Excessive flow through the information system means that not only are the data not trusted but they are not even looked at. Good planning requires early attention to eliminating from the information system all items not related to clear plan objectives and functional use.

In health planning, data customarily start with demographic information. The basic unit of health care is obviously the number of people to be served and their distribution. Because of the rapid rate of population growth in most developing countries, it is particularly essential to have as accurate population projections as possible.

The second category of information is epidemiologic, specifically information on the frequency and distribution of major health problems. In developing countries this is often very spotty. Because of the chronic difficulty of getting accurate mortality and morbidity information, an immediate need is oftentimes to organize some sort of sample survey. Certainly the patient selectivity factor makes hospital and other institutional reports of disease only minimally useful.

In many places the most serious deficiencies of planning information are in economic data. Most health people have little idea of what sort of information might be useful for economic analyses. The simplest type of information is usually accurate cost accounting of specific health activities, although the calculations become more complicated with the inclusion of indirect costs. Many of the more sophisticated measurements of items which would be useful in economic analysis, especially of the cost-benefit type, have still to be developed.

Another category of information which usually needs to be specially developed for planning purposes concerns the utilization of facilities and the functional patterns of work of various types of personnel. A recent international study shows remarkable uniformity in utilization systems under dissimilar health care systems (14). Planning can make its most dramatic contributions in short time periods by increasing efficiency of utilization. This requires careful attention to the process of setting work standards and performance budgeting. Without an adequate data system, such rationalization of the services is obviously impossible. A related type of information is basic administrative data on the availability and projection of both manpower and facility resources.

Finally, more sophisticated research is necessary to develop ways of measuring demand for various categories of services.

FOURTH STAGE—PRIORITY STATEMENT OF HEALTH PROBLEMS

Setting priorities is considered by most health administrators to be the heart of the planning process. The steps leading up to this point can in a way be considered preparation for the crucial decisions involved in priority setting. Once priorities have been set, the subsequent steps can be considered progressive moves toward implementation. In priority setting, judgment and wisdom are most needed, together with a unique ability to synthesize the numerous relevant details. It is the part of the planning process which is usually considered most intuitive. Priority setting, however, can perhaps benefit more than any of the other steps from being made an explicit and clearly defined exercise.

The greatest skill required in priority setting is to balance variables which have very different quantitative relationships and in fact lie in different dimensional scales. Too often, mistakes arise from giving undue stress to one dimension. The epidemiologist tends to view priority setting as primarily a matter of defining relative mortality and morbidity from specific health problems. This approach was overdone in the first versions of the "Latin American Method" of health planning (15). Social scientists, politicians, and the public tend to view priority setting as mainly a response to popular feelings about what is important. To them the important considerations are what the public wants done and what health programs will be acceptable. Administrators tend to view priorities mainly in terms of what the Latin American health planning method has called the "vulnerability" of particular health problems. The concern is with the availability of technical methods for controlling the diseases or conditions requiring attention. Perhaps the most serious limitation in developing countries, often even more restrictive than lack of money, is the question of whether there is an administrative framework to provide services and the necessary personnel.

Economists would lay particular stress on cost. This is usually the final constraint which determines what will be done, and the relative cost of various control programs must be balanced. The underlying policy in balancing costs in health planning generally is to put more stress on providing adequate care for the maximum number of people, rather than the highest quality care for a selected few.

The health planner must develop skills in all of the above disciplines sufficient to provide a balanced approach to each. Particularly needed are valid specific indices for both the quantitative and qualitative types of information implied in the above judgments. Even with all of his attempts at measurement and specific categorization, he will in the end have to rely on the indefinable elements of wisdom from experience or from evaluation of previous plans in making the final decisions.

FIFTH STAGE–PLAN OUTLINE WITH STATEMENT OF MAJOR ALTERNATIVE PROPOSALS

With the priority decisions in hand, it is necessary to begin to work out the alternative proposals which represent possible ways of coping with the health problems defined. A clear statement of alternative approaches provides a basis for deciding what should in fact be done. This involves actually specifying many of the underlying considerations which were gathered and balanced in the course of priority setting. The advantages at this stage of a clear outline for each alternative approach is that it provides a ready basis for comparison. Of the four approaches to analysis listed above under priority setting, the attention now shifts largely to the latter two: administrative and economic. Particular points to be included in the outline include: (1) a clear definition of the technical aspects of the program; (2) the organization framework required; (3) the personnel and facilities needed; (4) costs in comparable financial terms; (5) approximate benefits to be expected relative to priority of concern.

One of the more complicated issues at this stage is the problem of deciding between health activities that have multiple impacts on several health problems as compared with those that have only a single impact. Since decisions between alternatives must be based largely on a cost-benefit type of judgment, it seems that benefits should be greater in programs that have multiple health contributions. At this stage in planning methodology, however, these essentially intuitive and approximate cost-benefit judgments usually cannot be put into the economic formulations normally associated with cost-benefit analysis.

At this point, the difference between comprehensive planning, program planning, and project planning should be recalled. Comprehensive planning provides the general framework for development; it is particularly concerned with the problem of priorities and the relative stress to be given to various programs and projects. It provides the over-all conceptual structure within which program and project planning can be done. The most effective detailed planning, then, will be at the program and project level. Program planning is directed toward broad-impact activities that will affect a number of health problems. Project planning is the most focused and limited; it tends to be concerned with high-impact health activities directed against single health problems. It also tends to be more clearly limited in its time perspective.

SIXTH STAGE–DEVELOPMENT OF DETAILED PLAN WITH TARGETS AND STANDARDS

Construction of a detailed plan document is usually worked out in phases. Long-term goals are specifically stated, along with the proposed steps necessary to carry them out. Any programs requiring several years must be stated in flexible terms. Increasing detail and specificity can be introduced for more immediate periods, such as the next year.

As discussed in the next chapter on "Making the Plan Effective," one difficult issue to be decided is the balance between centralization and decentralization in the planning process. The probability of getting successful implementation of a detailed plan is proportionately increased with greater local involvement in the programming. If local units can be assigned responsibility for developing detailed programs on the basis of general procedures set up by the central unit, more spontaneous enthusiasm and active participation will be brought to the task.

In shifting the planning balance toward decentralization and local involvement, two major controls should be built in by central planning units. The first is the development of appropriate standards for performance. Since a good set of realistic standards can be evolved only out of experience, the initial set will necessarily have to be arbitrary and approximate. A major advance can be expected in subsequent cycles, however, if deliberate effort has been devoted to gathering the necessary information to permit more precise standard-setting as the plan is implemented.

Similarly, target-setting is an appropriate part of the central unit's responsibility. Targets should be specified according to quantitative indices of performance and within a clearly stated time framework. As with standard-setting, establishment of precise targets can be expected to improve with progressive implementation in successive plan periods. Both standard-setting and target-setting should be attempted from the beginning, however, in order to provide a rational basis for evaluation. Above all they should be realistic and based on the general human response that work effectiveness improves most if built on a reasonable experience of success. They should never be so likely to produce failure as to be punitive devices.

SEVENTH STAGE–IMPLEMENTATION AS PART OF THE PLANNING PROCESS

The concept of planning as a dynamic and continuing activity requires implementation to be included as an integral part of health planning (16). Early experiences in planning concentrated merely on the development of the plan as a document. Implementation was considered the responsibility of the service organizations responsible for particular activities. Enthusiastic planners sometimes seemed to take pride in developing plans which were so complicated and abstruse that they could not be understood by administrators and had little bearing on reality. No error in planning is more common or more serious than such a tendency to get lost in the planning process.

Implementation can be considered an important part of the planning process from two quite distinct points of view. Traditionally, comprehensive planning has been considered a process in which the entire health service should be involved; planning has been viewed as only a normal step in good administration. In this inclusive view, implementation is intimately associated with both planning and administration, so that the three aspects are not easily separated.

More recently health planning has gained recognition, at least potentially, as a discipline in its own right. Such a view clearly distinguishes the planner from those responsible for ongoing activities. If he is thus to be placed in an atmosphere of objective detachment, important questions arise concerning his role in the process of implementation. Clearly, the plan itself must incorporate detailed planning for implementation, but the health planner must set up the conditions which give the plan the greatest likelihood of being successfully carried out.

The first tactical step in plan implementation is to get the plan accepted. A completely innocuous plan which merely confirms existing conditions, of course, has the best chance for acceptance. The more innovative the plan proposal, the more difficulty there will be in getting political leaders, health personnel, and the public to agree. If a plan is to do some good, it should contain the seeds of progressive change.

The probability of acceptance of plan proposals increases proportionately with the extent to which health personnel, political leaders, and the consumer public participate in the planning process. The document produced will probably be less coherent and polished than one produced by planning technicians alone. Still, it seems wise to keep the balance as much toward decentralization as possible. Each particular situation will require an individualized determination of what this balance should be. These issues are discussed in greater detail in the following chapter, "Making the Plan Effective."

EIGHTH STAGE–EVALUATION

Evaluation is such an important part of the total dynamic process of planning that many functioning units are called "planning and evaluation units." At one time there was a conceptual problem growing out of the notion that we were dealing with three separate activities–planning, implementation, and evaluation. The modern view, however, is that it is all one process of a cyclic nature, with the evaluation step leading directly into the initiation of a new planning cycle (17).

Two fundamentally different types of evaluation must be distinguished: continuing evaluation for administrative purposes and a periodic, more focused evaluation specifically for plan revision. Particularly important to the administrator is continuing self-evaluation by local administrative health units. If the planning process can encourage local units to undertake systematic self-evaluation and provide them with appropriate know-how and mechanisms, this will be perhaps the best possible means of building in continuous improvement. In addition, a major role of the planning organization is to undertake continuing administrative evaluation to see that standards and targets are being met. One of the best ways for planners to establish their usefulness is to show that they can fulfill an important service role to the administrators. A natural service activity with great practical value to most senior administrators is a tough, frank approach to evaluation. In any centralized-decentralized balance, this naturally tends to continue as an important role of the central units.

The second major type of evaluation is more definitely related to the planning process. A centrally-directed activity has to be set up with the primary purpose of quantifying achievement in particular planning periods. Such activity tends to be timed to precede the evolution of a new major plan or the modification of an existing one. This kind of exercise should go considerably beyond mere measurement of achievement in terms of previous standards and targets. It should concentrate on assessment of such basic issues as whether the original goals and objectives were in fact appropriate; whether resource development is actually moving in the direction most suited to local conditions, both in terms of facilities and manpower; whether the priority setting was, in fact, justified by further experience; and especially whether the data gathering system is producing useful information. Such an evaluation does not spontaneously happen. It has to be worked out with as much ingenuity and innovative precision as any other part of the planning sequence.

A final comment must be made about the need for objectivity in evaluation. One of the more intractable obstacles to change is the innate human conviction that whatever one is used to doing must be right. Normal human pride of involvement leads to an almost uncontrollable subjective bias. Innovation requires both a willingness to give up even the most sacrosanct culturally accepted ways of doing things and an openness to the new.

REFERENCES

1. Waterston, Albert. *Development Planning: Lessons of Experience.* Baltimore: Johns Hopkins Press, 1967.
2. *National Health Planning in Developing Countries.* WHO Technical Report Series No. 350. Geneva: World Health Organization, 1967.
3. National Health Forum. *Planning for Health.* New York: National Health Council, 1967.
4. Conant, Ralph W. *The Politics of Community Health.* Washington, D.C.: Public Affairs Press, 1968.
5. Hochbaum, G. M. "Consumer Participation in Health Planning. Toward Conceptual Clarification." *American Journal of Public Health* 59:1698-1705, 1969.
6. Arnold, M. F. "Basic Concepts and Crucial Issues in Health Planning." *American Journal of Public Health* 59:1686-1697, 1969.

7. Government of India, Administrative Reforms Commission. *Study Team on the Machinery for Planning Final Report.* New Delhi: Government of India Press, 1968.
8. Hall, T. L. "Planning for Health in Peru—New Approaches to an Old Problem." *American Journal of Public Health* 56:1296-1307, 1966.
9. Blendon, R. J. and Gaus, C. R. "Problems in Developing Health Services in Poverty Areas: The Johns Hopkins Experience." *Journal of Medical Education* 46:477-484, 1971.
10. Kissick, W. L., editor. "Dimensions and Determinants of Health Policy." *Milbank Memorial Fund Quarterly* 46: No. 1, Part 2, January, 1968.
11. Kissick, W. L. "Health Policy Reflections for the 1970's." *New England Journal of Medicine* 282:1343-1354, 1970.
12. Kennedy, F. D. *Basic Concepts Required in the Development of a Planning Information System.* RM-OH-387-1. Research Triangle Park, North Carolina: Research Triangle Institute, November, 1968.
13. National Commission on Community Health Services. *Comprehensive Health Care: A Challenge to American Communities.* Washington, D.C.: Public Affairs Press, 1967.
14. Bice, W. and White, K. L. "Cross-National Comparative Research on the Utilization of Medical Services." *Medical Care* 9:253-271, 1971.
15. Ahumada, J., *et al. Health Planning: Problems of Concept and Method.* Scientific Publication No. 111. Washington, D.C.: Pan American Health Organization, 1965.
16. Waterston, Albert. "An Operational Approach to Development Planning." *International Journal of Health Services* 1:223-252, 1971.
17. *Methods of Evaluating Public Health Programmes.* Copenhagen: World Health Organization, Regional Office for Europe, 1968.

ADDITIONAL READINGS*

International

Ahumada, J., *et al. Health Planning: Problems of Concept and Method.* Scientific Publication No. 111. Washington, D.C.: Pan American Health Organization, 1965.
   A document of value as an indication of early efforts to develop a systematic analysis of health planning according to the "Latin American Method." Since then, emphasis on mortality in setting priorities has been reduced in recent years with more flexibility in adjusting field methods to local needs.
Arnold, M. F. "Basic Concepts and Crucial Issues in Health Planning." *American Journal of Public Health* 59:1686-1697, 1969.
   Philosophical dilemmas in planning are identified. Some special emphases are: an attempt to establish a difference between a "planned" and "planning" society, and the desirability of a political structure that allows citizens to participate in planning.
"Asilomar Conference on International Studies of Medical Care." *Medical Care* 9:193-290, 1971.

* Prepared by Harbans S. Takulia.

Papers from a workshop in August 1967, including topics of social epidemiology in the study of medical care systems, international perspectives of health planning and health manpower, cross-national research on medical services utilization, and research on comparative health service systems.

Baker, Timothy D. and Perlman, Mark. *Health Manpower in a Developing Economy: Taiwan, A Case Study in Planning.* Baltimore: Johns Hopkins Press, 1967.

An example of practical field research in developing a health manpower plan by using existing data and adding an innovative approach to estimating demand through household surveys.

Bice, W. and White, K. L. "Cross-National Comparative Research on the Utilization of Medical Services." *Medical Care* 9:253-271, 1971.

Background information on an important international study of utilization of medical care. Several theoretical and methodological problems are raised, with particular attention to relationships among research, evaluation, and decision-making.

Bryant, John. *Health and the Developing World.* Ithaca: Cornell University Press, 1969.

A comprehensive analysis of the health problems of developing countries leads into an attempt to rationalize the organization of health services. Among the issues discussed: priorities of whom should be served when resources are too scarce to serve all, the universal search for more effective institutional structures, the difficulties of adapting western medical education to developing countries, and the use of auxiliaries and the reluctance of professionals to accept them. Specific country case studies are included from Latin America, Africa, and Southeast Asia.

The Dawson Report on the Future Provision of Medical and Allied Services, 1920. Reprinted with the permission of H. M. Stationery Office. London: King Edward's Hospital Fund, September, 1950.

This document is the forerunner of many current ideas on regionalization of health care with the basic ideas still relevant for many parts of the world.

Field, Mark G. *Soviet Socialized Medicine.* New York: The Free Press, 1967.

This is a good introductory volume to the Soviet health system, the principles on which it is based, and the manner in which it operates.

Fry, John. *Medicine in Three Societies: A Comparison of Medical Care in the USSR, USA, and UK.* New York: American Elsevier Publishing Co., 1970.

Written by a practicing British physician, the book is "a very personal analysis" of the way medical care services in the USSR, USA, and UK cope with an acute heart attack, a brain-damaged child, a road accident, or a case of measles. General principles and practical provisions for first contact with a case, provision of specialist services, maternity and child care, and mental illness are discussed.

Government of India, Administrative Reforms Commission. *Study Team on the Machinery for Planning Final Report.* New Delhi: Government of India Press, 1968.

An evaluation of India's planning process, which represents in general an example of planning through expert panels and committees built on the existing ministry organization.

Grant, John B. *Health Care for the Community: Selected Papers.* Edited by Conrad Seipp. Baltimore: Johns Hopkins Press, 1963.

A collection of writings by an early and outstanding pioneer of health care organization. Three main topics are covered in this volume: regionalization as an administrative framework for health services; education of health manpower for community health care; and planning and development of health services as part of the process of community development. Illustrations are drawn from China, Southeast Asia, Puerto Rico, and elsewhere.

Griffith, D. H. S., Ramana, D. V., and Mashaal, H. "Contribution of Health to Development." *International Journal of Health Services* 1:253-270, 1971.

In defining the relationships between health and economic development three examples are included: health expenditures and production in Ceylon; effects of ill health on the growing of rice in Southeast Asia, and health benefits and cost-benefit ratios of malaria control in Thailand.

Hall, Thomas L. *Health Manpower in Peru: A Case Study in Planning.* Baltimore: Johns Hopkins Press, 1969.

A major research effort using multiple approaches to relating supply to demand, with particular effort being devoted to evaluating supply.

Hall, Thomas L. "Planning for Health in Peru—New Approaches to an Old Problem." *American Journal of Public Health* 56:1296-1307, 1966.

A description of the Latin American Method of health planning, emphasizing the importance of training courses in health planning for health personnel.

King, Maurice, editor. *Medical Care in Developing Countries: A Primer on the Medicine of Poverty and a Symposium from Makerere.* London: Oxford University Press, 1966.

The result of a conference on health centers and hospitals in Africa, this work evolved into a manual on the delivery of medical care as it is shaped by the constraints of poverty in developing countries. The practical issues discussed include: how a doctor can best use his time; the building and organization of hospitals; types of drugs and records; use of auxiliaries; and the organization of pediatrics, family planning, and maternity care.

Methods of Evaluating Public Health Programmes. Copenhagen: World Health Organization, Regional Office for Europe, 1968.

A symposium on methods and guidelines for evaluation of public health programs.

Myrdal, Gunnar. *Asian Drama: An Inquiry into the Poverty of Nations.* 3 volumes. New York: Pantheon Books, 1968.

A monumental work. Some appendices are particularly useful, especially those in which he discusses basic mechanisms of development and the structure of plans.

National Health Planning in Developing Countries. WHO Technical Report Series No. 350. Geneva: World Health Organization, 1967.

A basic publication giving the consensus of an Expert Committee on the fundamental components of the planning process.

Navarro, V. "Methodology on Regional Planning of Personal Health Services: A Case Study, Sweden." *Medical Care* 8:386-394, 1970.

Methods of estimating future demand and distribution of personal health services, specifically the "consumption unit index" by which Swedish health planners estimate demographic effects and geographic accessibility.

Popov, G. A. *Principles of Health Planning in the USSR.* Public Health Papers No. 43. Geneva: World Health Organization, 1971.

A review of how health planning works in the country with the longest experience.

Reinke, W. A., Taylor, C. E., and Parker, R. L. "Functional Analysis of Health Needs and Services." In: *Proceedings of the Sixth International Scientific Meeting of the International Epidemiological Association,* Primosten, Yugoslavia, September, 1971. (in press)

A field project developing a functional analysis methodology for local health planning emphasizing role definition and optimum utilization of health personnel.

Report of the Health Survey and Planning Committee. 2 volumes. New Delhi: Government of India, Ministry of Health, 1962.

The Mudaliar Committee Report is an example of a periodic effort to review progress following up the earlier classic, "The Bhore Report," of 1947.

Roemer, M. I. "General Physician Service under Eight National Patterns." *American Journal of Public Health* 66:1873-1899, 1970.

International comparisons of physician activity are placed in perspective.

Takulia, H. S., Taylor, C. E., Sangal, S. P., and Alter, J. D. *The Health Center Doctor in India.* Baltimore: Johns Hopkins Press, 1967.

An analysis of the elements of the health center concept with a review of the opinions of different groups of decision makers about the role of the rural doctor.

Taylor, Carl E., Dirican, Rahmi, and Deuschle, Kurt W. *Health Manpower Planning in Turkey.* Baltimore: Johns Hopkins Press, 1968.

A national manpower study attempting to interrelate specific relationships between professional and auxiliary categories with particular attention to educational implications.

Taylor, C. E. and Hall, M.-F. "Health, Population, and Economic Development." *Science* 157:651-657, 1967.

The interactions between components of development are summarized with a general review of available information.

Taylor, C. E. and Takulia, H. S., editors. *Integration of Health and Family Planning in Village Sub-Centers.* Narangwal, Punjab State, India: Rural Health Research Center, 1971.

A report of a village conference on organization of rural services for family planning and maternal and child health.

Training in National Health Planning. WHO Technical Report Series No. 456. Geneva: World Health Organization, 1970.

This report by an Expert Committee is devoted primarily to a consideration of the various elements in training for national health planning and a description of several programs for training different types of personnel for the practice of health planning. Several annexes give detailed explanations of courses in health planning which have been prepared by WHO Regional Offices.

Waterston, Albert. *Development Planning: Lessons of Experience.* Baltimore: Johns Hopkins Press, 1967.

A comparative study of planning for national development based on experiences of more than 100 countries in Asia, Africa, Latin America, and Europe. Part I emphasizes problems of plan formulation and plan implementation; in Part II, worldwide experiences in organization and administrative procedures in developmental planning are discussed.

Waterston, A. "An Operational Approach to Development Planning." *International Journal of Health Services* 1:223-252, 1971.
  Conventional planning approaches are questioned on the basis of practical experience and instead this paper presents arguments for "planning from below" as a workable alternative. Problems of plan implementation, particularly in developing countries, often reflect political instability, economic uncertainty, and a lack of political will and administrative capacity. Practical steps include relating investment to improved budgetary organization and emphasizing sector programs which provide feasible and viable projects.

Weinerman, E. Richard. *Social Medicine in Eastern Europe.* Cambridge: Harvard University Press, 1969.
  Focused on the national health services of three socialist countries (Czechoslovakia, Hungary, and Poland), this study gives particular attention to problems of organizing health care and professional training.

United States

Blendon, R. J. and Gaus, C. R. "Problems in Developing Health Services in Poverty Areas: The Johns Hopkins Experience." *Journal of Medical Education* 46:477-484, 1971.
  Description of an effort to get university involvement in an urban community program.

Blum, Henrik L. and Associates. *Notes on Comprehensive Planning for Health.* San Francisco: American Public Health Association, Western Regional Office, 1968.
  United States experiences in comprehensive health planning are summarized, emphasizing elements which must be considered in goal determination and in implementation, methods of measurement in gathering data on health services, health manpower planning, and organization of regional medical programs.

Conant, Ralph W. *The Politics of Community Health.* Report of the Community Action Studies Project, National Commission on Community Health Services. Washington, D.C.: Public Affairs Press, 1968.
  This study attempts to explain how some communities in the United States (specifically, Cincinnati, Ohio; Lincoln, Nebraska; Maryland State; Rochester, New York; and San Mateo County, California) have succeeded in providing acceptable health services for their citizens. The qualities of leadership needed in such endeavors are discussed.

Hilleboe, H. E. "Health Planning on a Community Basis." *Medical Care* 6:203-212, 1968.
  The local approach to health planning.

Hochbaum, G. M. "Consumer Participation in Health Planning: Toward Conceptual Clarification." *American Journal of Public Health* 59:1698-1705, 1969.
  Some problems of consumer participation in health planning are identified. Because of the many uncertainties, a plea is made for continuing evaluation of field experiences with particular need for the involvement of social scientists.

Kennedy, F. D. *Basic Concepts Required in the Development of a Planning*

Information System. Research Memo RM-OH-387-1. Research Triangle Park, North Carolina: Research Triangle Institute, November, 1968.

A memorandum written to describe a state planning information system.

Kissick, W. L., editor. "Dimensions and Determinants of Health Policy." *Milbank Memorial Fund Quarterly* 46: No. 1, Part 2, January, 1968.

This volume includes papers presented at a 1966 seminar organized by the Washington Institute for Policy Studies with the objective of reviewing the development of health policy in the United States as a major social concern and the need for mechanisms for governmental and private interaction in decision-making.

Kissick, W. L. "Health Policy Reflection for the 1970's." *New England Journal of Medicine* 282:1343-1354, 1970.

Health policy determination as part of health planning.

National Commission on Community Health Services. *Comprehensive Health Care: A Challenge to American Communities.* Report of the Task Force on Comprehensive Personal Health Services. Washington, D.C.: Public Affairs Press, 1967.

A highly readable report of changes in community health problems resulting from urbanization and the growth, movement, and aging of the population since World War II. It emphasizes the increasing needs of environmental health and the pressures to develop appropriate patterns of personal health services in the 1970's. The report discusses education in health sciences, poverty as a barrier to services, and special psychiatric, dental, and industrial medical needs.

National Health Forum. *Planning for Health.* New York: National Health Council, 1967.

Report of the 1967 Forum in which hundreds of leaders in the fields of health and medicine shared experiences and concerns and shaped some general guidelines for comprehensive health planning in the United States. Panel reports include the systems approach to health planning, performance measures, social goals, and community decision processes.

Sasuly, R. and Ward, P. D. "Two Approaches to Health Planning: The Ideal *vs.* the Pragmatic." *Medical Care* 7:477-484, 1971.

The pragmatic approach to health planning has been essentially a search for "what works" within the dictates of political needs. The ideal approach of "balancing needs with resources" has admittedly not always worked but better adjustment of theory to practice and more hard data are needed.

3

Making the Plan Effective

CARL E. TAYLOR

Failure in health planning is most commonly caused by inadequate attention to implementation. All too often, health planners have felt that their responsibility ended when they produced a plan document, thinking they could then turn over the actual work to health administrators. This tendency to stay isolated from the facts of real life and the process of implementation is responsible for the commonly heard criticism that health planners tend to be impractical and their plans irrelevant. While some administrative separation is necessary for the objectivity required for good evaluation, continuing involvement at the peripheral field level is absolutely essential for practical planning. In the perspective of cyclic planning, implementation must be viewed as the crucial activity toward which all the prior steps of planning build.

Some critical differences between the various types of health planning become most evident at the implementation stage. Based on the scope of subject matter covered, planning can be separated into comprehensive planning, program planning, and project planning. Comprehensive planning normally provides a framework for the other types and thus deals more with priorities than with details of implementation. Although concerned with practicality and feasibility, attention is on general considerations such as priorities and the relative contributions to be achieved by various types of health investment. A major interest is the balance between health services and the other important facets of socioeconomic development. With the increased specificity associated with program and project planning, greater attention to implementation, especially in relation to time scale and target setting, is obviously needed.

STRUCTURAL FRAMEWORK FOR PLANNING

In the interest of providing continuity between planning and implementation, an early decision must be made about the relative balance of planning responsibilities to be given to representative consultant groups and to a planning unit composed of full-time staff professionals. A spectrum of different arrangements may be necessary at various levels in the planning hierarchy. These range between two polar types which will be briefly discussed.

The process of bringing together appropriate groups of health officials, members of professional societies, interested voluntary agencies, and general consumer representatives under whatever title or terminology will be called for present purposes the "part-time committee approach." This approach is exemplified by the pattern of health planning developed in India in the preparation of the health components of the successive five-year plans (1). The National Planning Commission was composed of cabinet members and distinguished leaders representing many disciplines. The Health Panel of the Planning Commission similarly was composed of distinguished leaders interested in health services. Under this Health Panel there were numerous committees which had the primary responsibility for decisions required in formulating the plan. Staff work for all of this intensive committee work was performed mainly by officials from the Health Ministries, both Central and State.

In the other polar type of organization, planning has revolved around an elite full-time professional group of planners. The classic example is the Soviet system of planning (2, 3). As in India, a major burst of activity tends to occur during the preparation of a five-year plan; with a full-time professional group, however, planning tends to be done more on a continuing basis. The professional planners tend to work through their own hierarchy which reaches out from the center.

Evidence is increasing that the best planning requires an appropriate mixture of the committee approach and a full-time professional planning unit. In an analogy with political organization, the planning unit can be compared with the executive branch, while the various commissions, councils, and committees have functions which more nearly resemble legislative responsibilities. In general, an approximately equal balance of the two components is probably desirable in the central organization of planning. At the middle level, effective professional units are probably more important. At the local level, the committee approach becomes particularly important.

The balance of the two organizational components will also vary according to the type of planning activity. The committee approach is particularly necessary in comprehensive planning, while professional expertise is most needed in program and project planning. Perhaps this is one of the reasons why thus far project and program planning have been more effectively carried out than comprehensive planning.

The professional composition of the planning unit staff will be determined by the local situation and traditions. Certainly, nothing will cause planning to fall into disrepute among health personnel as quickly as a lack of health professionals in the planning groups. These health professionals should be respected for their practical experience and technical competence. Although a new specialty of health planning seems to be developing, it seems desirable that professionals who take this special training should first have had practical experience in general health programs. Of great importance in organizing the information system and undertaking the necessary analyses is strong representation of statistical skills. In view of the mounting evidence that the new techniques of systems analysis and operations research have much to contribute to health planning, some representation from this area should be incorporated, especially at the higher levels in the planning hierarchy. The planning team should also include someone with competence in health economics. Additional specialties which can profitably be included, perhaps through consultant arrangements, are public administration and the social sciences. Because of the tremendous importance of budgeting procedures in ensuring implementation, special expertise in budgeting and accounting is often valuable. Finally, as planning gets into particular substantive areas, such as the control of particular diseases or special subjects such as sanitation, the best technical experts in these areas must be available.

In setting up a smoothly functioning planning machinery, it is vital to define clearly the role of each member of the planning team (4, 5). Assigning technical responsibilities usually appears fairly obvious. Clear statements of responsibility are needed, however, to define the relationships between the professional planners and the innumerable other groups and individuals who should be involved in the planning process. Such liaison relationships may sometimes be shared among members of the planning team. Some of these, such as relationships with special consumer groups and professional societies; require the careful choice of appropriate individuals and delicate handling. For optimum implementation a direct linkage with all levels of the administrative hierarchy and with the institutions where health activities are carried out is also necessary. Some planners feel that they must have their offices located in direct proximity to the highest executive authority, even in the office of the president himself. Just as important in the long run, however, are good channels of access to all levels of the official hierarchy.

CENTRALIZATION-DECENTRALIZATION DILEMMA

No unresolved problem in the planning process recurs as continually as the question of the appropriate balance between centrally directed and peripherally initiated activities. One reason that this issue continues to be so aggravating is that generalizations are difficult. On the spectrum ranging between complete centralization or decentralization, the appropriate balance point in any planning situation must be determined by complex local considerations. In general, the most important determinants will be intangibles in the local political and social milieu. Popular participation is largely conditioned by tradition and culture. In those health programs where success is determined primarily by the extent to which individuals cooperate, it may be important for them to feel that the whole plan was their own idea in the first place. The extent to which people are willing to take direction from outside may also show great local variations. Judgment about such matters requires the experience that comes from practical involvement with particular groups of people.

A generalization derived from experience is that the usual tendency is to have too much centralization initially (6). This may be partly because most early efforts in planning were in situations which provided maximum centralized control, such as the typical United States corporation or the Soviet political system. This is certainly the most comfortable situation in which to plan. The planner works in a clear hierarchy. Assuming that he can convince the decision makers at the top about the appropriateness of his plan, he has the feeling that implementation will naturally follow. Reasonable as this may appear, the clearest evidence from past experience is that such reliance on central control does not work. Even the Soviets are finding that they have to move increasingly toward decentralization of their elaborate planning machinery.

Some mass health programs do tend to have highly centralized planning and implementation. This is usually most successful when activities are directed primarily toward changing the environment, with minimum need for modifying the habits of people. Sanitation and malaria eradication are examples that come to mind. Even in such programs, however, planners have found it wise to work hard at getting local participation and interest. Health activities more closely related to personal living require progressively greater decentralized involvement.

Enthusiasm in implementation is directly correlated with the extent of local involvement in planning. On the other hand, planning just does not happen spontaneously, and the move to decentralization can be carried too far. Certain responsibilities can be handled best from the center and others better at the periphery. An attempt will now be made to distinguish between some of the elements that need to be considered in this balance of functions.

Centralized Responsibilities

Early in the planning process aims must be defined, and this requires a large measure of central direction. Local units, of course, should have some opportunity to contribute ideas and suggestions. The real work of defining plan goals and balancing their importance, however, requires the highest level of responsible policy-making representation. A broad range of understanding is necessary, especially in relation to other aspects of development such as roads, communications, education, and economic growth.

Another major responsibility which must be primarily central is the specification of resource constraints. Planners must be told what the health services will have to work with, and then judgments must be made at the central level concerning limitations to be placed upon the funds and personnel which are centrally controlled. The central unit must also make over-all estimates of contributions expected from local participation, allowing for variation in what individual peripheral units actually decide to contribute to particular health activities; such local decisions will, however, usually be in the direction of expanding a particular project or program above the average for other local units.

A third responsibility which is primarily centrally controlled is adherence to basic plan priorities. This means that in the implementation process special central effort will have to be directed toward stimulating action in areas of deficiency.

Similarly, the establishment of the total organization and machinery of planning is primarily a central responsibility. The objective should be to have the planning machinery reach out as far as possible through the total range of public and private health services. The participation of private agencies is often one way to obtain the particularly important general objective of including representatives of all consumer groups. The significant organizational effort which is required to ensure this range of involvement must be initiated by the central planning unit. Efficiency demands a certain degree of standardization in relationships.

Another central responsibility must be the review of project plans and area plans prepared by peripheral groups. Local judgments based on knowledge of specific situations must be transmitted through a progressive screening process. Final approval, then, must be at some appropriate regional or central level where a sufficient range of proposals can be studied to give a balanced over-all view of priorities.

A final planning activity that is primarily a central responsibility is evaluation. Some continuing evaluation, of course, has to be built into the routine of any good local administration; the principal responsibility for evaluation as part of the planning process should, however, provide a considerable degree of external objectivity. An important part of such over-all evaluation is comparison with other areas and projects, and this can clearly be done best at the central level.

Decentralized Peripheral Responsibilities

Simply stated, the components of decentralized responsibility in planning are those residual functions not assumed by central authorities. The appropriate locus for the initiation of action in specified circumstances must be defined explicitly, however.

Effective data gathering is organized centrally, but the quality is obviously dependent on local involvement. If personnel at the periphery where the data originate know the purpose for which the data will be used, then there will be much more interest and precision in obtaining valid information. Any sort of feedback by which peripheral units can see the tangible contributions of their data will lead to an automatic improvement in validity.

Although general priorities usually originate in central planning groups, permitting considerable flexibility to local units in final determination of priorities has great advantage. Great effort can go into educating local groups to accept centrally chosen priorities. On the other hand, by taking care of problems which are already of local concern, it is frequently possible to get communities to move on to other priorities of which they were at first not aware.

Particularly important is that planning detailed programs be done by peripheral units (7, 8). Nothing promotes successful implementation as much as having communities feel that the planning hierachy has been set up mainly to help them with their own planning. At the local level there is often little awareness of the amount of effort that central and regional health planners put in to make the local unit's work effective. The most successful planners create a feeling of spontaneity in peripheral units so that credit for achievement is also decentralized.

Even more than other parts of the planning process, final implementation should be worked out at the local level. One of the more important considerations in implementation is allocation of responsibility for particular functions; this obviously requires knowledge of and accommodation to local organizational pressures and personal claims. More positively, implementation is mainly a process of finding the right persons to do particular jobs and this can be best done locally with appropriate opportunity for self-selection.

At the local level, success in plan implementation depends on the participation of several diverse groups (9, 10). Perhaps most important are the local professionals who are directly responsible for health services. No other group can so completely block the implementation of a plan. This may happen even when they agree with the concepts and practical decisions proposed. If they were left out of earlier stages of the planning process and feel that something is being imposed on them, they can obstruct implementation just by withholding support. Obtaining effective participation of professionals is usually not difficult if it becomes evident to them that this is the best way of protecting their own interests and status. The proliferation of professional associations of doctors, nurses, midwives, all ranges of specialists, and numerous paramedical groups may seem too complex to make it worth the trouble of maintaining liaison. One advantage of keeping in touch with all groups, however, is that those who are most cooperative can influence the others. It should even be possible to develop a desirable spirit of competition among professional groups who realize that they might be left behind.

Efforts to include lay and consumer groups in the planning process will also facilitate effective implementation. A major benefit is that such involvement can provide direct access to major gaps and areas of deficiency in services. Consumer participation is most essential in programs which have a large component of personal services. Since identifying appropriate community leaders is usually difficult, simply including representatives of interested agencies, especially those that are voluntary, is tempting. This does not necessarily ensure representativeness of consumer groups, however, and it is usually necessary deliberately to reach out to include those most in need.

As a local planning unit undertakes implementation of plans, it is important to recognize that a major ingredient of success is the art of capturing the right moment. Since implementation requires the simultaneous interaction of multiple forces, a high degree of opportunism is needed. Transitory shifts in opinion or personnel and temporary availability of funds may produce openings that require alert implementation even if all planning details have not been worked out.

USE OF PILOT AND DEMONSTRATION PROJECTS

Planning should not only improve existing ways of doing things, it should also open up entirely new approaches to the solution of problems. The planning process, of course, will reveal many areas in which existing technical knowledge and administrative experience can be translated directly into detailed plans for implementation. There will be certain other areas, however, in which gaps and deficiencies in technical and administrative competence are so great that the appropriate course of action is unclear. Good planning should not wait for new methods to develop spontaneously; instead deliberately planned field trials can sometimes demonstrate the feasibility of new ways of meeting high priority needs. In order to minimize the lag between new research knowledge and its application, the planned use of pilot projects is almost essential.

Local situations vary so much that any attempt at direct implementation based on experience from other countries or cultural situations is usually inadvisable. In adapting any sort of health program for local implementation, it is wise to use pilot and demonstration projects.

Because of the rigidity of most administrative structures, any change that is to be introduced into an administrative pattern should be tried out first on a pilot basis. Appropriate publicity given to the pilot study will then serve to get more traditional administrators thinking about the new approach and increase their willingness to try it. Especially complex are problems of manpower mix and job allocation. Because of the innumerable unpredictable elements in manpower relations, a rational approach requires the precaution of experimental trials. Multiple modifications of manpower utilization either in parallel or in series provide practical experience from which judgment can be made.

It is a truism that pilot and demonstration projects will produce better results than when mass programs are eventually implemented (11). Recognition of this fact can save disappointment later. It is important to build into general implementation plans sufficient latitude to allow for a normal fall-off in performance. The fall-off occurs not only because special projects have the advantage of selected personnel but also because they benefit from the motivational intangibles or "halo effect" of innovative efforts. This is not a disadvantage, since such highly motivated individuals will tend to raise standards in ways that will improve the mass programs.

Another advantage of pilot and demonstration projects is that their personnel and facilities can be used to establish training centers when wider implementation takes place. Selection of staff for the special projects should include consideration of the possibility of such training responsibilities.

PLANNING AS AN EDUCATIONAL PROCESS

Implicit in this discussion of implementation is the concept that planning is primarily an educational process. The planner's efforts will be proved effective not so much by what he does himself as by what he gets others to do. In spite of all that is said about the difficulty of educating the public, planners often need to concentrate even more educational effort on administrators and health personnel. The opinions of health workers are often harder to modify than public attitudes because of their greater personal investment in traditional ways of doing things.

A simple definition of organized planning is: the use of systematic approaches to enable diverse individuals to agree on mutually satisfactory ways of carrying out complicated activities. Left to themselves, individuals naturally do things in their own way. They feel that methods they have learned or worked out are naturally best. Much mutual education occurs, along with friction, when individuals from different backgrounds work together. With the increasing complexity of health services such friction can be more disruptive than spontaneously educational. Good planning should facilitate smoother mutual learning. Like most educational efforts, this should be realistically recognized to be a slow process.

Developmental change is primarily dependent on improved motivation. Public motivation starts with an interest in the immediate benefits of medical care. Professional guidance is needed in adjusting to a time scale of expected health improvements in which the public learns to think beyond immediate needs for curative services to the greater, though delayed, benefits of preventive activities.

Health personnel and administrators tend to be somewhat ambivalent in their approach to planning activities. Their investment in traditional activities and personal career goals makes them suspicious of planned change. A favorable motivation to change can be induced most readily by deliberate manipulation of incentives. Career and monetary rewards can be related directly to demonstrable improvements in services offered. An educational approach to plan implementation should be characterized by efforts to promote cooperation rather than to impose coordination.

REFERENCES

1. Government of India, Administrative Reforms Commission. *Study Team on the Machinery for Planning Final Report.* New Delhi: Government of India Press, 1968.
2. Field, Mark G. *Soviet Socialized Medicine.* New York: The Free Press, 1967.
3. Popov, G. A. *Principles of Health Planning in the USSR.* Public Health Papers No. 43. Geneva: World Health Organization, 1971.
4. Takulia, Harbans S., Taylor, Carl E., Sangal, S. Prakash, and Alter, Joseph D. *The Health Center Doctor in India.* Baltimore: Johns Hopkins Press, 1967.
5. Reinke, W. A., Taylor, C. E., and Parker, R. L. "Functional Analysis of Health Needs and Services." In: *Proceedings of the Sixth International Scientific Meeting of the International Epidemiological Association,* Primosten, Yugoslavia, September, 1971. (in press)
6. Waterston, A. "An Operational Approach to Development Planning." *International Journal of Health Services* 1:223-252, 1971.
7. Hochbaum, G. M. "Consumer Participation in Health Planning: Toward Conceptual Clarification." *American Journal of Public Health* 59:1698-1705, 1969.
8. Blendon, R. J. and Gaus, C. R. "Problems in Developing Health Services in Poverty Areas: The Johns Hopkins Experience." *Journal of Medical Education* 46:477-484, 1971.
9. Conant, Ralph W. *The Politics of Community Health.* Washington, D.C.: Public Affairs Press, 1968.
10. National Health Forum. *Planning for Health.* New York: National Health Council, 1967.
11. Taylor, Carl E. and Takulia, Harbans S., editors. *Integration of Health and Family Planning in Village Sub-Centers.* Narangwal, Punjab State, India: Rural Health Research Center, 1971.

ADDITIONAL READINGS

The list of readings will be found at the end of Chapter Two.

4

Methods and Measurements in Evaluation

WILLIAM A. REINKE

Planning without implementation leads to nothing, and implementation without evaluation can conceivably make matters even worse. On the contrary, in a conscientiously conducted evaluation process, the most valuable insights are gained concerning ways in which planning can be improved and performance upgraded. While this endorsement of evaluation is perhaps as acceptable as a kind word for motherhood, the fact remains that in practice evaluation is often considered too late and then only lightly.

ROLE OF EVALUATION IN PLANNING

Evidently this is the result of failure to understand the important roles of evaluation in planning: (1) to provide a means for continuing self-study and (2) to offer periodic external review. No one enjoys being policed; moreover, most of us exhibit greater energy in contemplating the future than in mulling over the past. Thus, when evaluation is looked upon as little more than a search for past failures, it is not surprising that little enthusiasm is generated, especially among those whose wrists may get slapped in the process.

In contrast, when the notion of continuing self-study is recognized to connote current and private surveillance designed to keep an individual or an agency in line with objectives—or perhaps to help explain why this is impossible to do—then the merits of evaluation begin to be appreciated. Further, when the review of accomplishments is designed for future improvement as well as past assessment, evaluation is likely to become still more palatable.

SCOPE OF EVALUATION

Related to the role of evaluation is its scope. In the strictest sense it asks: what *has been* done? More dynamically, however, it asks: what *is being* done? Most appropriately it enters the scene early to ask: what *can be* done?

When we seek to know what has been done, we are really drawing attention to two considerations. First, we are implying that a problem existed that reflected a sufficient departure from some norm to be considered important. Thus, inherent in evaluation is the notion of problems, goals, and priorities. Second, action to alleviate the problem is implied. Hence, evaluation inherently involves a measurement of resources and activities. Presumably these resources and activities are embodied within particular organizational relationships and responsibilities. The true importance of organizational interrelationships is recognized, however, only when we express the more dynamic concern for what is being done. Then evaluation begins to incorporate the notions of feedback, adjustment, and adaptability. Finally, when evaluation enters the picture early enough to consider what can be done, we sense the availability and the importance of controllable alternatives in place of the fatalistic recording of accomplished fact.

GENERAL PRINCIPLES

As we have considered the subject of evaluation in conceptual and rather imprecise terms, we have stumbled upon a number of important aspects. We have seen that it concerns the movement toward goals in an effort to alleviate priority problems. This search for the satisfaction of objectives is accomplished with tangible resources and measurable activities. Moreover, the organizational framework within which the resources and activities are mobilized is likewise important. In particular, organizations are made up of individual decision makers who contemplate the alternatives under their control and are held accountable for the results achieved from the courses of action they select.

Hopefully, we shall fit these various aspects together in a more systematic and precise manner before we are through. Our discussion thus far has proceeded to the point, however, where a number of principles of evaluation should be recognized and enunciated.

1. Evaluation must be *forward looking,* recognizing that planning, implementation, evaluation, and control comprise a unified dynamic feedback mechanism rather than a series of independent stages of a process. The evaluation aspect must be continuing and productive of guidelines for future changes as well as a record of past accomplishments and failures.

2. Evaluation must exhibit adequate concern for the *relationship between ends and means.* If implementation consists of the mobilization of resources and activities to accomplish certain objectives, then evaluation must incorporate measurements both of the levels of input (i.e., the action taken) and of output (i.e., performance).

3. To be effective, evaluation must consciously relate to the *centralization-decentralization* dilemma. When we add to the second point above recognition that action is taken through organization, evaluation clearly must be focused upon areas of responsibility. The advantages of decentralization can be fulfilled only to the extent that standards and measurements are feasible. Under such conditions the evaluation mechanism can be sufficiently powerful that the span of control can be loosened and lengthened.

4. Effective evaluation depends upon the existence of a good *information system*. Good information systems are not automatically those that produce the greatest volume of data. Indeed, as evaluation programs are extended the danger is that increased demands for information will be self-defeating. Instead, great care must be exercised to provide for the acquisition of limited amounts of truly useful information at the *right place* and the *right time*.

SPECIFIC ELEMENTS

Turning to the more specific elements of evaluation programs in practice, we identify four basic aspects: appropriateness, adequacy, effectiveness, and efficiency (1). *Appropriateness* comes into focus first as one asks critically whether the contemplated program is really directed at an important problem. Superficially, this appraisal may appear to be quite straightforward, but in fact it is sometimes difficult to be objective with respect to parochial interests that carry the ability to marshal a seemingly strong case and to present it vigorously. On the other hand, a good argument can be made for permitting a highly qualified and motivated organization to tackle a problem of only moderate community importance rather than to assign an important task to an indifferent agency with talents foreign to the job.

Once it is clear that attention is indeed being directed toward a problem of considerable magnitude, the question arises whether the contemplated program is *adequate* to make much of a difference. This aspect of evaluation is simply the determination of whether the mountain is to be removed through the use of teaspoons or bulldozers. Alternatively, it serves to guard against the attempt to assemble fine watches with the aid of pipe wrenches and sledge hammers.

The third aspect of evaluation, *effectiveness,* lies at the heart of the present discussion. Effectiveness has been defined as "the extent to which pre-established objectives are attained as a result of activity" (1, p. 324). Program *efficiency* in turn is defined as "the cost in resources of attaining objectives" (1, p. 323). Together, effectiveness and efficiency make up program performance. Thus, shortcomings in performance can be analyzed to determine the extent to which the unit costs of inputs were excessive and the extent to which inputs, regardless of how efficiently mobilized, failed to produce the anticipated results.

THE STRUCTURE OF EVALUATION

The evaluation measurements must be timely, and they must be made at the critical points in the program. Taking the family planning area for illustration, the official position might be that the eventual aim of the various family planning activities is a reduction in birth rate to a level of, say, 25 per 1,000 per year. This would be the *ultimate objective.* A particular program, however, may have the more immediate objective of prompting, say, 75 percent of a certain group of women to use some acceptable form of contraception. This identifies the *program objectives* which, as we can see, may or may not coincide with the ultimate objective. Normally the program objective cannot be achieved in the absence of the attainment of certain prior conditions which define the so-called sub-objectives. In our example, the use of contraceptives presupposes knowledge on the part of the women concerning their existence, a desire to make use of them, and actual availability of the contraceptives, as well as positive action by the women to obtain them.

By linking together the various sub-objectives to the program objective as well as with each other, we not only obtain a clearer understanding of the key elements of the program but we provide for *timely* appraisal of the degree of accomplishment of these key elements. This appraisal can begin even before implementation. For example, let us suppose that, in reviewing the various sub-objectives, we decide first that we cannot expect more than 90 percent of our target population to have or acquire knowledge about contraception. We might conclude in turn that at most 80 percent of those who know about it can be motivated to desire it. Further, problems of logistics may prohibit availability to more than 95 percent of the target population. Finally, we may anticipate that of the women who have knowledge of and desire for contraception and who have acceptable methods available to them, not more than 90 percent will actually become users. When we multiply each of these preceding percentages together, we find that the product is 62 percent, which falls short of our original goal of 75 percent usage. Thus, this more thorough advance appraisal has permitted us to understand better the various program components and their interrelationships and, as a result, has permitted us to establish more realistic objectives.

In the actual conduct of the educational portion of the program, it may turn out that dissemination of knowledge reaches only 80 percent of the target population. We can then calculate that even if the remaining sub-objectives were achieved we could not hope to end up with more than 55 percent of the target population as users. Through this early recognition of an impending departure from our 62 percent target, we can identify the source of the trouble and perhaps do something about it. For example, we can judge whether it would be worthwhile to allocate more resources to the educational component of the program.

We assume that specific sets of activities are directed toward the achievement of each sub-objective. We suppose further that resources are expended to support the performance of these activities. The measured association between activities conducted and degree of attainment of the sub-objectives characterizes program effectiveness. The comparison of projected resource expenditures with possible accomplishments constitutes cost-benefit analysis. Then, over-all program efficiency involves a comparison of actual accomplishments and resource expenditures relative to the bench mark established by the cost-benefit analysis. Efficiency studies can also be entertained to answer questions about the relationship between the extent of attainment of objectives and the number and kinds of activities conducted, as well as between the number and kinds of activities conducted and the resources expended.

Conceptually, the evaluation format that we have described has the major advantage of permitting the analysis of all the program linkages. Failure to achieve the program objective can be traced back to a failure of one or more of the prerequisite sub-objectives. These failures in turn can be traced back to the associated activities and resources. Either the required inputs were not forthcoming or else their anticipated contribution to the corresponding sub-objectives was not realized.

While the evaluation format has these obvious advantages, it presupposes a well-defined measurable system of linkages. In practice, of course, the contribution of each of the various components to the program objective is not always so clear. Even where the relationships are well understood, measurement can be a stumbling block. Consider the following elementary example. An attempt was made to immunize 80 percent of a certain preschool population against smallpox. Subsequent records reveal that in fact 60 percent of the population had been vaccinated. Apparently the program was 75 percent effective. This is an oversimplification, however, for it could be shown that one-fifth of the population would report for immunization regardless of the existence of a program. In reality, then, the program was designed to reach an additional 60 percent of the population, whereas it succeeded in adding only 40 percent. The true program effectiveness, therefore, was 67 percent.

REFERENCES

1. Deniston, O. L., Rosenstock, I. M., and Getting, V. A. "Evaluation of Program Effectiveness." *Public Health Reports* 83:323-335, 1968.

ADDITIONAL READINGS
Primary

Caro, F. G., editor. *Readings in Evaluation Research*. New York: Russell Sage Foundation, 1971.
    Review of recent progress in evaluation research.
Deniston, O. L. and Rosenstock, I. M. "Evaluating Health Programs." *Public Health Reports* 85:835-840, 1970.

Excellent concise exposition of methods for setting time-phased objectives and relating them to quantified program activities.

Deniston, O. L., Rosenstock, I. M., Welch, W., and Getting, V. A. "Evaluation of Program Efficiency." *Public Health Reports* 83:603-610, 1968.

Discussion of measurements of efficiency in contrast to those of program effectiveness.

Schulberg, H. C., *et al. Program Evaluation in the Health Fields.* New York: Behavioral Publications, 1969.

A classic as a compilation of the work of many authors in specific techniques and program areas.

Suchman, E. A. *Evaluative Research.* New York: Russell Sage Foundation, 1967.

A comprehensive, scholarly exposition of the subject.

WHO Technical Report Series No. 472. *Statistical Indicators for the Planning and Evaluation of Public Health Programmes.* Geneva: World Health Organization, 1971.

The product of a WHO Expert Committee directing attention to the body of information necessary for evaluation, as well as guides for its interpretation.

Secondary

Agency for International Development. Office of Program Evaluation. *Evaluation Handbook.* Washington, D.C.: Government Printing Office, 1971.

Borgatta, E. F. "Research Problems in Evaluation of Health Service Demonstrations." *Milbank Memorial Fund Quarterly* 44:182-200, No. 4, Part 2, October, 1966.

Kelman, H. R. and Elinson, J. "Strategy and Tactics of Evaluating a Large Scale Medical Care Program." *Medical Care* 7:79-85, 1969.

Methods of Evaluating Public Health Programmes. Report of a Symposium, Kiel, 1967. Copenhagen: Regional Office for Europe, World Health Organization, 1967.

Ortiz, J. and Parker, R. "A Birth-Life-Death Model for Planning and Evaluation of Health Services Programs." *Health Services Research* 6:120-143, 1971.

Osterweil, J. "Evaluation: A Keystone of Comprehensive Health Planning." *Community Mental Health Journal* 5:121-128, 1969.

Parker, A. H. and Shellard, G. D. "Measures of Health-System Effectiveness." *Operations Research* 18:1067-1070, 1970.

Sanazaro, P. J. "Comprehensive Health Care and the Researcher." *Journal of Medical Education* 45:486-489, 1970.

Schulberg, H. C. and Baker, F. "Program Evaluation Models and the Implementation of Research Findings." *American Journal of Public Health* 58:1248-1255, 1968.

Sheps, M. C. *Assessing Effectiveness of Programs in Operation.* Transactions of the Fourth Conference on Administrative Medicine. New York: Josiah Macy Jr. Foundation, 1956.

Steele, J. H. "Glossary of Evaluative Terms in Public Health." *American Journal of Public Health* 60:1546-1552, 1970.

Turban, E. and Metersky, M. L. "Utility Theory Applied to Multivariable System Effectiveness Evaluation." *Management Science* 17:B817-B828, August, 1971.

II

The Health Planning Base

5

An Overview of the Planning Process

WILLIAM A. REINKE

Health planning can be considered effective only to the extent that it produces a greater contribution to health status per unit of resources expended than would have been achieved in the absence of planning. Since resources are limited and some problems are more vulnerable to attack than others, the planner is challenged to develop a rational, practical, and efficient allocation of the scarce resources based upon realistic objectives and sensible priorities.

CONCEPTUALIZATION OF THE HEALTH SERVICES SYSTEM

General: Figure 5.1

Conceptually, we take the approach portrayed in Figure 5.1, where we note that health services draw upon resources in response to certain health problems for the purpose of producing an output, or result, in the form of improved health status (1, pp. 28-43). Such a broad conceptualization is, of course, of little practical value in coming to grips with real conditions. We must look more carefully, therefore, at each system component in turn.

People and Their Health Problems: Figure 5.2

Health problems are identified in relation to the population at risk in the planning area. Effectively, then, they have epidemiologic numerators, demographic denominators, and geographic bounds. The last item depends upon the mandate of the planning body, the location of health resources, political jurisdictions, transportation and communication patterns, and population concentrations.

Demographic considerations are based upon the fact that different segments of the population vary in the type and magnitude of their health needs, as well as in their utilization of health services. A planner is especially interested in identifying important population characteristics that are likely to change in relative importance. As a minimum, the population breakdown should include

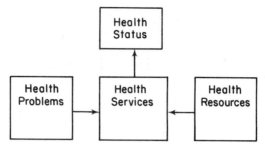

Fig. 5.1. Health care system overview.

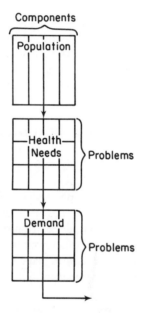

Fig. 5.2. Detailed view of health problems.

age, sex, and place of residence. Frequently, it is advisable to add social class and/or educational attainment, race, and participation in health insurance programs. Precautions must be taken, however, to avoid classifying the population into so many small subgroups that reliable enumeration becomes too costly.

Within each relevant population group, the planner must identify the nature and importance of individual health needs, as well as the extent to which these needs are currently translated into demands for health services. Assessment of problems should allow for both cause and effect. Consider, for example, the finding that at ages one to five months the white and nonwhite mortality rates in the United States are 4.2 and 12.0 per 1,000 live births respectively, whereas at one to five days the rates are much more similar, namely, 6.0 and 8.6 (2). This information is quite helpful in pointing to the problem as community-based rather than hospital-based.

In general, of course, gross mortality rates provide too crude a measure of health problems. Instead, identification of problems according to the *International Classification of Diseases* may be useful. Furthermore, within this classification system a planner will probably be concerned with morbidity or loss in productive capacity as well as mortality. In this regard, for example, the Division of Indian Health has developed a Health Problem Index (Q) that emcompasses lost time for in-patients and out-patients, in addition to productivity losses due to premature death (3).

Classification of health problems by disease not only provides information on effects in terms of mortality and morbidity, but also suggests specific disease agents as causal factors. In addition, more general environmental sources of health problems should be identified, including water supply sources, sewerage and waste collection systems, food protection mechanisms, housing conditions, air pollution, recreational sanitation, and vector control.

Health Resources: Figure 5.3

In considering health resources, the planner must separate human, physical, and financial components. He must determine the available quantities and locations of different kinds of health manpower, inventory existing facilities of various kinds (including insurance schemes, government support of health programs, and private contributions of various kinds). This breakdown of the health resources box is shown in Figure 5.3.

In some respects, an inventory of health resources lacks meaning apart from the services developed from those resources. Knowledge of the number of physicians in a country is of limited value without corresponding information about the number and types of patients seen by these doctors. Still, the fact that a country averages one physician per 3,000 population does convey something about the health potential of that country. Detailed information about the maldistribution of practitioners between the urban and rural areas is likely to be even more relevant for planning purposes.

Manpower resources must be viewed with respect to, first, existing supplies and, second, the training infrastructure as it could affect future levels. From among the many existing categories of health manpower, the planner will wish to concentrate on physicians, dentists, nurses, pharmacists, and certain auxiliaries and indigenous practitioners who may be relatively numerous in the particular area. In addition to numbers, the planner will be interested in the age and sex distribution, the affiliation, and the type and location of practice.

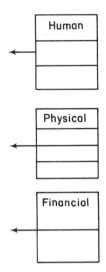

Fig. 5.3. Detailed view of health resources.

In assessing the training base for developing future manpower, the planner must consider the financial, physical, and teaching constraints of institutions for health training. In some areas, he may also need to survey the potential of general educational institutions, for the health field may be hard pressed in the competition with other professions for scarce secondary school graduates.

As manpower data are assembled, the planner has to make some judgment concerning the effect of geographical maldistribution, differences between the distribution of physical and human resources, and relationships among categories of health workers. Suppose, for example, that three regions of equal population have 100, 50, and 25 doctors, respectively. Is the effective gap between the second and third region more or less than that between the first two? How much would the judgment be altered if it were learned that the third region has more nurses? How would one look upon the fact that the third region has no hospital to serve additional physicians that might be attracted to the area?

Like manpower, physical facilities fit into a number of categories which must be separately identified and inventoried. These include hospitals, dispensaries, clinics, and private sources of personal care, as well as water, sewerage, and other environmental systems.

The degree of detail embodied in the information depends upon the availability of data and the uniqueness of given resources. Apart from the detail with which records are maintained, the essential criterion of interest to the planner is the degree to which facilities can be substituted for one another. Thus, he requires a geographical breakdown in order to recognize differences in population groups served. Distinctions are also made on the basis of differences in diagnostic and treatment facilities; consequently, information is assembled with respect to short-term general, long-term rehabilitation, and mental institutions, along with the·availability of various clinical and laboratory services within the institutions. Frequently, distinctions must be made on the basis of the goals of individual health agencies which arise from different sources of sponsorship, and these distinctions may be reflected in the financial structure and organization of the agency; hence, the planner is likely to distinguish among government, proprietary, religious, and other types of institutions.

Once the planner has appropriately classified a facility, he must place a value on it, usually in both physical and monetary terms. For example, a hospital might be identified as a 200-bed institution with a certain replacement cost. In looking to the future, the age of existing installations is an important factor, just as the age distribution of physicians is an important manpower consideration.

Although categorization is necessary to the inventorying of resources, attention must also be given to coordination and interactions among categories. Existing referral patterns must be recognized, along with the impact that such things as increased dependence upon extended care facilities would have upon the need for beds in short-term general hospitals.

Health Services: Figure 5.4

Figure 5.4 depicts schematically the structure of health services that develops from the organization of resources to satisfy health demands. The figure also shows the impact of these services upon health status. Although in a systems sense the health services "process" is distinct from the health status "output," in practice in the health field these two elements are not so easily separated. Indeed, the generally fuzzy relationship between the process and the result causes health planners and administrators at times to measure service units, such as annual physician visits per capita, as if they were endpoints or outputs.

In any event, Figure 5.4 shows health services to include diagnostic, treatment, and rehabilitative components. From the standpoint of planning and evaluation, these services should be viewed in functional rather than organizational terms. Thus, these three boxes are each subdivided vertically into the various categories of activity of which these services are comprised. These activities are directed in varying degrees toward particular health needs which are separated schematically by the horizontal lines. In other words, the planner must understand the present health services structure in terms of the performance of certain functions, each of which is a specific combination of human, physical, and financial resources organized to satisfy to some extent one or more existing health demands.

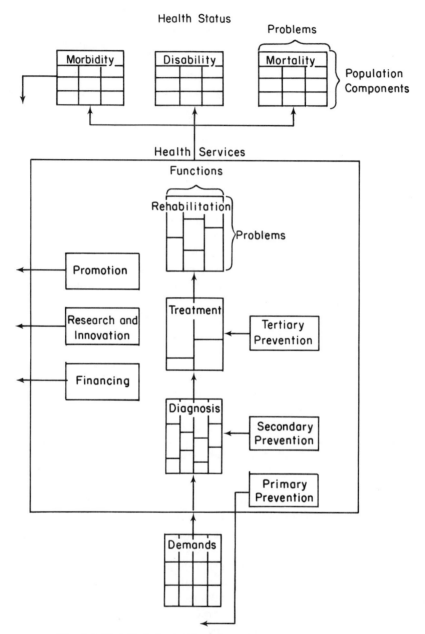

Fig. 5.4. Detailed view of health services and health status.

Prevention

In viewing the health services structure, explicit recognition should be given to the preventive aspects. Primary disease prevention, such as immunization, has an impact extending beyond the health services box to the basic needs box of Figure 5.2. Secondary prevention as a category of service, such as early detection of cervical cancer, has its major effect at the diagnostic stage, whereas tertiary prevention occurs largely at the treatment stage, as in the case where stroke patients are treated in a manner which minimizes muscular deformities and subsequent problems of rehabilitation.

Supply and Demand

The health field is unique in the extent to which supply and demand interact. This is exemplified by contentions that physicians largely create a demand for their own services and the utilization of hospital beds is in large measure determined by their availability. A complete and realistic appraisal of the health services structure, therefore, must include factors that influence demand for services. Three such factors are shown in Figure 5.4. First, we include the various forms of health education and professional influence that come under the general heading of promotion. Second, since demand for health services depends in large part upon the extent to which health problems are vulnerable to attack, we must include medical research and other innovative activities that affect the state of the art of medicine. Finally, we must recognize the role of the health services structure in extending effective demand beyond what it would be with private financing alone. For example, the health planner must know about training institutions that, in the interests of medical education, offer free services to the medically indigent.

Measurement

Actual measurement of services rendered should include, to begin with, a compilation of resource utilization data such as the annual number of physician visits and hospital discharges and durations of hospital stay. These figures must be related, of course, to the demographic and epidemiologic characteristics of the population served. Likewise, recognition of the key role of financial mechanisms in determining the nature of services actually provided is important, and a planner must know a good deal about the costs and sources of funding such services. In a broader sense, he should be cognizant of the current magnitude of health expenditures relative to the size of the total economy, along with future trends in both.

Besides measuring the mere utilization of resources, a health planner may construct indices describing services provided by certain types and quantities of resources. Molina and Noam have developed such a list of service indicators for Puerto Rico (4). From this list (Table 5.1), for example, we can see that the

Table 5.1
Selected Indicators of Health Services, Puerto Rico, 1940-1960

Indicators	1940	1950	1960
Health Services			
Number of inhabitants per physician	3,672	2,355	1,181
Number of hospital beds per 1000 inhabitants	–	4.7	5.1
Number of prenatal consultations per live birth	0.7	1.13	1.18
Number of well baby consultations per live birth	1.42	1.55	2.20
Percent of population with potable water	31.0	47.0	75.0
Percent of births occurring in hospitals	10.0	37.7	77.5
Percent of deaths with medical certificate	–	47.0	68.9
Annual per capita health expenditure (1958 dollars)	8.4	27.5	48.5

SOURCE: Molina, G. and Noam, I. F. "Indicators of Health, Economy, Culture in Puerto Rico and Latin America." *American Journal of Public Health* 54:1193, 1964.

number of well baby consultations per live birth increased substantially between 1940 and 1960. Therefore, Puerto Rico should be prepared in the future to allocate additional health resources in this area, quite apart from any future increases in the number of births. We can observe further that the percentage of births occurring in hospitals has been increasing. This has implications not only with respect to resource utilization in the future, but in addition suggests possible improvements in the health status of infants and mothers.

Health Status: Figure 5.4

For schematic purposes, health status can be considered in terms of mortality, disability, and morbidity. Morbidity is linked to population, indicating that the entire health system is dynamic. That is, we are interested in the ability of the health services to modify and improve health status and to return healthy individuals to the population. This suggests further that each health status component (mortality, disability, and morbidity) should have the same subdivisions by population groups and health problems (see Figure 5.2). As a result, a planner must identify not only the major sources of health needs but also areas in which these needs are not being met satisfactorily.

Important as health services indicators are, they are not substitutes for measures of health status. This point has been made rather dramatically by Peterson and his associates in a compilation of health statistics from the United States, the United Kingdom, and Sweden (5). Their data, some of which are presented in Table 5.2, show no consistent associations among the various measures of health status and health services.

Comparison of Health Levels and Health Services

HEALTH STATUS | HEALTH RESOURCES AND SERVICES

Country	Life Expectancy at Birth		Infant Mortality per 1000 Live Births		Health Expenditures as Percent of GNP	Physicians per 100,000 Population	Annual Per Capita Doctor/Patient Contacts
	Males	Females	Males	Females			
United States	66.6	73.4	28.4	21.9	5.2	137	5.3
England and Wales	68.0	73.9	23.7	18.4	4.7	127	4.7
Sweden	71.3	75.4	17.4	13.2	4.7	106	2.7

HEALTH RESOURCES AND SERVICES: SHORT-TERM HOSPITAL STATISTICS

	Admissions per 1000 Population	Mean Length of Stay (Days)	Beds per 1000 Population	Bed Days per 1000 Population	Bed Utilization Rate (Percent)	Nonmedical Staff per 1000 Patient Days
United States	134	7.7	3.7	1032	76.4	241
England and Wales	82	14.8	4.4	1217	76.6	?
Sweden	127	12.5	6.0	1588	72.5	138

Source: Peterson, O. L. et al. "What is Value for Money in Medical Care?" *The Lancet* 1:771-774, 8 April 1967.

62   /   *Reinke*

Impact of Planning: Figure 5.5

These health system components and linkages exist regardless of the role that health planning may play. Planning does, however, carry with it the potential for improving the performance of the system. Inherent in the notion of improvement is the specification of goals, or norms, toward which conscious

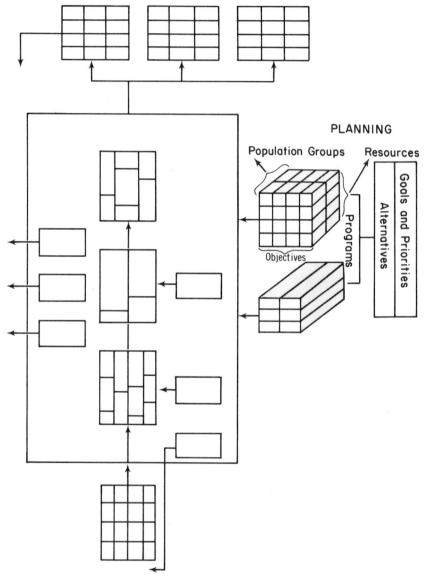

Fig. 5.5. Detailed view of health services and health status with planning.

effort is to be directed. The core of planning, then, is the analysis of alternative means of moving toward identified health goals in the light of specified priorities and existing constraints. The selection process results in a variety of program packages. Each program, which is directed at one or more health problems, is designed to achieve specific measurable objectives through a certain combination of resources oriented toward particular population groups. These program packages vary, depending upon whether objectives are limited or more comprehensive, whether the programs are simple or require complex organizations, and whether they are general in scope or directed toward a small population segment, such as mentally retarded children.

The Total Picture: Figure 5.6

Finally, all the health system components are brought together in Figure 5.6. This figure is a restatement of Figure 5.1, but is considerably more detailed and expressly incorporates the role of planning into the schematic representation.

THE ESSENCE OF PLANNING

As we focus upon the planning process itself, we reiterate that the core of planning is *analysis* (in the face of constraints) of alternative means of achieving established *goals* ranked in some order of *priority*. These two factors—goals and analysis—form the base of our attention in the remainder of this overview.

Goals and Priorities

We must first define and distinguish among the terms mission, goal, objective, and target (6). Although other terms might be employed, the notions inherent in these four must be a part of rational planning and decision-making.

Mission describes an organization's reason for existence, the general functions or services it performs, and the limits of its jurisdiction and authority. The mission of a state or local health department might be the protection and advancement of the public health of the population of that state or community within certain legally specified limitations.

A goal is a long-range specified state of accomplishment toward which programs are directed. It is not cast in terms of current availability of resources or a fixed time for achievement, but it must be consistent with the mission. In the health field, the goal is usually stated in terms of completely overcoming a health problem or reducing it to the extent the state of the art permits.

An objective is stated in terms of achieving a measured amount of progress toward a goal. It must include a specification of:

1. *What:* the nature of the situation or condition to be attained;
2. *Extent:* the quantity or amount of the situation or condition to be attained;

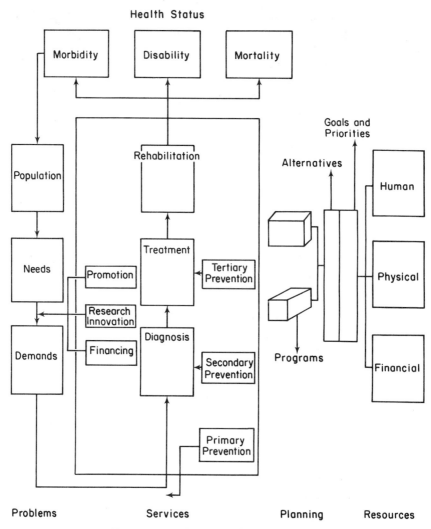

Fig. 5.6. Detailed view of health system.

3. *When:* the time at or by which the desired situation or condition is intended to exist;
4. *Who:* the particular group of people or portion of the environment in which attainment is desired;
5. *Where:* the geographic area to be included in the program (7).

A target establishes a measured amount of progress toward a health objective via a specific program activity. In order to appreciate the difference between an objective and a target, consider a plan to deal with the problem of influenza. The objective might be "to decrease mortality from influenza throughout the state to

50 per 100,000 population per annum by the end of two years," regardless of how this might be achieved. With this objective in mind, a target might be established "to immunize 80 percent of high-risk individuals against influenza during the next year."

Alternatives and Constraints—A Functional Framework

It follows that targets can be established only after particular programs have been selected from a set of alternatives. Moreover, reasonable objectives can only arise from a consideration of the costs and resources required to achieve the benefits that underlie contemplated objectives. For example, one could not automatically argue that an influenza mortality rate of 40 per 100,000 population represents a better objective than one of 50 per 100,000 population. It might be that the reduction from 50 to 40 would require an unconscionable drain on resources. Specifications of aims, then, is intimately bound up with the analysis of alternatives, even though we discuss the two aspects separately.

To be most effective, consideration of program alternatives should proceed within the framework of the health functions of particular concern. To illustrate, one agency has established the following nine study areas: reproduction, nutrition, dental and oral health, infectious and communicable diseases, trauma and safety, chronic diseases, handicapping conditions, mobility, and mental disorders (8). Other planners might prefer a breakdown in terms of personal preventive, curative, and rehabilitative activities, environmental sanitation, mass campaigns against communicable diseases, and so forth. These functions could be analyzed further with respect to such important dimensions as age or urgency of need (emergency, acute, and chronic conditions).

Regardless of the classification scheme employed, the planner then seeks to identify the activities and resources currently mobilized in pursuit of each of these functions. At the same time, he will seek to determine associated standards of performance. Particular combinations of resources assembled according to certain standards for specific purposes have been designated as "instruments" by the Latin American planners (9). The cluster of activities involved in the utilization of this set of resources is known as a "procedure." Each procedure then is made up of a sequence of individual tasks or operations.

To illustrate the concept of functional analysis in planning, consider its application by Yankauer to maternal and child health activities in Latin America (10). Within the function of well child care, Yankauer has listed four broad classes of action: (1) screening for early "unrecognized" disease and referral for care; (2) anticipatory guidance for parental education (including nutrition education) designed to prevent future disease; (3) dietary supplementation; and (4) immunization. Each of the four classes of action embodies a series of different tasks; for example, BCG immunization is a specific preventive task of tuberculosis control. Then

> . . . the "instrumentation" of all these specific tasks involves the human and material resources of a health-care service for mothers and children integrated into the general health-care services of a community. Thus, in the context of a health planning framework . . . . well child care . . . . can be defined as the sum of all specific preventive tasks to be included within a health-care service for mothers and children (10, p. 753).

By structuring his thinking in this way, a planner can gain a broad understanding of the relative importance currently attached to each of the health functions, the demands made by each upon scarce resources, and the methods employed in carrying out the functions. Consequently, as health programs are developed in an effort to improve the functioning of the health services system, the projected impacts upon functional emphasis and demands for scarce resources become more visible. For example, one study of pediatricians revealed the limited amount of time spent with patients and further showed that one-half of the patient time was spent with well children and another 22 percent treating those with minor respiratory problems (11). This kind of concrete information gives more solid support to whatever intuitive notions one may have regarding benefits to be derived from the use of pediatric auxiliaries.

The preceding exposition has developed the framework within which planning alternatives are to be analyzed. This framework is shown schematically in Figure 5.7. To begin with, broad goals are establshed consistent with the over-all mission of the enterprise. Then, specific quantified objectives are developed with the aim of effective functioning of the health services system. Progress toward the achievement of these objectives is made by means of health programs. These programs, which organize activities (procedures) for the efficient utilization of combinations of resources (instruments), have certain targets. Although a given program may affect more than one health function, individual targets most probably will not. An MCH program, for example, may have both a family planning and a well child care function, but the program target to immunize 80 percent of the preschool population against measles would apply only to the latter function. Planning takes place, then, in the belief that a measurable correspondence exists between resources expended and activities performed. It further assumes that a meaningful comparison can be made between the activities performed and the degree of attainment of targets and objectives.

Analysis of Alternatives

Within this framework, planning involves the specification and analysis of alternatives—that is, alternative problem priorities and alternative programs or

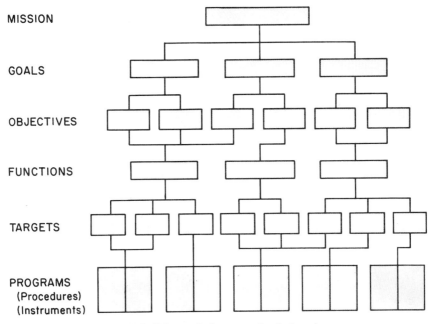

MISSION

GOALS

OBJECTIVES

FUNCTIONS

TARGETS

PROGRAMS
(Procedures)
(Instruments)

Fig. 5.7. Schematic framework of planning.

techniques for coping with the problems, with due consideration for the many physical, environmental, technological, social, cultural, and political constraints.

In particular, certain problems are not yet vulnerable to attack. In these cases, the planner has no choice but to provide for the allocation of resources required to treat the problems as they inevitably arise. Leukemia and many of our chronic diseases tend to fall into this category. Then, some problems are recognized by the population to such an extent that the effective demand for services cannot be ignored by the planner; he can only entertain alternative means of satisfying the need. Malaria, with its curative and preventive alternatives, illustrates this class of problems. Finally, certain health needs occur of which at least some individuals in the population are either unaware or are financially unable to satisfy. Realizing that health resources are limited to begin with and are further reduced by demands generated from the first two problem areas, the planner is forced to make some critical decisions concerning problem priority and resource allocation in the third category.

The traditional response has been "to select and justify programs on the basis of intuition or tradition, plan and budget in terms of object and activity, and evaluate in terms of effort" (12, p. 45). Hopefully, the future will witness an increasing degree of quantification to accompany the always important factor of experienced intuition. We can expect the planner to be guided by a priority indexing system and cost-benefit analyses where appropriate. Moreover, the planning-programming-budgeting concept should serve to unify the entire planning process through implementation, evaluation, and control. Since experimentation with alternatives in an operational setting is not feasible, the planner should make maximum use of operations research techniques involving the mathmatical analysis or computer simulation of true-to-life models.

In more specific terms, the analysis of alternatives must include consideration for *what* is to be done and *when* it is to be accomplished, and *where, for whom,* and *how* it is to be carried out.

The questions of what and when are, of course, interrelated. Objectives can stress either that fixed levels of attainment will be reached in minimum time or that results will be maximized over a fixed time horizon. For example, the intent may be to have one doctor for every 1,000 members of the population as soon as possible, or it may be to train the maximum number of physicians in the next decade. Clearly, the appropriate courses of action may differ according to the emphasis of the objective. Also, the course of achievement will likely follow a sigmoidal curve over time. Early in the planning period, progress may be slow, followed by an acceleration and then a leveling off as a saturation point is approached. Naturally, the extent of progress will then depend upon the points in time selected for the initial and final measurements. Finally, we must appreciate the fact that definitions of acceptable health standards vary, not only by community and nation, but over time within a geographical region. Our present standards are not what they were in 1920; present norms cannot simply be projected into the future, ignoring changes in aspirations and capabilities.

The questions of where, for whom, and how the planned activities are to come about must also be considered jointly. If special attention is to be given to rural areas, then a much different population will be served than if urban areas were emphasized. Furthermore, serious limitations in the quantity and kinds of health workers and facilities in the rural areas may lead to an entirely different service program there than in the cities, apart from any differences in health needs. For example, the rural program may have a heavy input of dietary supplementation, immunizations, and other productive activities that can be carried out by auxiliaries with a minimum of supervision.

SUMMARY

Planning initially requires the identification of health problems as major deviations from broad goals and of the causal and contributing factors associated with the problems. Second, alternative plans of action are specified in light of imposed constraints. Particular courses of action are selected from among the alternatives on as rational a basis as possible. Objectives are then assigned to appropriate points in the plan of action along with the activities (procedures) and resources (instruments) required to achieve the objectives.

Application of the Planning Process

To illustrate the approach, let us consider its application specifically to the problem of respiratory diseases in a given state. In his consideration of the matter, a health planner might assemble the following information pertaining to the problem itself, plans of action, and the objectives of the action (6).

Nature of the Health Problem

Pneumonia (excluding pneumonia of the newborn) accounts for over one-half of the deaths from respiratory diseases. Influenza accounts for one-fifth, and emphysema another one-tenth of the deaths in this category. Other URI are responsible for 1,175 days of restricted activity per 100,000 population annually.

Factors Related to the Causes

Some important factors related to the causes of respiratory diseases are common to all populations where socioeconomic levels prohibit an adequate standard of living to provide a suitable home environment. The incidence of these diseases and death and disability are directly related to such factors as overcrowded home conditions, inadequate housing resulting in exposure to climatic extremes, poor nutrition, inadequate knowledge of modern health practices, inadequate medical care, and low immunization levels. In at least two metropolitan areas of the state, air pollution has been shown to be a factor in contributing to, if not actually causing, some respiratory problems. Weed pollen is also a factor in this health problem, especially with regard to the restricted activity days.

Plans of Action (Selected from Alternate Plans)

1. Conduct monthly immunization clinics at each local health department.
2. Conduct television and radio education programs through a series of one-minute spot announcements daily on each television and radio station in the state.
3. Eliminate all open burning of refuse in two metropolitan areas by the state air pollution control authority.
4. Extend weed control programs to cover 60 percent of the urban areas in the state by the state department of agriculture.
5. Replace 3 percent of the substandard homes in the state through long-term, low-interest home mortgages in a program conducted by the state housing authority.

Health Objectives to be Achieved at the End of Two Years (Rates per 100,000 Population)

1. Decrease mortality to 50.
2. Decrease days of hospitalization to 25.
3. Decrease out-patient visits to 340.
4. Decrease days of restricted activity to 1,140.

Activity Targets
1. Immunize 80 percent of high risk individuals against influenza.
2. Provide monthly public health nurse visits to 80 percent of economically deprived homes.
3. Reduce air pollution (in terms of SO_2 level) in two metropolitan areas by 10 percent.
4. Reduce average pollen count by 15 percent.

REFERENCES

1. For a related approach, see: Kennedy, F. D. *Basic Considerations Essential to the Design and Development of Community Health Service System Simulation Models.* RM-OU280-3. Research Triangle Park, North Carolina: Research Triangle Institute, 1967.
2. National Center for Health Statistics. *Infant and Perinatal Mortality in the United States.* U.S.P.H.S. Publication No. 1000, Series 3, No. 4. Washington, D.C.: Government Printing Office, 1965.
3. *The Principles of Program Packaging in the Division of Indian Health.* Silver Spring, Maryland: Department of Health, Education, and Welfare, Bureau of Medical Services, 1966.
4. Molina, G. and Noam, I. F. "Indicators of Health, Economy, Culture in Puerto Rico and Latin America." *American Journal of Public Health* 54:1191-1206, 1964.
5. Peterson, O. L., Burgess, A. M., Berfenstam, R., Smedby, B., Logan, R. F. L., and Pearson, R. J. C. "What Is Value for Money in Medical Care? Experiences in England and Wales, Sweden, and the U.S.A." *The Lancet* 1:771-776, 8 April 1967.
6. Michael, J. M., Spatafore, G., and Williams, E. R. "An Approach to Health Planning ." *Public Health Reports* 82:1063-1070, 1967.
7. Deniston, O. L., Rosenstock, I. M., and Getting, V. A. "Evaluation of Program Effectiveness." *Public Health Reports* 83:323-335, 1968.
8. *Health Goals for Greater Cleveland: Summary.* Cleveland: Health Goals Committee, 1966.
9. Ahumada, J. *et al. Health Planning: Problems of Concept and Method.* Scientific Publication No. 111. Washington, D.C.: Pan American Health Organization, 1965.
10. Yankauer, A. "National Planning and the Construction of Maternal and Child Hygiene Norms in Latin America." *American Journal of Public Health* 57:751-761, 1967.
11. Bergman, A. B., Dassel, S. W., and Wedgwood, R. J. "Time-Motion Study of Practicing Pediatricians." *Pediatrics* 38:254-263, 1966.
12. Wagner, C. J. "A Systems Approach to Health Planning." In: *Planning for Health: Report of the 1967 National Health Forum.* New York: National Health Council, 1967.

ADDITIONAL READINGS

Primary

Ahumada, J. *et al. Health Planning: Problems of Concept and Method.* Scientific Publication No. 111. Washington, D.C.: Pan American Health Organization, 1965.

Description of the original CENDES/PAHO planning method developed for use in Latin America.

Anderson, Odin W. and Kravits, Joanna. *Health Services in the Chicago Area: A Framework for Use of Data.* Research Series No. 26. Chicago: University of Chicago, Center for Health Administration Studies, 1968.

An attempt to show how existing data might be arranged to reveal the structure and functioning of a health services system.

Bauer, Raymond A. *Social Indicators.* Cambridge: M.I.T. Press, 1966.

A beginning effort toward the quantification of social indicators to match the construction of economic indicators.

Blum, Henrik L. *Notes on Comprehensive Planning for Health.* San Francisco: Western Regional Office, American Public Health Association, 1968.

An extensive set of readings on health planning, oriented to the United States.

Division of Hospital and Medical Facilities. *Procedures for Areawide Health Facility Planning. A Guide for Planning Agencies.* U.S.P.H.S. Publication No. 930-B-3. Washington, D.C.: Government Printing Office, 1963.

Sourcebook on facilities planning.

Fanshel, S. and Bush, J. W. "A Health-Status Index and Its Application to Health Services Outcomes." *Operations Research* 18:1021-1066, 1970.

A practical attempt to develop a scalar measure of health level.

Gentry, J. T. *The Availability of Cost-Effectiveness Data for Uses in a Community Health Service System Simulation Model.* RM-OU280-2. Research Triangle Park, North Carolina: Research Triangle Institute, 1967.

Companion to the Kennedy document (see below) citing actual sources of data.

Kennedy, F. D. *Basic Considerations Essential to the Design and Development of Community Health Service System Simulation Models.* RM-OU280-3. Research Triangle Park, North Carolina: Research Triangle Institute, 1967.

Proposed framework for assembling and analyzing health information.

National Commission on Community Health Services. *Action Planning for Community Health Services.* Washington, D.C.: Public Affairs Press, 1967.

Sourcebook on community assessment for health planning.

The Principles of Program Packaging in the Division of Indian Health. Silver Spring, Maryland: U.S. Public Health Service, Bureau of Medical Services, 1966.

Description of the framework for planning, developed in the Division of Indian Health.

Zemach, R. "A Model of Health Service Utilization and Resource Allocation." *Operations Research* 18:1071-1086, 1970.

Another model for health services analysis.

Secondary

Altshuler, Alan. *City Planning Process: A Political Analysis.* Ithaca: Cornell University Press, 1966.

Battistella, R. M. and Weil, T. P. "Comprehensive Health Care Planning. New Effort or Redirected Energy?" *New York State Journal of Medicine* 69:2350-2370, 1969.

Bureau of Health Services. "Classification of Health Activities with Related

Output Measures (Tentative)." Washington, D.C.: Department of Health, Education, and Welfare, January, 1967.

"Guidelines for Organizing State and Area-Wide Community Health Planning." *American Journal of Public Health* 56:2139-2143, 1966.

Hilleboe, H. E. "Health Planning on a Community Basis." *Medical Care* 6:203-214, 1968.

Holder, L. and Deniston, O. L. "A Decision-Making Approach to Comprehensive Health Planning." *Public Health Reports* 83: 559-568, 1968.

Kissick, W. L., editor. "Dimensions and Determinants of Health Policy." *Milbank Memorial Fund Quarterly* 46: No. 1, Part 2, January, 1968.

National Center for Health Statistics. *An Index of Health—Mathematical Models.* U.S.P.H.S. Publication No. 1000, Series 2, No. 5. Washington, D.C.: Government Printing Office, 1965.

Pifer, A. "The Health Care Dilemma—New Directions for Medical Education. I. A New Climate." *Journal of Medical Education* 45:79-87, 1970.

Sasuly, R. and Ward, P. D. "Two Approaches to Health Planning: The Ideal vs. the Pragmatic." *Medical Care* 7:235-241, 1969.

Somers, A. R. "Goals into Reality: The Challenges of Health Planning." *Hospitals* 43:41-49, August 1, 1969.

Strauss, M. "Health Care Planning." *Hospitals* 43:105-108, April 1, 1969.

U.S. Department of Health, Education, and Welfare. *Toward a Social Report.* Report of the Panel on Social Indicators. Washington, D.C.: Government Printing Office, 1969.

6

The Political Aspects of Health Planning

THOMAS L. HALL

Politics is concerned with relationships of power or of influence, generally within the context of government (1, p. 2). A change in these relationships is apt to be either a prerequisite for or a consequence of successful health planning. This chapter reviews some aspects of the interface between health planning and the political process in the nonsocialist economies and suggests ways in which the planner can turn an understanding of this process into improved chances for implementation. Illustrative cases and references are based primarily but not exclusively on American experience. In a field as broad as the one under consideration, the planner must carefully assess the validity of the various observations made here in the light of the local situation in which he works.

THE POLITICAL CONTEXT OF HEALTH PLANNING

Health planning antedates by many years the formal organization of planning units. As long as organized health agencies have existed, systematic efforts have been made to improve the delivery of health care. Regrettably, they have not been accompanied by parallel attempts to record and understand the political context within which health authorities operate (2).

This situation has at last begun to change. In the United States various observers have commented on the adverse effects of political factors on plan implementation (3-5); the National Commission on Community Health Services explicitly recognized this when it entitled one of its monographs *The Politics of Community Health* (6). This study, directed at learning more about what contributed to successful community health planning, reported on the five rather modest "success stories" which were all the investigators were able to gleen from the two dozen nominations received nationwide. Other investigators

The valued comments and suggestions of my colleagues in the Department of International Health at the Johns Hopkins School of Hygiene and Public Health and of Drs. Abel Wolman, M. G. Wolman, C. Torrey Brown, A. Peter Ruderman, and Mr. Peter Marudas are gratefully acknowledged.

have begun to study the determinants of planning outcome and the results of their work are discussed below. Despite the as yet very incomplete nature of their findings, there is general agreement that the planner's ability to understand and turn the political process to his advantage is a prime determinant of success.

In the United States at least, the failure of many planners and health authorities to give adequate attention to the political component of their jobs has perhaps not had as adverse an effect on their activities as could have been anticipated. Various authors have pointed out past tendencies of politicians and the public alike to defer to the health professions in all matters pertaining to health care (2, 7, 8). Within the limits of the resources made available to him, the health administrator has had greater freedom from outside influence to dispose of such resources as he thought best than have his counterparts in other sectors such as education, welfare, and housing.

Health authorities have tended to foster such deference by presenting a public image of dignity and aloofness to controversial matters which extend beyond their immediate professional concerns (8, 9). The reluctance of health professionals to participate in the rough and tumble of program and interagency politics, or their perpetuation of the myth of the nonpolitical character of public health, has meant many lost opportunities for constructive action or has needlessly generated conflicts through ignorance of the political process (10).

All this is not likely to be the case in the future, for the situation has changed drastically in recent years. The spontaneous rise in community activism, reinforced by legislation promoting consumer participation in matters of public policy, and the growing awareness of the inability of the health professions to provide comprehensive care at reasonable cost have combined to bring the public and politicians into the debate on health policies more than ever before. Whereas in the past health officials *received* a mandate to discharge the traditional public health responsibilities, they now find themselves obliged to *generate* one for the expanding responsibilities of providing medical care.

Even more than the health administrator, the planner has sought to insulate himslf from the vagaries and hazards of the political process. To minimize interference with his work, he has experimented extensively with the organizational chart in an attempt to find an administrative location with the utopian combination of proximity to the sources of power as well as independence from "politics." Based on his extensive experience in the World Bank, Waterston believes that "...it is impossible for a planning agency to be both autonomous and effective. A plan which is to have a good chance of being implemented must be a joint project of those who have to carry it out and must express their coordinated aspirations in the context of a common goal. Moreover, the very essence to planning, indeed the very decision to begin planning, is political. There is no way of avoiding this, even if it were desirable" (11, p. 477).

The planner's desire to disassociate himself from the political process reflects a misunderstanding of his primary responsibilities, which have been succinctly defined, as first, "the illumination of choices for the political decision maker," and second, as a natural consequence of the first, the "persistent restraint and prevention of the foolish, the wasteful, and the cynical" (12, p. 148). As the planner strives for an improved world and not a perfect one, he must accept the impossibility of simultaneously satisfying all the values present in any political system. The extreme expression of the planner's ultimate value (that no proposal should be compromised) must inevitably clash with others such as those of radicalism (all proposals should be adopted), conservatism (no proposal should be adopted), checks and balances (the distribution of authority should be wide), and democracy (all actors are autonomous) (13, p. 323).

Effective planning is unavoidably controversial and indeed many planners underestimate the degree to which the public and politicians oppose planning (3,14,15). Allocation of scarce resources necessitates the unpopular task of deferring the attainment of lower priority objectives. Most people accept the need to plan their own affairs but are reluctant to allow others to plan for them because of the loss of independence that this may entail. Moreover, planning implies change, a difficult and unpleasant process for both individuals and societies. To induce planned change, health planners in many nonsocialist countries can offer neither strong incentives nor sanctions as means to ensure implementation (3,16). Often they may not even have much occupational security or visibility and as their actions progressively extend into the field of medical care, they come into direct conflict with the antiplanning sentiment of most private physicians. They must, therefore, make efficient use of what little power they have and capitalize on the convergent interests of others.

POLITICS AND PLANNING: PRACTICAL CONSIDERATIONS

Up to this point the discussion has focused on the inescapably controversial nature of planning and on the importance of political factors in determining planning effectiveness. The remainder of this chapter considers some practical implications of these factors as they relate to getting the planning process underway for the first time and to developing appropriate relationships between planning agencies and other participants in the planning process. Since planners are more apt to exercise their craft through intermediaries such as administrators, consumers, and professional groups than through direct contact with politicians, primary attention will be given to how they can best utilize these groups to assess the political feasibility for change and to promote plan implementation.

Getting Started

The first few months for a new health planning unit are apt to be the most difficult. Expectations are high and perhaps unrealistic, planning staff must be recruited and trained, and many division chiefs within the health agency may view the advent of planning with apprehension, if not open hostility. The way the first few planners approach their task during this period will do much to determine their eventual effectiveness.

The Will to Plan

A first and crucial question to be answered, particularly in countries which have only recently started to plan, is whether a discernible "will to develop" exists and, by inference, a "will to plan." According to Waterston, insufficient government support is the prime reason why most plans are never carried out successfully (11, p. 340).

No conclusive test exists of the will to plan, although various indicators can provide suggestive evidence. The planner can begin by examining the following questions. Is the country's ideological framework congenial to planned change? Are political and other leaders committed to change and what tangible evidence exists of this commitment? Do matters relating to internal politics consume an excessive amount of leadership time? Do graft and corruption siphon off an inordinate proportion of the resources necessary for plan implementation? To what extent have previous plans been oriented primarily toward meeting short term political objectives or obtaining international assistance rather than as part of a continuing developmental effort? Does the will to plan exist at both the policy-making and implementation levels? What priority is given to health programs and to what extent does a consensus exist regarding the major problems confronting the health sector?

For countries with a previous history of planning, perhaps the best test of the will to plan is the confrontation of past plans with subsequent performance (11, p. 345). The observed gaps between promise and performance can be considered a measure of political-administrative efficiency and provide the planner with a valuable correction factor for bringing theoretically feasible targets more in line with reality.

The will to plan is seldom monolithic; wide differences may exist in the readiness of health and other authorities to consider change, depending on the policy area under consideration. When the over-all planning environment is relatively unfavorable, the planner can begin with those policy areas where the opportunities for improvement are greatest. Conversely, when commitment is generally high, the planner can complement his regular activities with efforts directed at increasing the awareness of and concern for problem areas not yet widely recognized.

The importance the planner attaches to one or another criterion of the will to plan will vary greatly depending on the country situation in which he finds himself. As in the development process itself, the minimal acceptable standards for getting started cannot be made too high or otherwise nothing will be done. Furthermore, if careful appraisal of the planning environment suggests that chances for success are slight, the planner should limit his objective to promoting the necessary preconditions to planning.

Staff Recruitment

A priority task for a newly created planning agency is the recruitment of staff. Competence and integrity must obviously take precedence over other selection criteria but candidates' political preferences may also have to be considered, particularly in an unstable or highly politicized situation. The top planning job will often be a position "of confidence" of the chief executive and hence dependent on the party in power. While the political affiliation of staff planners is not so important, experience suggests that planning effectiveness and continuity will be improved if staff members are drawn from all major political groups.

Characterization of the Organizational Milieu

Effective planners are generally those who can tailor their strategies to the specific characteristics of each organization involved in the planning process and to the incentives that maintain it (17). Correctly identifying the values and interests underlying the policies of the various institutional and professional entities which make up the health system is a basic element of organizational characterization (18). Knowledge of the hierarchial and power relationships can also be decisive in the successful negotiation of a new project, particularly within an international context.

The central questions the planner will want to answer are, who decides what, and why? Organizational charts depicting relevant intra- and inter-institutional relationships provide a useful but generally inadequate introduction to how the health system really functions. Numerous examples exist of persons or interest groups with power to influence policy quite disproportionate to their positions on an organizational chart; in some cases (for instance, Mrs. Mary Lasker in the United States), enormous power to shape policies may be held by persons who are nominally outside the health and political fields (19). Various methods based on such variables as reputation, participation, social activity, and position have been developed to identify and characterize community leadership, although the findings of comparative research suggest that different methods with ostensibly similar objectives may produce substantially different results (20,21).

Other, simpler procedures can provide valuable clues as to who counts in the decision-making process within a given organization. Senior staff at the division or section chief level may have an equal or greater role in setting agency policy, and determining the eventual success of implementation, than the top executive. The differential proximity of senior staff to the director's office, particularly in less established bureaucracies, may reflect their current standing in the hierarchy. Those frequently asked to prepare background documents, policy drafts, and speeches, or to accompany key authorities on trips, are in a favored position to influence policy. The ease with which different individuals or interest groups can gain access to top executives also suggests their relative importance in the health and political systems.

The history of how different organizations have responded to major policy issues in the recent past can provide the planner with useful insights into their internal dynamics. He must be cautious, however, in extrapolating past behavioral patterns to the future due to possible intervening factors which, as an outsider, he may not readily detect.

The planner should look behind the official objectives of each organization to see whether other, more personal objectives and concerns exist that are of equal or even greater importance in influencing policy decisions. To illustrate this point, Binstock cites a recent case in San Francisco where planners unsuccessfully tried to establish a multiphasic screening program for the elderly (17). Their rational arguments, based on demonstrations of the inadequacy of existing care, were directly contrary to those of the local medical society (then embroiled in opposition to Medicare), which maintained that the current private system of medical care for the aged was more than adequate, and perhaps no arguments could have enlisted the support of the medical society at that point in time (22). By recognizing what types of persuasion are most suited to the situation in hand, by avoiding hopeless battles, and by having a keen sense of timing, the planner can substantially improve his chances for success.

Knowing who makes the decisions and why is not enough; the planner must also assess the probability of successful plan implementation. An analysis of the organizational milieu and power structure can help suggest the degree to which the various institutional participants in the planning process will be effective in the implementation of policy. In addition, such analysis may aid in determining whether one group will be more effective in mobilizing community support and growth and development than another, and why (23, pp. 368-404).

Broadening the Support for Planning

As he begins to apply his knowledge of organizational dynamics, the planner should try to avoid excessive dependence on only one or several persons, no matter how important they may be at a given point in time. Occupational vulnerability tends to increase as one nears the top levels of an organization's hierarchy; in most organizations, the top job is the most vulnerable of all. Waterston sums up the practical dilemma confronting the planner in search of a desirable administrative location for the planning function. In a new or unstable situation, linking planning to the support of one of several strong officials may help ensure short term survival and prominence, though it may retard institutionalization of the planning process and ultimately decrease its long term effectiveness (11, pp. 470-475).

Various strategies may help to broaden support for planning. In Chile, national health planning was weakened during a recent four-year period due to five changes of Director General of the National Health Service, but planning at the regional and local levels continued relatively unaffected. Under such circumstances planners at the central level might have improved their effectiveness in an obviously unstable situation by cementing working relationships with the senior, more permanent technical staff rather than with the chief executive. Other measures useful for generating support of the planning function, *provided* the planners do not lose sight of their ultimate objectives, include: doing the odd tasks that no one else has the time or ability to perform; concentrating on the factual analyses in which many place so much faith; compiling, summarizing, and publishing statistics gathered by others; and, by means of the review process, devoting primary attention to providing additional support for the proposals of others in preference to working on the planning office's own and probably more controversial priorities (24, pp. 376-379).

Selecting a Planning Approach

Knowledge of the type outlined in the preceding sections will be decisive in determining the most appropriate planning approach for each situation. Basil Mott provides an excellent discussion of the limitations of two principal models of community health planning in the United States, the Rational Decision Model and the Community Action Model. In the first, planning follows the classical sequence of problem solving according to objective and rational procedures. He considers this approach politically naive because it fails to recognize that in the real world objectives and courses of action are often selected by an essentially nontechnical and highly subjective process. Any decision must ultimately rest on certain values, evident or unrecognized, and conformance of the planner's values with those of the other components of the health care system is by no means assured. Moreover, the organizational context of planning in many countries limits the ability of planners and planning agencies to implement their decisions. By ignoring these two factors—the largely subjective nature of the decision-making process and the limitations on planning agency powers—the rational decision model is prone to overlook a central issue in planning—namely, feasibility (25).

The main difference between the rational decision and community action models is that the latter approach calls for the active participation of all groups affected by the planning process. The development of a decision-making consensus is a central objective. Despite this laudable attempt to come to grips with the issue of feasibility, Mott believes this approach fails to recognize the political realities of group and organizational behavior. Fundamental differences among contending groups cannot be resolved by consensus since they arise from differing interpretations of health data, which are themselves rooted in divergent responses to potential changes in the health system. Based on his detailed study of one of the more powerful coordinating councils in the United States, Mott concludes that the only way to induce an organization to accept a decision that runs contrary to its interests is to bring such pressures to bear on it as to make it more costly to the organization to resist than to accept the decision (26).

In most situations both planning agency power and the validity of the rational decision model approach will vary directly with the amount of previous country experience with planning. Unfortunately, it is precisely in those situations where organized planning is newest and weakest that the planner most needs powerful incentives and sanctions to help him overcome the indifference or resistance of others to his efforts. In these cases the planner must be especially attentive to enlisting as much outside support as possible, often through a complicated and seemingly unholy alliance of convergent interests, before becoming involved in controversial issues.

Once the basic approach has been selected the planner must assess the potential feasibility of his specific preference goals and determine the pathways most apt to exert influence on and overcome the resistance of the target organization. In his classic work, *Political Influence*, Banfield postulates five distinct bases for exercising influence: "friendship," "obligation," "rational persuasion," "selling" (other than that based on rational persuasion), and "coercion" or "inducement" (13). Case studies, including some taken from the health field, have been accumulated to show how planners have succeeded or failed to utilize effectively the resources at their disposal (22).

In concluding this section, the planner and administrator would be well advised to keep in mind that the apparent political "givens" which act to constrain their present activities are in fact the products of negotiation and compromise that took place during some earlier period. Viewed in this historical context, policy makers may be more inclined to test and challenge the validity of these "givens" in the light of contemporary political realities.

Keeping Others Informed

A planning unit must devote considerable time to information and communication functions. Aside from their many outside contacts in connection with data gathering, planners will need to keep others continually apprised of the results of their studies, of parallel program and research efforts being carried out elsewhere, and of the implications of their work for future policies. They will also want to use these opportunities to learn of new developments and to gain continual feedback on the extent to which proposed plans are likely to be understood and accepted.

Before deciding what procedures to use, the planner would be well advised to clear them with his administrative superiors. It is not much of an exaggeration to say that he who controls an organization's access to and release of processed information is virtually in control of the organization itself. Moreover, plans and planning have to do with man's aspirations for the future, which in turn are the central concerns of the politician and senior executive. The planner is anxious to enhance his professional stature and to widen his power base beyond that afforded by his parent agency, and his control over specialized information affords a good opportunity to further these objectives. If pursued too openly, however, he may run into direct conflict with his superiors to the ultimate detriment of both planning and the planner. As will be discussed later on, it is especially important for planners to check with appropriate authorities before discussing with outside interest groups major study findings or policy issues.

Dissemination of Information

Many planning units have found it advantageous to prepare periodic bulletins or newsletters for distribution to the persons and institutions with whom they come in contact. The examples of Peru and Chile are typical; in each country the planning unit sends to a large mailing list a monthly bulletin which (1) reviews developments in the field of health planning, (2) summarizes the principal findings of recent planning studies, and (3) reports on current activities of potential interest to the readership. Although such measures probably do little to change attitudes of others towards planning, they can assure the prompt, simultaneous, and low cost dissemination of information to a wide audience while at the same time keeping others aware of the planning unit's existence.

Conferences, round tables, workshops, presentations before interested groups, and other similar direct contacts between planners and their constituencies represent effective ways of exchanging information with diverse interest groups. While the use of these mechanisms will be discussed more fully as they relate to the involvement of others in the planning process, several observations are relevant here. First are the elementary rules for meetings such as clarity, conciseness, relevance of the presentation, avoidance of professional jargon, and provision of sufficient time for audience discussion of the points raised. A particularly troublesome obstacle to effective communication is the extended time scale used in planning. By referring to target dates five, ten, or more years in the future, or to implementation strategies notably out of phase with governmental periods in office, the planner may find his audience either quite disconnected from the realities of the present or, alternatively, annoyed with the planner's apparent lack of concern with the problems of today. At each step in his presentation, the planner must convey a sense of immediacy of his concerns and he must emphasize that the shape tomorrow takes will be determined in large part by what is done today.

Timing the Release of Information

The potentially controversial nature of planning means that the release of information must be carefully timed. A recent experience in the Chile health manpower study graphically shows the extent to which the planning process can be complicated by a premature and hastily prepared exposition. In early 1970, planners were still about eight months from completing their preliminary analyses and projections of the health manpower situation. On short notice the planning group was asked to make a presentation before the National Health Advisory Council. At that time planners had just begun to analyze the probable demand for professional midwifery personnel and first estimates suggested that the supply of midwives might exceed the effective demand by a substantial margin within a few years. In their wish to provide the Health Council with a striking example of some of the more surprising study findings, the planners neglected to consider the possible impact of a projected "surplus" of midwives on the midwifery profession.

The actual presentation was dramatic and the sequelae equally so. Invited leaders of the midwifery profession were shocked at the findings, which seemed to contradict the conclusions of all their earlier studies which had showed a large deficit of midwifery personnel and thus had led to a rapid increase in enrollments over the past five years. Important issues such as the capacity of the sector to absorb the new graduates, the economics and feasibility of assigning professional midwives to attend the obstetrical needs of small rural populations, and the possible effects on demand of a recently inaugurated nurse-midwife training program were all quickly lost from view in the debate that followed, and relations between the manpower study staff and the profession became strained thereafter.

In this case, planning office findings were bound to disappoint the midwifery profession: with a large number of graduates about to enter the labor market the supply was soon going to increase close to seven times faster per year than the potential client population, a situation which could not continue indefinitely. Nevertheless, a more gradual, diplomatic, and imaginative presentation of these findings could have helped direct energies toward a common ground between the planners and the profession. Above all, if the findings of the planners were certain to meet with great resistance, they should have done much more to strengthen their arguments, to develop counterproposals potentially acceptable to segments of the opposition, and in other ways to marshall support before actually entering the arena.

A final observation relating to the information function hardly needs emphasis—namely, the potential danger of using planning information for partisan purposes. No clear lines exist between what type of information use is acceptable and what is not. Moreover, in an agency subject to the over-all direction of the government (and political party) in power, a planning unit cannot ignore the requests of administrative superiors for special analyses, tabulations, or other materials of potential political value. To the extent that the planner keeps the risks in mind, he can take measures to avoid being unduly partisan in his professional capacity.

Involvement of Others in the Planning Process

It is commonly accepted that those who are to be affected by planning should be directly involved in the planning process. In this way planners can help ensure that the priorities have been properly identified, that the plan is feasible, and that, most importantly, the implementation phase will enjoy broad support.

There is much less unanimity as to the ways in which meaningful involvement can be attained. Indeed, in a highly politicized or controversial situation, planners may conclude that early involvement of the contending interests would aggravate rather than improve relationships, and in any event be too demanding on their time. While such arguments occasionally may be valid, the planner should recognize that he is only postponing controversy, not eliminating it, and that failure to confront the issues early may lead to unrealistic assumptions regarding plan feasibility.

Comparison of experiences in Turkey and India suggests the benefits that may accrue to planners who attain early involvement and participation of those being planned for. The Turkish study was concerned with all major health manpower categories at the national level (27), but the planners did not have any mechanism for ensuring a continuing involvement of representatives of the health professions or the educational institutions in the planning process. The conclusion of the study was a one-day meeting of more than 100 persons representing major interest groups. An intense and at times acrimonious debate took place over the study design as well as the findings, as many conferees tried to soften the study's possible impact on their own interests by undermining its over-all legitimacy and validity. Emotions gradually cooled and many of the study findings eventually contributed to policy formulation, but it was felt that the study did not attain its full potential, due in large part to the failure to achieve early and extensive involvement of those to be planned for.

In India, attention was directed at a detailed evaluation of the obligatory rural internship for physicians. The procedures used there were quite different from those in Turkey. Each year during the five-year project, over 50 key authorities from medical schools, the Ministry of Health, and other interest groups were invited to the village of Narangwal (Punjab State) for a week-long conference. The first Narangwal conferences were similar to the Turkish experience, in that the debate was intense and participants challenged the study team at every juncture. Since the project was still in its early stages, the investigators could incorporate most of the suggestions into the study. Later, attention turned to data analysis and conferee attitudes became more positive. The successful internalization of the study and its policy implications among conference participants was clearly demonstrated in the last year (1966) when participants from the Third World Conference on Medical Education in New Delhi were invited to attend the Narangwal meeting, at which they raised many, and frequently critical, questions about the study design and findings. By this time, however, the Indian health officials who had participated in the yearly meetings were so identified with the project that they gladly assumed the principal role in resolving the doubts and questions of the newcomers. More importantly, when the time came to translate project findings into new educational and service policies, a broad degree of consensus about what had to be done existed.

Who Should Participate in the Planning Process?

One of the more difficult tasks for the planner is deciding who represents the "community" of consumers and providers and how should he make this "representation" operative. Which is preferable, to have persons able to interpret accurately the interests of the groups they represent, even though they may have little power to influence policy, or to have persons with the potential of power even though they may be poor interpreters of current group thinking? These attributes—power and the ability to interpret group interests—are not necessarily found in the same persons. The planner will also want to know how best to balance the representation of health service providers, other direct interest groups, and consumers. How many participants can he realistically accommodate in the planning process? Too few will result in poor representation; too many will either frustrate active participation or lead to a parcelization of council responsibilities among many subcommittees (resulting in a tendency for professional specialists to dominate subcommittee deliberations). Who should take the initiative in selecting interest groups to be represented? When does the planning process call for consulting interested parties about common concerns and when does it call for their more direct involvement and continuing representation on appropriate planning bodies? These issues have only recently been studied systematically with reference to health planning; even though certain trends are evident, conclusions remain tentative.

Blum identifies at least 13 interest categories which must be involved in health planning: political interests; technical interests; government agencies in the subject area; voluntary agencies; other government and voluntary agencies in the same geopolitical area; planners; special interests (e.g., agriculture, labor); consumers; special need groups; specifically vested groups; experts; operatives; and policy-making persons (28, pp. 15.4-15.6). With respect to voluntary agencies, professional associations, and other interest groups not a part of the regular governmental health system, he suggests that allowing each participating organization to self-select its own representative holds too many risks for the planner. The planner is apt to find himself committed to providing comparable organizations (e.g., PTA's, labor unions) with equal representation with a consequent imbalance of membership. Alternatively, he may get organizational representatives who are either uninterested or unprepared to contribute to the tasks at hand. The planner may want to seek an equality (or neutralization) of special advocacy groups such that, for example, representatives from certain voluntary agencies who are known to use their position on a health planning council as a forum for promoting their own special interests are counterbalanced by representatives of competing special interests (29).

Selection and Training of Consumer Representatives

The consumer or citizen role in shaping health plans and policies in the United States has been the subject of much study in recent years. New legislation and growing consumer activism have impelled health authorities to seek better ways to achieve meaningful involvement. The Comprehensive Health Planning Act (P.L. 89-749), with its requirement for setting up planning bodies with substantial consumer participation, has been a powerful force for change. The potential value of such participation is still in doubt; in some cases consumer involvement even may lead to a deterioration in the quality of care, due to lowered standards and the need to make frequent compromises between contending interest groups (30). Although the ultimate value of consumer participation in the planning process is still unclear, the planner is usually obliged to consider it as one of his "givens." Exceptions to this rule may be those countries where local systems of representation have not yet undergone sufficient development or where the degree of illiteracy is high (31).

Selection of consumer representatives is especially difficult, particularly when differences between the social, cultural, and economic backgrounds of consumer and provider groups are marked. Unfamiliar with the organization and dynamics of working class or agricultural communities, the planner tends to assume that persons with leadership roles in familiar institutions such as schools, churches, and businesses are also leaders in the greater community of which they are a part. "Leaders" so selected are not anxious, for obvious reasons, to alter this image, although the politics of confrontation in recent years suggests that these leaders often are out of touch with the felt needs of their presumed constituencies and have limited power to affect policy (32, 33).

Some alternatives used by health planners to select consumer representatives are, to say the least, unconventional. Despairing of any formula for identifying true community leaders in the fluid context of the modern urban poor, some planners have eliminated bias in the only way possible, i.e., by selecting consumer membership randomly from a communitywide sampling frame. While this provides a miniature cross-section of community interests on the health planning council, the planner will have to ensure that such consumer representatives are trained to discharge their functions, lest their unfamiliarity with the health field and the dynamics of working in groups leads them to defer to other more experienced advocates.

Another approach which has yielded mixed results is to select consumer representatives from among those who have gained recent prominence as community dissidents, however defined. Although such consumer representatives may guarantee spirited council meetings and a quick ventilation of community grievances, there is no assurance that persons who have come to public notice by virtue of their ability to oppose policies they do not like are qualified to represent the greater community to which they belong or to propose constructive alternatives to what has been the target of their criticisms.

Once consumer representatives have been selected, and regardless of the planner's innermost doubts about the validity of the choices, he should treat them as in fact representative until they prove otherwise. The dynamics of the unfettered political process will permit a successful challenge to be made by other, more appropriate representatives and leaders, if the initial choices were poor. Moreover, if the initial selection provides only a core of representatives, the remainder to be selected by the community and the core representatives together, the planner's potential for error will be minimized.

Experience with indigenous consumer representatives (as differentiated from established civic and business leaders) in the planning process suggests the importance of providing them with training for their new role if they are to be effective. According to Lewis, a first phase of developing a functional advisory council is to convert all consumers into semi-professionals so that all sides are equipped with equal weaponry in the debate over health policies (14, p. 776). He foresees a shift to advocacy planning in which consumers, guided by sympathetic professionals (who in some cases may be assigned directly by the planning agency to provide the consumers with technical backstopping), will enter into conflict with the Establishment. In view of the multiple interests and values involved, he believes that the adversary system of the political process should be used in an overt manner, with a health council being charged to select the best plan based on all proposed alternatives rather than seek what can be considered virtually unobtainable—a "unified" plan. To qualify consumer representatives for this unaccustomed role, the University of Cincinnati (in cooperation with the Ecumenical Council for Continuing Education) began in 1968 to provide courses for consumers who would be acting as change agents in community development (34). Each consumer selects the field of functional specialization (such as health, welfare, or education) where he expects to spend most of his time, even though he will plan to interrelate with other consumer team members specializing in other fields.

Planning Councils

The diversity of community interests and the obligation to provide adequate numerical consumer counterbalance to the many provider groups which must be accommodated in the planning process will usually force the planner to work with planning councils larger than might otherwise be considered desirable. Blum, while recognizing the problems of large, unwieldy planning councils which tend to become rubber stamps to smaller executive subcommittees, believes that a council membership of fewer than 150 would probably not provide the planner with the necessary breadth of interests for community involvement at more than the local level (28, pp. 15.6-15.8). In order to have the benefits of a council of this size, without its obvious disadvantages, he suggests that a much smaller planning body be operationally enlarged by the creation of standing *ad hoc* committees heavily composed of nonmembers (to the planning council) who represent the various council elements in each discipline or policy area under consideration. He also foresees the growing use of polls, surveys, and public hearings as ways to sample the many and changing shades of community opinion on health policy. Such procedures were used to good avail in Cleveland to extend the outreach of a relatively small Health Goals Committee of 50 lay and professional members; over a five-year period the Committee was able to involve 43 health agencies and more than 700 persons in the health planning process (35).

A planning council's effectiveness will be determined largely by the care with which its functions have been defined. A crucial issue centers on the extent of its powers: will it have an advisory role only or will it have some of the attributes of a policy-making board? The concept of a hospital board with a policy role is well established; but only recently has this function been considered as possibly appropriate for a planning council extending beyond a single institution. At least for small geographic areas, planning councils with consumer representation should probably have policy-making functions over matters of direct concern to them. Relegating consumer representatives to advisory status is to invite feelings of deception and frustration which may result in council ineffectiveness or dissolution. Few comparative studies have been made of how planning councils work under diverse frames of reference, although preliminary evidence from a survey of 27 consumer groups active in OEO-assisted health center planning and operation suggests that they can function well either as a board or as an advisory group (36).

Many other aspects of a planning council's pattern of operation will need to be considered besides the extent to which it can decide policy. In Blum's excellent review of the functions and capabilities of planning bodies, he stresses the importance of providing them with freedom of operation. He lists some 11 "freedoms" which can help ensure that a planning council will be able to exercise its unique ability to provide planners with an insight into community needs and pave the way for eventual plan implementation (28, pp. 14.1-14.29). Other helpful guidelines for setting up community health boards are discussed by Brieland in relation to maximum feasible participation of community representatives (33).

Anticipating a Change in Government

The importance of political factors to the planning process is never so apparent as when a hotly contested election or other governmental change draws near. If the electoral outcome is uncertain or if an unexpected nonelectoral change occurs, the planner may find his normal rhythm of work completely interrupted and, in some cases, much of his earlier work invalidated. These risks are unavoidable but much can be done to soften the effect of governmental change on the planning process and even to facilitate the new government's prompt formulation and implementation of new policies.

An obvious first step is to minimize the political vulnerability of both the planning process and the planning office. For example, one of the earliest casualties of a change in government will be those plans whose primary rationale is to promote partisan objectives. Moreover, the planning process will be less vulnerable politically if, as already noted, the political affiliations of planning office staff are roughly comparable to those found in the society as a whole.

Where the planner is able to anticipate a possible governmental change he should, to the extent allowed by his administrative superiors and consistent with his country's political system, maintain informal contact with the health representatives of the major contending political parties. At these meetings he can keep them informed of the main problems affecting the sector and of planning office work in progress, in return for the chance to learn of party objectives regarding the provision of health care. Naturally, the planner should exercise discretion to avoid being accused of engaging in partisan politics.

One of the better guarantees of plan and planning survival from one governmental administration to the next is built-in plan flexibility. If the planner is prepared to show at each stage of the planning process the general resource and benefit implications of major policy alternatives, he can quickly recast his projections depending on election outcome. Confronted in Chile with a three-way presidential race between candidates of widely differing views, this was the course followed by health manpower planners (with as yet unknown success) as they completed the first phase of the health manpower plan for that country (37). The use of flexible models in which the several input variables can be modified easily and independently of each other can facilitate greatly this task. It may be desirable also to prepare a "perspective plan" that can be used by the several contending parties prior to the election and, more importantly, by the victor during the early months of his new administration. This type of plan provides an outline of the probable course of events—health problems, health resource requirements, and the effects of health services—under several different sets of hypotheses, one of these being the continuation of present policies. Programming, fiscal, and other details are elaborated once the priorities and goals of the next governmental administration have been defined.

It should be remembered that the main objective is to ensure the survival of the planning process from one governmental administration to the next, and not necessarily the survival of specific plans or the positions of the health planners. Indeed, senior health planning authorities may well be expendable when a major governmental change occurs, even though their jobs are not usually considered political. Irrespective of his own occupational tenure, a top planner can take pride if his attention to the political aspects of planning has helped ensure that the incoming government maximally benefits from work done in prior administrations.

SUMMARY

The central arguments of this chapter have been that (1) the political process is often of decisive importance in determining the outcome of plans and planning, and (2) there is no effective way of isolating planning from the political process. Good planning is inevitably controversial since it introduces technical analysis and an explicit value system for decision-making into a process which heretofore has relied largely on personal judgments and the politics of power. The planner, therefore, must be continually alert to opportunities to incorporate into his planning efforts such measures as will help assure eventual acceptance by political and administrative authorities.

An obvious, although frequently overlooked, first question the planner must answer is whether a "will to plan" exists. Past performance in planning and plan implementation, supplemented by an appraisal of the present political and administrative climate, will help the planner keep his recommendations within the range of political feasibility.

The planner should be well acquainted with the organizational milieu within which he must operate. The formal administrative structures of the organization involved in the delivery of health care tell only part of the story; the planner also must know the informal decision networks which are often of equal or even greater importance. The recent history of how and by whom key decisions were made can provide valuable clues as to an organization's true objectives and internal power structure.

The information collected on the organizational milieu will guide the planner in his selection of a planning approach and incentives and sanctions appropriate to the local situation. By aligning his goal preferences as much as possible with those that already exist among the principal actors on the health scene, he can facilitate plan implementation. This information will be useful also in suggesting where the planner can seek natural allies within the health system so that he does not become overly dependent on only one source of support.

The planner's access to, and control over, multiple sources of information are powerful tools in the furtherance of his objectives. Conversely, injudicious use of information can make effective planning difficult, or even impossible. Examples of the latter alternative include use of information for overt partisan purposes, untimely or premature release of information, and release of information in ways and in terms ill-suited to the intended audience.

An increasingly important determinant of the eventual political acceptability of a plan is the degree to which planners are successful in achieving meaningful consumer and provider involvement in the planning process. Many problems face the planner in carrying out this objective: how soon should large scale involvement begin; who should be involved, how should they be selected, and in what proportion should different groups be represented; should the role of citizen groups be primarily advisory, or should they also have policy-making roles; and how can consumer representatives be trained for their new role so that they do not end up as rubber stamps to the decisions of health experts. Although these questions have only recently come under study, certain preliminary answers are beginning to emerge, and these are discussed in the chapter, particularly as they relate to consumer involvement.

The close relationship between planning and politics is never so evident as during the change of governmental administration, particularly if the change is unexpected and the new administration's policies diverge sharply from those of its predecessor. The planner can help soften the impact of such changes on the planning process, even though he may be unable to guarantee his own job security. Obvious precautions include avoiding plans based on predominantly political criteria, or planners selected according to party affiliation. Moreover, the planning methods used should allow the planner maximum flexibility in the variations of those inputs and assumptions most apt to be affected by the electoral outcome. In highly politicized situations the planner may find it useful to develop alternative "perspective plans" which show the major consequences of each party's position as it relates to health. Moreover, within the constraints imposed upon him by superiors usually identified with the party in power, the planner can help ensure that the contending parties have access to basic planning data and are kept apprised of the major decisions apt to confront the new administration.

Only some of the many aspects of the interaction between politics and planning have been considered in this chapter, and, unlike the situation in the physical and biological sciences, the lessons learned in one location can be applied only with great caution in another. Like many professions, planning is both an art and a science. As in many other emerging fields, planners have tended to concentrate on the latter component to the detriment of the former, which in most cases can be equated with the political aspects of planning and plan implementation. This chapter will have accomplished its objective if it has helped stimulate the planner to redress the balance.

REFERENCES

1. Key, V. O. *Politics, Parties and Pressure Groups.* New York: Thomas Y. Crowell Company, 1942.
2. Kaufman, H. "The Political Ingredient of Public Health Services: A Neglected Area of Research." *Milbank Memorial Fund Quarterly* 44:13-34, No. 4, Part 2, October, 1966.
3. Feingold, E. "The Changing Political Character of Health Planning." *American Journal of Public Health* 59:803-808, 1969.
4. May, J. Joel. *Health Planning: Its Past and Potential.* Health Administration Perspectives No. A5. Chicago: University of Chicago, Center for Health Administration Studies, 1967.
5. Gordon, J. B. "The Politics of Community Medicine Projects: A Conflict Analysis." *Medical Care* 7:419-428, 1969.
6. Conant, Ralph W. *The Politics of Community Health.* Report of the Community Action Studies Project, National Commission on Community Health Services. Washington, D.C.: Public Affairs Press, 1968.
7. Elling, R. H. "The Shifting Power Structure in Health." *Milbank Memorial Fund Quarterly* 46: Suppl.: 119-143, Part 2, January, 1968.
8. Bernstein, B. J. "Public Health—Inside or Outside the Mainstream of the Political Process? Lessons from the Passage of Medicaid." *American Journal of Public Health* 60:1690-1700, 1970.
9. Hilleboe, H. E. "Health Planning on a Community Basis." *Medical Care* 6:203-214, 1968.
10. Schaefer, M. "Current Issues in Health Organizations." *American Journal of Public Health* 58:1192-1199, 1968.
11. Waterston, Albert. *Development Planning: Lessons of Experience.* Baltimore: Johns Hopkins Press, 1967.
12. Wolman, A. "Water—Economics and Politics." *Journal of the Water Pollution Control Federation* 37:145-150, 1965.
13. Banfield, Edward C. *Political Influence.* Glencoe, Illinois: The Free Press, 1961.
14. Lewis, C. E. "The Thermodynamics of Regional Planning." *American Journal of Public Health* 59:773-777, 1969.
15. Sasuly, R. and Ward, P. D. "Two Approaches to Health Planning: The Ideal vs. the Pragmatic." *Medical Care* 7:235-241, 1969.
16. Snoke, A. W. and Glasgow, J. M. "Regional Planning: Pious Platitude or Practical Implementation." *Inquiry* 7:17-25, September, 1970.
17. Binstock, R. H. "Effective Planning through Political Influence." *American Journal of Public Health* 59:808-813, 1969.
18. Colt, A. M. "Public Policy and Planning Criteria in Public Health." *American Journal of Public Health* 59:1678-1685, 1969.
19. Drew, E. "The Health Syndicate: Washington's Noble Conspirators." *The Atlantic:* pp. 75-82, December, 1967.

20. Hawley, Willis D. and Wirt, Frederick M., editors. *The Search for Community Power*. Englewood Cliffs, New Jersey: Prentice-Hall, 1968.
21. Arnold, Mary F. and Welsh, Isabel. "Political Decision-Making and Health Planning." In: Henrik L. Blum and Associates. *Notes on Comprehensive Planning for Health*. San Francisco: American Public Health Association, Western Regional Office, 1968.
22. Morris, Robert and Binstock, Robert H. *Feasible Planning for Social Change*. New York: Columbia University Press, 1966.
23. Presthus, Robert V. *Men at the Top: A Study in Community Power*. New York: Oxford University Press, 1964.
24. Altshuler, Alan A. *The City Planning Process*. Ithaca: Cornell University Press, 1965.
25. Mott, B. J. F. "The Myth of Planning without Politics." *American Journal of Public Health* 59:797-803, 1969.
26. Mott, B. J. F. *Anatomy of a Coordinating Council: Implications for Planning*. Contemporary Community Health Series. Pittsburgh: University of Pittsburgh Press, 1968.
27. Taylor, Carl E., Dirican, Rahmi, and Deuschle, Kurt W. *Health Manpower Planning in Turkey*. Baltimore: Johns Hopkins Press, 1968.
28. Blum, Henrik L. and Associates. *Notes on Comprehensive Planning for Health*. San Francisco: American Public Health Association, Western Regional Office, 1968.
29. Fifer, E. Z. "Hang-ups in Health Planning." *American Journal of Public Health* 59:765-769, 1969.
30. Hochbaum, G. M. "Consumer Participation in Health Planning: Toward Conceptual Clarification." *American Journal of Public Health* 59:1698-1705, 1969.
31. *National Health Planning in Developing Nations*. WHO Technical Report Series No. 350. Geneva: World Health Organization, 1967.
32. Wilson, James Q. "Planning and Politics: Citizen Participation in Urban Renewal." *Journal of the American Institute of Planners* 29:242-249, November, 1963.
33. Brieland, D. "Community Advisory Boards and Maximum Feasible Participation." *American Journal of Public Health* 61:292-296, 1971.
34. Henry, P. "Pimps, Prostitutes, and Policemen: Education of Consumers for Participation in Health Planning." *American Journal of Public Health* 60:2171-2174, 1970.
35. Barry, M. C. and Sheps, C. G. "A New Model for Community Health Planning." *American Journal of Public Health* 59:226-236, 1969.
36. Sparer, G., Dines, G. B., and Smith, D. "Consumer Participation in OEO-Assisted Neighborhood Health Centers." *American Journal of Public Health* 60:1091-1102, 1970.
37. Ministerio de Salud Pública y Consejo Nacional Consultivo de Salud, Republica de Chile. *Recursos Humanos de Salud en Chile: Un Modelo de Analysis*. Santiago: National Health Service Press, 1970.

ADDITIONAL READINGS

Anderson, D. M. and Kerr, M. "Citizen Influence in Health Service Programs." *American Journal of Public Health* 61:1518-1523, 1971.

This preliminary report of a study of citizen participation in community health groups focuses on observation of group interaction, a poll of group members on who should have responsibility for given activities, and a review of the group's formal documents.

Banfield, Edward C. *Political Influence.* Glencoe, Illinois: The Free Press, 1961.
This book provides an excellent exposition of the multiple ways in which political influence can be exerted, and of the problems that arise in identifying the value premise which best reflects the public interest. The many case examples used include one drawn from hospital planning.

Barry, M. C. and Sheps, C. G. "A New Model for Community Health Planning." *American Journal of Public Health* 59:226-236, 1969.
An interesting model of how many diverse groups can be brought together around the common task of defining community health goals. The appendices include examples of the forms used in the Cleveland Health Goals Committee Project.

Blum, Henrik L. and Associates. *Notes on Comprehensive Planning for Health.* San Francisco: American Public Health Association, Western Regional Office, 1968.
A number of the chapters of this book discuss either directly or indirectly matters related to the political ingredient of health planning. Chapter 5 considers such questions as the community power structure, citizen participation, and the process whereby decisions are made, Chapers 14 and 15 examine the functions, capabilities and organization of different types of planning bodies, and Chapter 16 touches on the political and other factors which limit the effectiveness of comprehensive health planning.

Brieland, D. "Community Advisory Boards and Maximum Feasible Participation." *American Journal of Public Health* 61:292-296, 1971.
This article provides a good review of the uses for community advisory boards and guidelines to setting them up. The author presents comparative experience from various cities with the operation of such boards and considers in some depth the difficulties encountered in selecting community representatives and ensuring their participation in the planning process.

Burke, E. M. "Citizen Participation Strategies." *Journal of the American Institute of Planners* 34:287-294, September, 1968.
This article provides a good review of the alternative strategies open to the planner to resolve some of the dilemmas caused by the basic conflicts which arise between participatory democracy and professional expertise. By recognizing and adopting a strategy of participation designed to fit the role and resources of the particular organization, the planner can help encourage citizen participation in decision-making. Five strategies are discussed: education-therapy, behavioral change, staff supplement, cooptation, and community power.

Clavel, Pierre. "Planners and Citizen Boards: Some Applications of Social Theory to the Problem of Plan Implementation." *Journal of the American Institute of Planners* 34:130-139, May, 1968.
The article presents a good discussion of the problems encountered by nonpartisan citizen boards in utilizing expert planning advice. If the citizen boards do not count among their membership persons with the requisite time, training, and experience to use expert advice, a state of inequality between experts and boards exists which will limit the extent to which the

experts can be used. Moreover, this inequality may lead to a defensive reaction on the part of the boards which will tend to reject the expert advice and reaffirm traditional institutions.

Conant, Ralph W. *The Politics of Community Health.* Report of the Community Action Studies Project, National Commission on Community Health Services. Washington, D.C.: Public Affairs Press, 1968.

This book describes in detail five case examples of successful health planning, in large part attributable to the ability of the planners involved to use the political process to their advantage. The presentation of these examples is complemented by a general discussion of some politically related reasons for planning successes and failures.

Hawley, Willis D. and Wirt, Frederick M., editors. *The Search for Community Power.* Englewood Cliffs, New Jersey: Prentice-Hall, 1968.

This reference details the problems inherent in identifying who has real power in a community. The four methods of locating leaders in local communities described yielded different types of leaders with varying roles in the decision-making process. The potential hazards of the widely-used "reputational approach" are demonstrated.

Hochbaum, G. M. "Consumer Participation in Health Planning: Toward Conceptual Clarification." *American Journal of Public Health* 59: 1698-1705, 1969.

Useful orientation is given in this article to the problems and potential of consumer participation. Examples are described of the conflicts apt to arise between consumers and health professionals due to problems of communication, overlap in their decisional territories, and differences in their social and cultural backgrounds.

Jonas, Steven. "A Theoretical Approach to the Question of 'Community Control' of Health Services Facilities." *American Journal of Public Health* 61:916-921, 1971.

This well documented article considers the extent to which community control of health institutions, within the context of the United States socioeconomic system, can contribute to the improvement of health care. It distinguishes between the health service "institution" and the health service "system," and discusses where the locus for the real control of each resides. The article concludes by considering the implications of the struggle for community control on the provision of health care and on the role of the professional.

Kaufman, H. "The Political Ingredient of Public Health Services: A Neglected Area of Research." *Milbank Memorial Fund Quarterly* 44:13-34, No. 4, Part 2, October, 1966.

This reference provides an extensive review of political science and public health literatures through 1965, and amply documents the importance of the political dimension in public health.

Marmor, T. and Thomas, D. "The Politics of Paying Physicians: The Determinants of Government Payment Methods in England, Sweden, and the United States." *International Journal of Health Services* 1:71-78, 1971.

The authors present and test an explicative hypothesis for the various methods of physician payment that have developed in the three countries under consideration. This article, and the references it cites, provide useful insights into the options open and not open to health planners as they consider alternative policies affecting sensitive matters such as remuneration.

Morris, Robert and Binstock, Robert H. *Feasible Planning for Social Change.* New York: Columbia University Press, 1966.

> This volume presents an excellent discussion of the ways in which the planner can assess the potential feasibility of his preference goals and the pathways most apt to exercise influence on and overcome the resistance of the target organization. The San Francisco case is reviewed in detail as are case studies in health planning and social welfare planning taken from other communities in the United States. The authors give abundant examples of how the planner can operate to maximize the effectiveness of the resources he has at his disposal.

Mott, Basil J. F. *Anatomy of a Coordinating Council: Implications for Planning.* Contemporary Community Health Service. Pittsburgh: University of Pittsburgh Press, 1968.

> This book provides a good review of the evolution of one of the more powerful coordinating councils operating at the state level in the United States. The reasons for its successes and failures on major policy matters over the years are analyzed in detail.

"The Politics of Health Planning: A Symposium." *American Journal of Public Health* 59:795-813, 1969.

> The four papers presented in this symposium are concerned with the inseparability of politics from planning, the changing nature of the political component in health planning, and ways of using political influence to advantage in the planning process. This issue (May) also provides several other articles of direct relevance to the politics of health planning.

Waterston, Albert. *Development Planning: Lessons of Experience.* Baltimore: Johns Hopkins Press, 1967.

> This book is a gold mine of accumulated world experience in planning. Although most of the case examples are drawn from development planning, they frequently illustrate principles equally relevant to health planning. The political ingredient of planning is considered, directly or indirectly, in many sections of this reference.

Wilson, J. Q. "Planning and Politics: Citizen Participation in Urban Renewal." *Journal of the American Institute of Planners* 29:242-249, November, 1963.

> This article gives an excellent discussion of the problems of identifying the real community, and of the differences between the value systems of government authorities and of inner city neighborhoods.

7

General Economic Considerations

A. PETER RUDERMAN

INTRODUCTION: ECONOMICS AND ECONOMISTS

Before discussing the general economic considerations involved in health planning, we should explain why some economists are deeply involved in planning, while others consider it to be a dirty word.

One of the better textbook definitions of economics is ". . . the study of how men and society *choose,* with or without the use of money, to employ scarce productive resources to produce various commodities over time and distribute them for consumption, now and in the future, among various people and groups in society" (1). Economics, then, is largely concerned with making choices, hopefully sensible choices. The grounds for economic decision are often weak, however, because of poor statistics, insufficient information, and lack of complete understanding of why things happen in economic life. Since economists are nevertheless under pressure to make decisions, a number of schools of economic thought have come into being in which doctrine and conjecture can, up to a certain point, be used in lieu of facts to justify the economist's recommendations.

What is sometimes termed "classical economics" of the Anglo-American school has its historical roots in the eighteenth century doctrine of laisser faire (leaving things to work themselves out) and in the business experience and relatively crude statistics of the nineteenth century. It starts from the belief that the interaction of supply and demand under conditions of perfect competition in free markets will ensure that optimum choices are made. The chain of reasoning runs as follows: People engage in activity in order to satisfy their wants; greater wants reflect themselves in the willingness to pay higher prices; high prices induce people to produce more of the wanted goods and services. The role of Government in this system is held to a minimum—to maintain public

Parts of this chapter have appeared in somewhat different form in: A. P. Ruderman. "Economic Aspects of Health Planning." In: W. Hobson, ed. *The Theory and Practice of Public Health.* Third Edition. London: Oxford University Press, 1969. Other portions were adapted from an unpublished paper, "Measurement Implications of Economic Assessment," by William A. Reinke.

order and to insure the least possible impediment to the working-out of free market forces.

Contemporary adherents of this "free enterprise" school have departed from the purely classical doctrine of their forbears in view of clear statistical evidence of the imperfections of the market and of the price mechanism as allocators of resources. They have come to believe that market forces must be supplemented and guided. These liberal economists hold that the management of economic life by socially responsible Governments, using instruments such as tax policy and control of the rate of interest to influence factors such as the amount of investment and the distribution of income, will assure that market forces lead in fact to the best possible choices. This, incidentally, is the prevailing economic doctrine in the United States today. An occasional American economist can still be found who professes to believe in old-fashioned free enterprise. Professor Milton Friedman of the Universtiy of Chicago is a leading example.

The major rival of the Anglo-American school is the Marxist. Karl Marx based his original doctrine on the same statistics and observations of the same nineteenth century business world that influenced Alfred Marshall and others of the Anglo-American school. He merely came to different conclusions. Through the historical evolution from Marxism to Leninism and the "thaw" of the 1960's that produced some concessions to the role of the price system and the profit motive, members of this school continued to place their main reliance on the comprehensive planning of economic life (now a very much more sophisticated and computerized process than in earlier years) to ensure that socially desirable choices were made.

When we move from general theories that attempt to explain the working of the economy as a whole to specific applied areas such as the economics of farms, road transport, or health services, we find less doctrine and more emphasis on statistical studies and scientific inference on the part of economists of all schools. There is a tendency to avoid emotionally overloaded words such as "Communist" and "Capitalist" and to classify economic systems, and individual sectors of economic activity, by the relative preponderance of "market" or "command" elements—that is, by the degree to which free market forces operating through the price mechanism, or the decisions of planners made effective through an administrative structure, bring about the allocation of resources.

Health planners should recognize, however, that the advice economists give them is inevitably affected by the school to which they belong. For example, an economist of the free enterprise school is likely to recommend that the recipient pay directly at least part of the cost of medical care or of drinking water, while economists of other persuasions would feel that health services should be absolutely free to the beneficiary in order to be fully accessible. The response of a "command" economist to the problem of physician service in rural areas or urban ghettos is to require a period of such service, while "market" economists would suggest incentives such as higher pay. Each side can mobilize some logical arguments and some evidence in support of its position, but neither side can deny that it is influenced by its underlying moral philosophy as well.

HEALTH ECONOMICS AS A SPECIFIC DISCIPLINE

A general nonspecific relationship typified by the "vicious cycle of poverty and disease" has been recognized for many years, and attempts to calculate the cost of sickness and premature death go back at least to the 1920's. Serious attempts to establish health economics as a formal discipline, however, date only from the 1950's.

One reason for the slow growth of health economics is that other areas (economic theory, econometrics, finance, and so forth) provided more rewards for the professional economist in terms of peer group recognition. In addition, market-oriented economists of both the laisser faire and money management persuasions found conceptual difficulties in applying to health a body of theory based on the assumption that prices reflect wants and lead in turn to the satisfaction of wants. Health authorities, certainly, preferred to talk about "needs" rather than "wants" in any case. Furthermore, theories based on the interaction of buyers and sellers in free markets clearly could not explain what happened in the market for health services. Consumption of hospital bed-days or prescription drugs did not respond to price like the consumption of beef or beans because the consumers did not necessarily want to be hospitalized or drugged, because the consumers knew less about these commodities than they did about common market items, because the suppliers were not always in business to make a profit, and because a third party, the physician, often interposed himself between buyer and seller and made the real decisions by signing a hospital admission slip or writing a prescription.

Economists in command economies did not have this theoretical difficulty, but the market-oriented economist was faced with a genuine dilemma—whether to ignore health services because they did not follow market rules or to ignore the body of market doctrine in order to explain the working of health services realistically. The solution, in free enterprise countries like the United States, has generally been to adopt a view of health services as a "command sector" in a market economy, just like other areas of public interest (education, communications, transportation) where government intervention had to be recognized despite an emotional commitment to the free market. From this, it follows that comprehensive planning of health services by governments is both necessary and desirable even when the allocation of resources to satisfy the majority of consumer desires can be left to the market place.

Economic analysis of health services is usually broken down into two main areas, microeconomic and macroeconomic, that require different methods of study. *Microeconomics* is concerned with the individual producing unit—the hospital, the health center, the doctor's office. It is concerned with the efficiency of operation in human and money terms, with problems of cost and utilization, and of the scale of operations. It involves managerial cost accounting rather than social statistics. Microeconomic analysis is more important in the administration of the individual producing unit than in the planning of the health sector as a whole, although microeconomic data also provide the basis for more general cost calculations in comprehensive health planning.

Macroeconomics of health is concerned first with summing up the individual producing units into aggregates and then with the relative share of resources going to health services as an aggregate as compared with those allocated to other branches of economic activity. Macroplanning for health involves considerations of the relative return to society from investment in health services, from investment in education and other so-called "social" sectors, and from investment in directly productive activities such as agriculture and industry. Within the health sector, broad considerations of regional geographical balance, of the rural-urban distribution of services, and of the relative returns from investment in curative versus preventive services or in-patient versus out-patient care can be studied in much the same way on a macroeconomic basis.

MICROECONOMIC ANALYSIS

A number of useful concepts can be borrowed by the health planner from the general field of microeconomics. Of these, perhaps the most widely applicable is the concept of *marginality*. In any economic calculation, the *next* value on any given scale is referred to as *marginal* from the point of view of the observer. For example, let us assume that a physician under specified circumstances can attend five patients per hour in one examining room, eight patients per hour if he uses two examining rooms, ten patients per hour if he uses three examining rooms, and also that he finds that using four examining rooms does not enable him to attend more than ten patients per hour (Figure 7.1). In economic language, for a physician with one examining room, the marginal product is three patients per hour; that is, by adding the next examining room his output is raised from five to eight patients per hour. For a physician with two examining rooms, the marginal product of the next room is two patients per hour. For a physician with three examining rooms, the marginal product of the next room is zero. If we were to assume that the physician had to use every examining room provided, then if a fifth examining room were provided he would begin to spend more time moving from room to room and less time seeing patients, so that with five examining rooms he could perhaps attend only nine patients per hour. In

Patients Seen per Physician per Hour

Number of Examining Rooms	Patients Seen per Hour (Average Product)	Increase in Patients Seen per Hour, Obtained from Adding Another Examining Room (Marginal Product)
1	5	3
2	8	2
3	10	0
4	10	-1
5	9	*

*Not known. This figure would depend on the change in average product from 5 to 6 examining rooms.

Fig. 7.1. Illustration of average and marginal product.

this case, we would say that for a physician with four examining rooms the marginal product of a fifth examining room would be negative, since he would see one patient less per hour than with four rooms.

This illustration also depicts the so-called "law of diminishing returns," sometimes spoken of as diminishing output per unit input, since, for successive additions to input (number of examining rooms) the output (patients seen per hour) first rises rapidly, then less rapidly, then ceases to rise, and finally declines. Depending on the technical characteristics of the production unit studied, some such relationship can usually be seen. Some inputs, however, do bear a steady rather than a diminishing relationship to output; an example would be the relationship between quantity of vaccine and persons vaccinated. Examples of increasing returns can also be found; before one reaches the lethal dose LD_{50} of an insecticide, for instance, successive increases in dosage can have more than proportional effects.

The value of marginal analysis is that it develops a way of looking at the matter being studied—always remembering, when economic measurements are being made, that the existing level of the inputs (resources, manpower, and others) will affect the output obtained from subsequent increments to input.

Need, Want, and Effective Demand

Markets respond to wants while health service planning is often oriented to needs. The health planner nevertheless finds it important to study wants and the market mechanism because these serve to explain the prices of many of the goods and services purchased by health agencies.

In brief, the way wants make themselves felt in the market place is through demand. What the economist terms "effective demand" is the combination of wants and the money to pay for them. Thus, if the officials of a health service want to have a jet injector, the mere desire does not constitute a market force. When money is authorized in the operating budget for this purpose, the want is translated into effective demand in the market for jet injectors.

Demand is not considered apart from money, and Figure 7.2 shows two demand curves (also known as demand schedules)—curve A showing a commonly encountered relation between demand and price, and curve B showing a similar relation between demand and income. Both curves involve the *ceteris paribus* assumption (other things being equal) in that the relation between demand and price is usually studied on the assumption that income is constant, and the relation between demand and income on the assumption that a given price prevails. The ideas expressed are quite simple—buyers tend to buy less when prices are high than when prices are low, and, for any given level of price, buy less when incomes are low than when incomes are high.

In real life, prices and incomes change over time and market statistics are gathered hourly, daily, weekly, etc. In theoretical economics, the demand schedules are considered to exist at a single instant of time; they represent the amounts that would be consumed *if* one price or another, or one level of income or another, prevailed. No movement takes place from point to point on the curves, but each curve as a whole is viewed as the line depicting a set of alternatives. An empirical demand curve based on market statistics over time would not reflect this assumption, but would still be useful as a guide to the approximate amounts that would be consumed if prices or income were at one level instead of another.

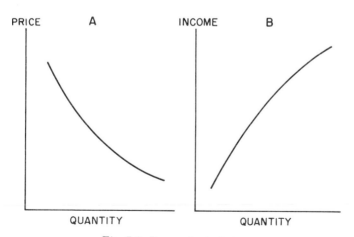

Fig. 7.2. Demand schedules.

Clearly, the relation between price and consumption will be different for different goods and services. Figure 7.3 illustrates the demand for two different goods. Curve A might represent a luxury and curve B a necessity. In the case of a luxury, demand is very sensitive to price changes. If the price is a little higher much less may be bought, and if it is a little lower much more may be bought. Demand in this case, illustrated by a flat curve, is called *elastic*. At the other extreme, the price of a basic necessity may change quite a bit; whether it be high or low, consumption cannot be expected to change very much. This is the case of *inelastic* demand, the steep curve B. Observation has confirmed to some degree the generally held belief that the demand for many health services is relatively inelastic. It should be understood that the demand curves do not relate to a single individual and should not be considered in a personal sense. Do not ask, "Will I buy more diamonds if the price goes down?" A sharp change in demand at different price levels occurs because more individuals make decisions to buy or not to buy at that price, not because each individual decides to buy more or less of the goods in question.

The concept of elasticity is important in health planning because, in countries where health is a command sector in a market-oriented economy, it helps the planner appraise the likely market repercussions of command decisions. Not only the amount demanded but the amount offered for sale (supply) will show differences in the elasticity of response to changes in price. Administrative decisions in health services also make use of the concept of elasticity when financial deterrents or incentives are being considered. For example, the imposition of a prescription charge by the National Health Service in England was based on the assumption that the demand for prescription drugs as a whole was sufficiently elastic to respond to an increase in price by declining to some extent. Actually, demand proved less elastic than had been hoped.

Underlying the demand curve is the relationship between wants and the

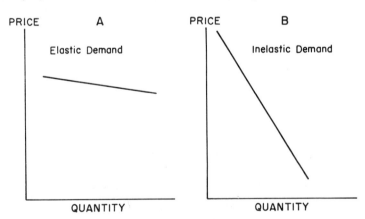

Fig. 7.3. Elasticity of demand.

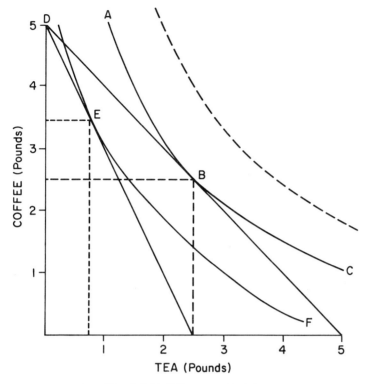

Fig. 7.4. Indifference schedules.

money available to satisfy wants. Price theorists in the nineteenth century were very much concerned with explaining just why different amounts of goods and services would be desired. They introduced a concept of the *utility* or usefulness of goods to the consumer and brought into play the idea of diminishing marginal utility (e.g., after drinking a glass of water the utility of the next glass of water is less than that of the first to a thirsty man) to explain why the price-consumption relationship illustrated by demand curves was not perfectly linear. The only problem with the concept of utility was that it could not be measured, but *substitution* between different goods which appeared in markets at different prices could be measured. "Indifference curves" such as those shown in Figure 7.4 enabled economists to infer from observed (or at least observable) behavior the nature of consumers' wants and their changing response to price.

A consumer, for example, might be indifferent to different combinations of tea and coffee that yielded the same total satisfaction. Indifference curve ABC indicates that equal satisfaction would be obtained from 5 pounds of coffee and 1 pound of tea, 2.5 pounds of each, 1 pound of coffee and 5 pounds of tea, and points in between. If both tea and coffee cost $1 per pound and the consumer has an available income of $5 to spend, he would get maximum satisfaction from buying 2.5 pounds of coffee and 2.5 pounds of tea, indicated by point B where the "price line" is tangent to curve ABC. Any other combination he could afford would be on a lower curve (i.e., would yield less total satisfaction). Now if the price of coffee remains $1 per pound but the price of tea rises to $2 per pound, an income of $5 could buy either 5 pounds of coffee or 2.5 pounds of tea and combinations in between. The greatest possible satisfaction would then result from buying about .75 pounds of tea and 3.5 pounds of coffee, as indicated by point E on curve DEF. The total satisfaction would, of course, be lower than before. Assuming different prices for tea (other things being equal), E and B would be found to be points on a curve that related the price of tea to the consumption of tea. This is how an indifference curve leads to a demand curve.

The curve also shows, incidentally, the relationship between changes in the price of tea and changes in the consumption of coffee. This concept is known as the "cross-elasticity" of demand, and is a useful tool whenever substitutable items are being considered. Whenever the argument is heard that the scarcity (and high incomes) of physicians justifies devolving more functions on nurses, for example, this exemplifies cross-elasticity of demand.

Supply, Demand, and Price Determination

For a market to exist, there must be sellers as well as buyers. Assume that the relation between wants and income leads to some demand curve DD' as shown in Figure 7.5. Assume further that a supply curve or schedule SS' also exists, which shows the amounts sellers would be willing to offer at different prices. Some point exists at which the demand and supply curves intersect, i.e., where buyers are willing to buy the amount sellers are willing to sell. This price (P) and quantity (Q) corresponding to this point are referred to as "equilibrium" price and quantity since demand and supply are in balance at that point. The equilibrium, such as it is, exists only in an instant of time, since the willingness to buy and sell at a given price change over time as supply, demand, and costs change.

In the nineteenth century, when market processes were less well understood than they are today, much attention was paid to equilibrium as if the achievement of equilibrium were a goal in itself and represented a desirable state of affairs. Modern economics tends to focus more on dynamic than on static aspects of markets and to emphasize growth and development rather than static equilibria.

One useful purpose of the supply and demand diagram of Figure 7.5, however, is that it focuses attention on the way prices are determined by the mutual interaction of the two variables. Behind the demand schedule lies a set of desires related to a set of prices (as described by Figure 7.4). Behind the supply schedule lies a set of costs of production. In analyzing costs, distinguishing

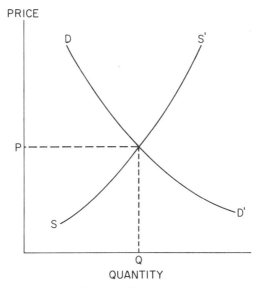

Fig. 7.5 Market price determination.

between fixed and variable costs has proved useful. As with any given scale of operations, fixed costs are those which do not change with the quantity produced, while variable costs do change. In air transport, for example, the cost of maintaining airport facilities is largely independent of passenger-miles travelled, and within limits is a fixed cost. Fuel, on the other hand, varies directly with the weight of the passengers transported and is clearly a variable cost. The aircraft is in an intermediate position—representing a fixed cost until it is full, when the cost of a second aircraft is incurred, and so on in a step-wise rather than continuous pattern as the number of passengers increases.

Figure 7.6 illustrates the relation of fixed and variable costs for a hypothetical laboratory devoted to the microscopic diagnosis of malaria. Costs are assumed to be of three kinds. The cost of the floor space, furniture, and microscopes is $10,000, charged at $5 per day over an expected working life of 2,000 days. This is a fixed cost for the period under consideration. The cost of disposable slides, stains, solvents, immersion oil, and electricity is variable, and is assumed to be 10¢ per slide. The payroll for microscopists and supervisor is $100 per shift.

The base line in Figure 7.6 is the variable cost which remains constant at 10¢ per slide. The broken line shows the fixed costs, which are all charged to the first slide if only one slide is examined, and reach a minimum when the assumed full output of 300 slides per day is reached. Finally, there are payroll costs which reach a minimum when 100 slides have been examined by the first shift of workers, jumps up again when the new shift starts work, reaches a second mimimum, jumps again when the third shift starts work, and reaches a final

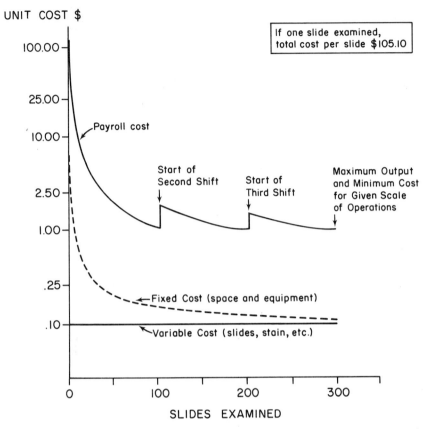

UNIT COST $

100.00

25.00

10.00 ·Payroll cost

2.50

1.00

.25 ←Fixed Cost (space and equipment)

.10 ↖Variable Cost (slides, stain, etc.)

If one slide examined, total cost per slide $105.10

Start of Second Shift

Start of Third Shift

Maximum Output and Minimum Cost for Given Scale of Operations

0   100   200   300

SLIDES EXAMINED

Fig. 7.6 Cost in a hypothetical laboratory for the microscopic diagnosis of malaria.

mimimum when all three shifts reach full output. The total cost per slide, which includes all three classes of cost, is indicated by the upmost solid line in Figure 7.6. Once 300 slides have been examined by the three shifts, we reach the limit of economies possible at this scale of operations. To go beyond this, we would have to incur new fixed costs for more space and more microscopes, and a similar figure could be drawn for larger and larger laboratories to show the differences in cost that might be involved at different scales of operation.

The higher the ratio of fixed to variable costs, the greater will be the economies that can be realized by planning for full utilization of facilities. Thus, the cost of leaving a major hospital half empty would be greater than the cost incurred by the same degree of underutilization of a rural health post staffed by a single nurse. In either case, however, full utilization is not necessarily within the power of the service unit to achieve. Careful study of prospective demand is essential in determining the size of the unit, and the ideal size is seldom reached.

Experience has shown that the introduction of new health facilities stimulates demand because of their education and demonstration effects. Add to this the unpredictable future course of population size and structure and causes of sickness and death, and it is clear that frequent reappraisals of demand and readjustments of plans may be required. Nevertheless, the closer the scale and organization of service approach the optimum, the greater will be the economies realized.

An upper limit to utilization is dictated by the nature of health services. In the case of physician services, for example, quality may be unimpaired as the average time spent per patient is reduced from one hour to twenty minutes when demand increases. But if utilization is so great that the physician cannot spend more than five minutes per patient, as has occurred in some instances, even the lower cost per patient attended will not justify the resulting reduction in quality of service. A growing number of agencies are seeking indices of quality as concern with the cost of medical care increases, and practicable indices hopefully will be developed to aid health planners in the future.

MACROECONOMIC CONSIDERATIONS

Knowledge of the criteria for allocating resources to health in the aggregate is important to health planners because these criteria guide national authorities at the highest level in deciding what share of total national resources should be devoted to the health sector. The basic national decisions may be made for a variety of political or economic reasons. Whatever the criteria, health services are often considered as a dependent sector of activity, expected to do the best possible job with the resources provided, but by no means provided with all the resources desired when higher priority is conceded to other "social infrastructure" areas such as education or to directly productive activity.

Relative Importance of Health Services in the Total Economy

Observers have found a certain rough consistency from country to country in the share of national resources spent for health. Illustrative figures for 14 countries are shown in Table 7.1. Despite their limited coverage, they serve to demonstrate the rather narrow range of variation in the share of gross national product devoted to health in rich and poor, large and small countries. Some slight change in the percentages is introduced when a roughly similar measure such as national income is used instead of gross national product as a basis for comparison; no matter what the divisor, however, a large element of potential error is introduced in countries where a significant portion of medical care is provided privately. Nevertheless, many countries devote about 5 percent of gross

Table 7.1
Percent of Gross National Product Going for Health and Health Share of
General Government Budgets, Circa 1961

Country	Total Current Expenditure on Health Services as Percent of Gross National Product	General Government Expenditure on Health Services as Percent of Total General Government Expenditure
Australia	4.9	25.8
Canada	5.5	17.1
Ceylon	3.7	14.9
Chile	5.6	16.4
Finland	4.3	18.8
France	4.2	25.4
Israel	5.9	9.0
Netherlands	4.5	18.7
Rhodesia and Nyasaland	4.1	13.2
Sweden	4.9	21.0
Tanganyika	2.5	11.8
United Kingdom	4.0	19.8
United States	5.5	7.0
Yugoslavia	4.4	21.3

Source: Abel-Smith, B. An International Study of Health Expenditures.
Public Health Paper No. 32. Geneva: World Health Organization,
1967.

national product to health care, although the percentage of government expenditure going for governmental health services varies over an extremely wide range because of their differing importance within total health care.

It is conceptually and administratively important, although statistically quite difficult, to distinguish clearly between expenditures on current account (payroll, drugs, supplies, etc.) and capital expenditures (buildings and grounds, durable equipment, and other nonrecurring or seldom-recurring items). While not all countries have yet adopted the practice, the establishment of separate current and capital budgets makes possible the separation of long-term considerations involved in planning capital investment (hospitals, roads, factories, etc.) from short-term budgetary forecasts of the cost of routine current operations.

In some countries, unfortunately, current and capital items are so mixed in accounting practice that it is not certain how much of the latter has been included in statistics of current expenditure. To the extent that the statistics of gross national product or national income for any country follow the Standard National Accounts system of the United Nations, the data cannot be compared directly with figures for countries that use the conceptually different Material Balance System (e.g., countries in Eastern Europe). In data referring to any single year, the signing of a contract for a single major facility, particularly in a small country, can introduce a decided shift in the ratio of health expenditure to total expenditure for that year.

Despite the reservations attached to the data, the "fact" that countries devote 5 percent of gross national product to health and the companion notion that 10 percent of government expenditure goes for government health services (based on an earlier WHO study of six countries) (2) have been interpreted as indicating the share of national resources that *should* be spent on health. Actually though, this seems to be the result of historical accident more than any other single factor. Even in the USSR, where considerable effort has been devoted to systematic health planning for more than 50 years, relative shares in the national economic plan appear to be set in accordance with a "law of proportional growth" and do not seem to represent much more than a convenient explanation for the absence of increased effort in any given branch of health activity.

In short, there is no objective way to determine what the relative share of resources for health should be. No method is known for comparing returns from expenditure on health, education, agriculture, manufacturing, and other activities, since the only common unit availabe to measure returns on a single scale is money. Many ingenious efforts have been made to guess at the money value of health activity, but even if it were possible to assign money values to improved health or longer life it is not always possible to identify the direct contribution of health services. Multiple causation must be taken into account, and such elements as higher incomes, more food, better housing, and higher levels of education are known to be positively correlated with lower infant mortality, higher life expectancy at birth, and other available health indices.

In the absence of any objective rule for determining the share of resources that should be spent on health, the economist is forced to concede second place, after historical accident, to political pressure. Health services are often oriented to satisfying needs rather than wants; wants, in the form of market demand working through the price mechanism, seem to have little direct influence on the supply of health services. In the absence of an organized marketplace, however, wants can influence the supply of health services when they are expressed politically as votes or by organized public opinion. Decisions as to public spending on health are often taken in response to such political pressures.

Political expression of wants necessitates even more the maintenance of the economic distinction between current and capital expenditures. Political decisions are often characterized by such short-run considerations as the tenure of an individual or a party in office, and their "time horizon" seldom runs beyond the period of foreseeable political power. This probably explains the common experience, in countries across the whole spectrum of economic and political structure, that it is easier to get administrative or legislative approval for investment in buildings and equipment than for added staff; and easier to get increased staff than improved wages and working conditions for existing staff. To many presidents and prime ministers, a hospital is a more satisfactory monument than an arch of triumph. Certainly, some of the unutilized and underutilized capacity in some of the less-developed countries results from the fact that politicians have decided to build hospitals and health centers without planning—without devoting sufficient thought to the manpower, supplies, equipment, and operating budgets that should go with the new construction.

Finally, in the absence of a precise formula for determining the shares of resources to be spent on health, the allocation of health funds involves a range rather than a precise figure. The lower limit to this range is the politically irreducible minimum, below which considerable difficulty could be anticipated by any government. In practice, this lower limit usually represents the level of service or expenditure per head of population at the time planning is introduced; it can be expected to increase over time as population and prices rise. The upper limit is the maximum amount that scientific argument and personal and political suasion can induce national authorities to concede. Economic and technical considerations are useful in determining allocations within the range thus established, even when they have been ignored in setting the upper and lower limits.

Input-Output Analysis

Interaction of supply and demand and individual demand curves were illustrated earlier (Figures 7.2-7.5). Supply and demand factors can also be analyzed in terms of national aggregates, and as such are also part of macroeconomics. The most common form of analysis is the input-output table. This type of analysis is based on the observation of actual flows of goods and money. The economy is composed of many individual sectors, each of which may supply inputs to the others and may in turn demand outputs from them. By fitting multiple regression lines, the intersectorial relations can be estimated and used for planning and forecasting.

For a concrete illustration, let us consider a very simple economy consisting of only three sectors, which are broadly classed as metals, fuel, and transportation. In addition to the sectorial relationships, of course, individuals provide the necessary labor and act as ultimate consumers. Finally, we assume that all activity can be translated into a monetary (dollar) common denominator.

Table 7.2 summarizes activity for a given year. We observe, for example, that of $276 million of transportation equipment supplied, $130 million went to ultimate consumers and the remainder became input as intermediate goods and services to the various sectors. We see further that the transportation product included $166 million worth of metals, $28 million worth of fuel, and $55 million in transportation, along with a $27 million conversion contribution for labor. In other words, the transportation product is roughly 60 percent metals (166/276), 10 percent fuel (28/276), 20 percent transportation input (55/276), and 10 percent labor (27/276). A similar view of the outputs of each of the sectors yields the set of so-called technical coefficients recorded in Table 7.3.

The table of technical coefficients (Table 7.3) gives some indication of what is required in the expansion of a given sector. The indication is not complete, however, because of the interrelationship among sectors. We note, for example, that an additional $100 worth of transportation output will require, among other things, an extra $60 worth of metals and $10 worth of fuel. These requirements in turn will force secondary expansions which will further increase requirements in all sectors. The total impact can be evaluated by a method developed by Leontief, whereby the technical coefficients and ultimate

Table 7.2
Input-Output Analysis: Activity for a Hypothetical Year (Millions of $)

Input	Metals	Fuel	Transport	Consumption	Total
Metals	54	23	166	20	263
Fuel	52	12	28	30	122
Transport	79	12	55	130	276
Labor	78	75	27		180
Total	263	122	276	180	841

Table 7.3
Input-Output Analysis: Technical Coefficients

Input	Metals	Fuel	Transport
Metals	.2	.2	.6
Fuel	.2	.1	.1
Transport	.3	.1	.2
Labor	.3	.6	.1
Total	1.0	1.0	1.0

consumption targets are combined into a set of simultaneous equations for solution (3).

To illustrate, let us propose to double the final consumption of fuel. Solution of the simultaneous equations produces the results presented in Table 7.4. In order to increase final consumption of fuel by $30 million, we find that total fuel output must increase by $39 million (from $122 million to $161 million) and that each of the other sectors must expand. Further, these expansions will require the availability and utilization of one-sixth more labor (rising from $180 million to $210 million in value).

Our input-output model has been unrealistically crude in a number of ways. For one thing, the input-output relationships as described by the technical coefficients have been assumed constant at all levels of activity. Moreover, labor input and final consumption were equal in value, thus allowing no room for savings and investment. Certain historical elements such as inventories and capital stocks were also ignored.

As we focus on economic measurements in the health sector proper, it should be borne in mind that three kinds of benefits can accrue from health programs. First, gains in economic output can result. The consequences of bad health were so clear to businessmen in British Guiana in the 1940's, for example, that malaria eradication was begun not by the government but by the sugar producers' association. Second, noneconomic personal benefits may be gained. Thus, treatment of disfiguring skin diseases may be justified largely in terms of increased personal comfort and self-esteem. Finally, use of health resources may result in savings. Introduction of antibiotics has, among other things, succeeded in reducing the duration of certain illnesses, thereby reducing the number of acute-treatment hospital beds needed.

In listing these benefits, we recognize health services as inputs which provide an output that has both investment and consumption components. Conceptually, then, we could add to input-output Tables 7.2 and 7.4 another row

Table 7.4
Input-Output Analysis: Activity After Doubling of Fuel Consumption

Input	Output				Total
	Metals	Fuel	Transport	Consumption	
Metals	56	32	173	20	281
Fuel	56	16	29	60	161
Transport	85	16	57	130	288
Labor	84	97	29		210
Total	281	161	288	210	940

representing the health sector input, with hopefully measurable contributions to the output of other sectors and to consumption in its own right.

Analyses similar to those of the input-output table have been applied to the flows between the different subsectors of health care (primary patient care, consultant care, hospital care, home care, and so forth) (4).

DECISIONS AND PRIORITIES IN HEALTH PLANNING

Seat of Decision-Making Authority

Consumer ignorance is much more of a concern in the health field than in most other fields because consumers often are unaware of their own needs. Beyond this, translation of a given need or want into an economic demand for specific health services is a technical matter which lay consumers are often unable to handle. Since the decisions are commonly made for the consumer by physicians and other professionals, these groups contribute much to the demand for their own services. Thus, "Roemer's Law" states in essence that if hospital beds are available they will tend to be utilized.* Similarly, some persons advocate a rather tight supply of physicians in order to restrict expenditures for their services to reasonable levels.

If the translation of health problems into tangible services is not clear-cut, the response to some related needs is even more cloudy. For example, while we recognize the desirability of eliminating excessive patient travel and inconvenience through the provision of readily accessible facilities and services, this involves important locational and organizational decisions which are not easily arrived at quantitatively.

The relationship between need and effective demand is influenced by the increasing acceptance of the principle that access to health services is a basic right rather than a privilege. This principle brings the question of ability to pay to the foreground and, when some classes of consumers are unable to pay for needed services, leads necessarily to government and third-party intervention in the health care system.

Intervention at this level provides the opportunity for more broadly based and technically sound decisions. To the extent that these decisions apply to personal health services, of course, utilization of services that are "good" for people requires the acceptance of these services by the potential beneficiaries, perhaps through financial underwriting by the government.

* As a matter of national pride, it is held in Canada that "Roemer's Law" is really "Roth's Law" since Professor F. B. Roth of the University of Toronto is reputed to have said it first when he was in charge of the hospital system in Saskatchewan!

If the planning and decision-making agencies can succeed in being truly representative of the community of individuals they serve, their breadth of view can be extremely useful. This is true primarily because so-called externalities typify many health service situations in the sense that the effects of a given action extend beyond the specific purpose intended. The *externality factor* can be considered at three levels: in connection with the actions of individuals, actions of institutions, and actions of government agencies. With respect to individuals, for example, immunizations and prompt treatment of communicable diseases can have a preventive impact upon other members of the community not receiving the services directly. At the institutional level, externalities may lead to a divergence of interest between the individual hospital and the community at large. The individual hospital is naturally concerned with over-all institutional strength and may exaggerate the effects of failure to establish a certain facility. The community, on the other hand, is interested in minimizing the total cost of a particular service and thus seeks to avoid duplication of facilities. At the government level, the actions of one arm of government often interact with those of another. Hence, the benefits of many national programs are hard to measure because of the rather uncertain ripple effect of increasing or decreasing corresponding local programs.

As we review in economic terms the research, training, and service elements of the health system, the interaction among the three must be taken into account. The research and training elements are institution- and government-based, so the service element can hardly escape such an orientation to some degree. Moreover, individual choice in the services area is not always the road to rational decision-making. This reinforces the conclusion that health planning in some form is essential. Fortunately, as Girard Piel forcibly pointed out at the 1967 National Health Forum, the potential benefits of planning have increased with the introduction of powerful new tools of systems analysis (5). Lest we fail to retain a balanced view, however, we must observe with Klarman that "if a planning agency is effective it reduces the risk of a multitude of small or moderate mistakes but it raises the risk of a few large ones" (6, p. 727).

Setting Priorities within the Health Sector

Wherever the decision-making authority may lie in health planning, numerous constraints operate to reduce freedom of choice. Certain activities (for example, vaccination to achieve given levels of immunity in the community) are essentially indivisible. Others (such as house connections for drinking water) lend themselves to the imposition of a charge on the identifiable user. Funds for some general promotional activities such as health education may be assigned to school budgets, or water and sewer construction to over-all public works budgets, and are thus beyond the decision-making authority of the health services. Above all, popular demand for medical care (in the sense of curative services) usually means that 90 percent or more of all health expenditures—the portion commonly devoted to medical care—can become part of the politically irreducible minimum. Possibilities exist for affecting the delivery of medical care services and influencing both quantity and quality through efficient planning, but this does not affect the constraint on expenditure as a whole. This leaves only expenditure on a limited number of community-wide preventive and promotional activities in the full discretionary power of health planners, although influencing medical care services to some degree is often possible, especially when the financing system promotes public awareness of costs as well as benefits.

Econometrics

Within the health authorities' area of discretion, available resources commonly fall far short of satisfying all identifiable needs. This in turn imposes the need for establishing priorities, which can often be stated in mathematical terms.

Application of mathematics and statistics to economics is called econometrics. This discipline has flourished in the past three decades, and the econometric approach was introduced in health planning in the early 1960's. Basic considerations in establishing priorities can be expressed in the vocabulary of mathematics in the simple relationship:

$P = f(M, I, V, C)$, in which

P stands for relative *priority;*

f means that the priority is a function of (bears an identifiable but unspecified relation to) each of the other variables;

M stands for the *magnitude* of the disease or other condition under attack, commonly measured by statistics of mortality and morbidity, alone or in combination;

I represents the relative *impact* or *importance* of the disease; in the present state of health economics it cannot be measured with precision, and is usually given an arbitrary numerical value based on the relative incidence among children, the aged, and persons of working age, or some similar factors;

V is the *vulnerability* of the disease to attack by known and available means; like importance, it cannot be measured with precision, so that arbitrary rating scales based on expert consensus must be used;

C is the *cost* of the proposed activity; it can be measured with a fair degree of accuracy, as can morbidity and mortality.

The specific formulation of these factors is an arbitrary decision but one that should have a common sense basis. In Latin America, the relationship

$$P = MIV/C$$

has been widely used. Naturally, a multiplicative formula is likely to produce a different ordering or priorities than one based upon the notion of additivity or some other relationship.

EXAMPLE OF AN ECONOMETRIC PLANNING MODEL FOR ONE DISEASE

Mathematical models are being proposed with increasing frequency. The following example, where the Latin American planning formula appears in a new guise in terms of a set of linear equations, is based on the econometric approach. The model was developed by Hector Correa, and the following version is taken with minor modifications from his article "Health Planning" (7). The reader is referred to this source for a discussion of refinements of the linear model presented, of nonlinear models, and of dynamic models that involve data for different periods of time.

The Basic Model

P represents the susceptible population;
B = the total number of people affected by the disease, i.e., that become sick;
T = the total number of deaths due to the disease;
E_1 = total expenditure on prevention of the disease;
E_2 = total expenditure on treatment of the disease;
R = total resources available to the health service; and

$$R = E_1 + E_2 \tag{1}$$

The number of people who get the disease is assumed to be a linear decreasing function of the total expenditure on prevention. Specifically,

$$B = P - a_1 E_1 \tag{2}$$

where a_1 is a parameter that represents the number of cases that can be prevented with an expenditure of one dollar.

Next, the number of deaths is assumed to be a linear function of the number of sick people and the expenditure on treatment,

$$T = B - a_2 E_2 \tag{3}$$

where a_2 is a parameter that represents the number of deaths that can be avoided with the expenditure of one dollar.

With equations (1), (2), and (3), the problem of minimizing the number of deaths takes the following form: Minimize

$$T = P - a_1 E_1 - a_2 E_2 \tag{4}$$

subject to

$$R = E_1 + E_2 \qquad (5)$$

and $T \geqslant 0$.

Since in practice the amount of resources R will not be enough to reduce deaths T to zero, attention has to be concentrated on getting T down to some low value. Solving (5) for E_2 and combining with (4), it follows that

$T = P - (a_1 E_1) - (a_2 [R-E_1])$,
$T = P - (a_1 E_1) - (a_2 R - a_2 E_1)$,
$T = P - (a_1 E_1) - (-a_2 E_1) - (a_2 R)$, and finally
$T = P - (a_1 - a_2)E_1 - a_2 R$, and $\qquad (6)$
$0 \leqslant E_1 \leqslant R$.

Hence, T will be a minimum if

$E_1 = R$ when $a_1 > a_2$ and
$E_2 = R$ when $a_1 < a_2$. $\qquad (7)$

The result obtained (i.e., that all the resources should be devoted to the measure that gives the higher return per dollar) corresponds with common sense.

A More Realistic Model and Numerical Example

The main limitation of the basic model is that it does not include any indication of the method that should be used to evaluate the parameters a_1 and a_2 using statistical data. The following more elaborate system of equations was proposed by Correa to remove this limitation.

P   is the susceptible population
N_1 is the number of people who have to be protected by preventive measures such as vaccination in order to minimize deaths
N_2 is the number of people who do not have to be protected
$P = N_1 + N_2$ $\qquad (8)$

b_1 is the morbidity rate among the people protected
b_2 is the morbidity rate among the people not protected
B   is the total number of cases of the disease, and
$B = b_1 N_1 + b_2 N_2$ $\qquad (9)$

M_1 is the number of cases that have to be treated in order to minimize deaths

M_2 is the number of cases that do not have to be treated

$$B = M_1 + M_2 \tag{10}$$

t_1 is the mortality rate among cases treated
t_2 is the mortality rate among cases not treated
T   is the number of deaths, and

$$T = t_1 M_1 + t_2 M_2 \tag{11}$$

c_1 is the cost of protecting one person
c_2 is the cost of treating one person

E_1 is the amount that should be spent on prevention in order to minimize deaths
E_2 is the amount that should be spent on treatment
R   is total resources available, and

$$R = E_1 + E_2 \tag{12}$$
$$E_1 = c_1 N_1 \tag{13}$$
$$E_2 = c_2 N_2 \tag{14}$$

The problem is to determine E_1 and E_2 so as to minimize T. The following transformations are required.

From (10) and (11)

$$T = (t_1 - t_2)M_1 + t_2 B \tag{15}$$

From (8) and (9)

$$B = (b_1 - b_2)N_1 + b_2 P \tag{16}$$

From (15) and (16)

$$T = t_2 b_2 P + t_2 (b_1 - b_2)N_1 + (t_1 - t_2)M_1 \tag{17}$$

And from (13), (14), and (17)

$$T = t_2 b_2 P + t_2 (b_1 - b_2)E_1/c_1 + (t_1 - t_2)E_2/c_2 \tag{18}$$

The problem then reduces to minimizing T in (18) subject to condition (12). This problem corresponds to the one in equations (4) and (5) of the earlier model, with

$$-a_1 = t_2 (b_1 - b_2)/c_1 \quad \text{and} \quad -a_2 = (t_1 - t_2)/c_2 \tag{19}$$

With a_1 and a_2 obtained from (19), the solution of (7) in the earlier model can be applied.

From equation (18), it should be clear that a_2, as defined in (19), is the number of deaths that can be avoided by spending one dollar on treatment, while a_1 is the number of deaths that can be avoided by spending one dollar on prevention of the disease, but without treating those who fall sick. It is possible to verify directly the meanings just given to a_1 and a_2 with the following approach:

First, from (11) we have

$$\Delta T = t_1 \Delta M_1 + t_2 \Delta M_2 \tag{20}$$

in which Δ indicates "increment to." Thus, ΔT represents an increment to T, the initial number of deaths.

From (10), since B is assumed to remain constant, we have

$$0 = \Delta M_1 + \Delta M_2 \tag{21}$$

Hence, from (20) and (21)

$$\Delta T = (t_1 - t_2)\Delta M_1 \tag{22}$$

From (22), with $\Delta T = 1$, we obtain

$$-\Delta M_1 = -1/(t_1 - t_2)$$

as the number of people to be treated to avoid one death. Since c_2 is the cost per person treated, the cost to avoid one death by treatment is

$$- c_2/(t_1 - t_2).$$

Its inverse, a_2, is the number of deaths that can be avoided with the expenditure of one dollar. A similar analysis can be made for prevention with respect to a_1.

Correa was able to give his model empirical content by using the PAHO data on whooping cough in Northern Santiago, Chile, in 1963 (Table 7.5). With the numerical data, formula (18) becomes

$$T = 0.018P + (-a_1 E_1) + (-a_2 E_2) = 0.018P - a_1 E_1 - a_2 E_2.$$

Since $a_1 = 0.015$ and $a_2 = 0.00069$, the formula then becomes
$$T = 0.018P - 0.015E_1 - 0.00069E_2.$$

Since $a_1 > a_2$, the maximum reduction of deaths will be obtained by concentrating all resources on prevention, with $E_1 = R = 31.317$ and $E_2 = 0$. In this case, the total number of deaths that could be avoided is $a_1 R = 470$.

Since the actual distribution of resources in Santiago was $E_1 = 7.158$, $E_2 = 24.159$ and the number of deaths prevented was 124, Correa was able to assert that, with a planning approach based on his model, a total of 346 additional deaths could theoretically have been avoided.

Table 7.5
Numerical Illustration of the Correa Econometric Model

Symbol	Definition	Value
b_1	Morbidity rate in protected population	0.45
b_2	Morbidity rate in unprotected population	0.60
t_1	Mortality rate with treatment	0.01
t_2	Mortality rate without treatment	0.03
c_1	Cost of protecting one person	0.30
c_2	Cost of treating one person	28.86
R	Total resources available (Escudos)	31.317

SOURCE: Ahumada, J. *et al. Health Planning: Problems of Concept and Method.* Table 7, p. 39. Washington, D.C.: Pan American Health Organization, 1965.

HEALTH IN THE SERVICE OF NATIONAL DEVELOPMENT POLICY

Up to this point, the allocation of funds within the health sector has been discussed in terms of the kinds of decisions that health authorities make when they set priorities for that portion of health expenditure over which they have discretionary power. Even within this area, however, occasions may arise when considerations other than M, I, V, and C will override the calculated priority for a given activity. A country may be faced with the need to meet development targets in another sector, to economize on foreign exchange because of an adverse balance of payments, or simply to adjust to the fact of poverty by adopting systems and classes of health service consistent with their ability to pay rather than with "ideal" patterns observed in richer or more advanced countries. Under these circumstances, the health authorities may be called on to abandon the planned priorities for the sake of other goals.

A case in point is the use of social security or social insurance mechanisms to provide health services in poor and underdeveloped countries, a trend that has been evident since World War II. It usually means that in the first instance health services are made available to employed wage earners in the major cities, spreading only slowly thereafter to cover family dependents and workers in small towns and rural areas. In a period of urbanization and industrialization, this means concentrating health services not in the area of greatest need (morbidity and mortality may well be higher from all causes in rural areas) but in the area considered to be of greatest importance for the future economic development of the country. If it were possible to identify the importance for national development of individual health programs, this factor could be rated on a numerical scale and introduced in the I term of the priority formula. Without this possibility, it becomes a matter for political or administrative decision. The political desire to establish a social security system may result in ignoring altogether the question whether some other form of health service would be more efficient.

In Peru, for example, the national health plan presented to the Congress in 1965 recognized the overriding national priority given to development of the Amazonian region by specifying that new construction of health centers in the plan period would be concentrated in that region. The importance for development of the projected Andean highway was recognized by the Ministry of Health in special health provisions recommended for road workers (and eventually colonists) in the high mountains. As another example, in Buenaventura, Colombia—an important transshipment point on the Pacific coast—the most active and best-financed health center (as of 1966) was not part of the Departmental Network of the Cauca Valley, but was a dependency of the national government, operated by the port authorities for the benefit of the dock workers and their families.

Economic development involves more than the growth of urban industry and trade, however. Some countries rely heavily on agriculture to feed the domestic population, provide export earnings, and accumulate a surplus for investment in nonagricultural development projects. The health services that grew up on sugar estates and banana plantations in the early twentieth century constituted tacit recognition of the need for a healthy, stable, and productive agricultural labor force. More recently, many of the newly self-governing countries of the world are attempting to create rural health services with similar aims (and the satisfaction of increasingly vocal demand) in mind.

Allocating resources to health services on the basis of other than health considerations does, of course, run counter to the commonly accepted views of universality (the right of all persons to health care) and of the importance of maintaining the highest possible quality standards. But when the money does not stretch to cover the need, arguments of equity are countered by the scarcity of resources. Allocating equal funds to all areas and all classes of the population would often mean inadequate health services for all instead of adequate services for a select (hopefully, productive) few.

THE USE OF HUMAN AND PHYSICAL RESOURCES WITHIN THE HEALTH SECTOR

Human Resources

One might imagine that the decision as to priority ratings for programs within the health sector determines once and for all the priority ratings for the allocation of manpower to the different programs. This is not so because labor and capital are substitutable to a certain extent, because some categories of labor may be substituted for each other, and because health programs differ from one another in their capital and labor requirements.

Substitutability

The substitutability between labor and capital is illustrated by the use of the jet injector in mass smallpox vaccination programs. A single operator trained in the use of this rather costly piece of equipment can vaccinate as many persons in an hour as several vaccinators using the conventional scarification technique can vaccinate in a day with far cheaper instruments. The jet injector, then, is a substitute for the additional vaccinators. This example also serves to underscore the importance of utilization; if only a few persons have to be vaccinated, or if the year's work-load can conveniently be spread over many working days, vaccination with the jet injector may prove more costly than the manual technique. Other things being equal, if sustained high numbers of persons are to be vaccinated and the jet injector can be used for many hours each day and many days in the year, the cost per vaccination will be lower by this method.

Deciding whether to substitute capital for labor will depend in each case on the volume of service to be provided and the relative cost of capital and labor. In the less developed countries where work-loads are uneven, unskilled labor is cheap and abundant, and capital equipment is imported, scarce, and expensive, it may well prove economical (and have the political advantage of helping to maintain employment) to refrain from the introduction of labor-saving capital equipment even when the volume of service would justify such substitution.

Much the same considerations underlie the basic decision whether to emphasize in-patient or out-patient care in planning the over-all system of health services. Elaborate hospitals with modern diagnostic and treatment aids are expensive to build and require a variety of skilled professionals to provide a full range of services. An equal number of people could be cared for in lower-cost health centers by preponderantly semiskilled and auxiliary personnel. In this case, the choice of system and the kind of capital investment undertaken can be said to predetermine to some extent the kinds of manpower needed, and a "reverse feedback" would be to take the cost of the different kinds of manpower into account in planning the kinds of facilities to be constructed. Clearly, alternative systems of health service may take care of equal *numbers* of people, but not necessarily the *same* people. One individual may die of peritonitis when there is no hospital where an appendectomy can be performed, while at the same time the life of another may be saved at low cost simply by rehydration of an infant with diarrhea performed in a local health center.

The problem of substitutability has been studied in a wide variety of settings. Countries experiencing manpower shortages (and shortage relative to demand exists even in affluent societies) have commonly seen a planned or spontaneous devolution of functions from the physician to the trained nurse and from the trained nurse to the nursing auxiliary. A variety of intermediate professional categories—the Feldsher in the USSR, the Assistant Doctor in Fiji, the nurse with responsibilities that approach the general practice of medicine in northern Canada—have been established. An even more important development has been the growing awareness of the possibilities of ensuring better utilization of physician time on professional tasks by using various combinations of professional and supporting personnel as a team. To the economist, this is a somewhat tardy rediscovery of the eighteenth century doctrine that economies and efficiency arise from the appropriate division and specialization of labor, but it is no less fruitful for being delayed. Nevertheless, without good management practices and full utilization of personnel, even an "ideal" team may be inefficient and expensive.

Differences in Capital and Labor Requirements

Divergences between money and manpower requirements of health programs often arise because of the varying requirements of the programs themselves. Perhaps the problems of manpower substitution and combination have been studied too much in the context of medical care, with a resultant lack of emphasis on the differences between kinds of health programs. When the whole spectrum of health activity is studied, medical care of the sick obviously makes the greatest demands on skilled. professional manpower, while mass preventive and promotional activities rely far more heavily on subprofessional or nonmedical skills.

In advanced countries, the greatest demand for hospital beds, for individual attention by physicians, and for skilled nursing care usually exists in the relatively small, if growing, group of individuals suffering from the chronic and degenerative diseases of old age. In the less-developed and poorer countries, in contrast, most deaths occur at earlier ages and are attributable to the general group of infectious and parasitic diseases. The so-called "vertical" or "penetration" campaigns against such diseases as smallpox, yellow fever, and malaria rely heavily on unskilled labor—drivers, spraymen, warehousemen, and vaccinators and microscopists with specific limited skills. Far smaller numbers of physicians, nurses, or, for that matter, parasitologists and entomologists are employed.

Environmental sanitation activities—whether for the provision of potable water or for the disposal of excreta or refuse—principally involve digging, drilling, earth moving, and pipe laying. These activities call for far more unskilled labor than foremen or supervising engineers. At least in the early stages of health program development, unskilled labor in preventive, promotional, and environmental programs may contribute more to over-all health in terms of death and illness avoided than physicians and nurses contribute by treating those already sick. In such cases, high money allocations may well be associated with low demand for professional medical manpower.

To summarize, the problem of manpower in health planning is to obtain the highest output of services for a given cost by selecting the most appropriate combinations of capital and labor, the optimum mix of personnel skills, types of capital, and health technology, and the mix of programs that best reconciles manpower availability in the different categories with the targets set for the health services.

In a perfectly competitive market economy, money costs usually provide a good measure of real cost; in the health industry, with its curious mixture of philanthropy, government subsidies, imperfect labor markets, and contributed labor time, concentration on money costs alone may frequently be misleading. Good decisions about the allocation of resources require information about the real costs involved. For example, the establishment of increased numbers of nursing homes would presumably lead to an increase in the number of licensed practical nurses, who would receive substantial money wages. It is possible, however, that these and other necessary attendants might be selected from among the unemployed and trained briefly. In this case, the real economic cost would be relatively low.

Finally, the relation between human resources utilization and the cost—as well as the quantum—of health services must be explored. The argument has been advanced in the United States, for example, that the large personal service component in health care prevents the kinds of gains in productivity that can be obtained in sectors such as manufacturing through rationalizing production processes. As a result, hospitals have not been able to offset wage increases with productivity gains and this is thought to explain at least in part why the price of hospital care has risen faster than the general level of prices.

With regard to many goods and services, where the possibility of consumer ignorance is considerable, the competitive behavior of the producers affords some protection to the consumer. When competition is vigorous among producers, they may very well (among other practices) inform the consumer of the merits of their products as compared with those of their competitors. When middlemen such as wholesalers and retailers are involved, one of their functions is commonly to provide some kind of product information. These putative safeguards do not exist in the field of health care. Severe restrictions on entry are imposed by licensing requirements in the health professions and for the operation of hospitals. Advertising and price competition are frowned on.

Critical comment concerning the output of competitors, particularly in the case of physicians, is regarded as unethical. Numerous arguments can be advanced in support of the restrictive practices of the medical profession, but in the present context such practices merely mean that the output and performance of health care services cannot be appraised by economists on bases that might be appropriate to a more competitive industry (8). In addition, since the benefits produced by specific activities within the field of health care are more difficult to measure than those arising from the production of most other goods and services, industrial engineering-type studies are less likely to provide clear-cut recommendations for the optimal allocation of manpower than they do in manufacturing industry.

Physical Resources

In dealing with facility planning, five special features of the health field deserve attention: the waste of resources occasioned by a low rate of occupancy, the problem of adaptation to random variations in admissions, the scale of operations, the life of the physcial plant, and population changes.

Occupancy Rates
Hospitals are characterized by high overhead costs despite the fact that about two-thirds of total cost represents payroll. Thus, large numbers of unfilled beds are generally considered to be a serious threat to the financial stability of the institutions, since the unfilled beds reflect substantial losses of income without corresponding declines in expenditures. Clearly, then, carefully coordinated planning is needed to satisfy future requirements without duplication of facilities. Bed occupancy rates must not be taken too literally, however, for they are closely associated with duration of stay. One institution may be very efficient in limiting duration of stay but thereby increase its bed occupancy management problems, while another institution may take advantage of third party prepayment schemes to keep its beds filled. This suggests that, in addition to bed occupancy rates, one must consider turnover rates and the purposes for which the beds are utilized.

Variability of Admissions
An important reason for less than 100 percent occupancy of medical care facilities is the random nature of admissions. Although this may seem to be simply one aspect of the preceding bed utilization question, it must be analyzed separately because of the number of devices that have been developed through operations research and other techniques for reducing the degree of randomness. These have included such things as improved scheduling of elective admissions, replacement of large wards with small bedrooms, designation of swing beds between intensive and intermediate care units in progressive care facilities, and

occasional attempts to end the physical separation of maternity patients from others.

Scale of Operations

The appropriate scale of operations for a given facility depends in the first instance upon the nature of the cost curve, which has often been held to be U-shaped, as noted earlier in this chapter. On the one hand, specialization and division of labor result in declining unit costs as the scale of operations increases. Beyond a certain point, however, complexities of management intrude to hamper coordination of efforts, and consumers are subjected to increased travel times and inconvenience. As a result, unit costs may rise again once a certain point is reached. Some authorities, however, do not believe that the turning point is critical in the case of hospitals.

Even if the decision is to stop short of the very large, high cost scale of operations, the problems of indivisibility of equipment and teams are likely still to be present. Cobalt bombs for radiation therapy, renal dialysis units, and teams for open heart surgery are obviously facts of life, although hopefully not for every individual institution. Avoiding the duplication of these expensive facilities and services requires recognizing the importance of selective duplication of staff appointments for physicians.

Life of Physical Assets

The buildings and equipment used to provide health services tend to have long physical lives, which create problems in two ways. First, improving technology may cause obsolescence to be an important factor, thus making economic life far shorter than potential physical life. It is very difficult to convince a health official that a still-sturdy building and functional piece of equipment may be economic liabilities worthy of replacement from seemingly scarce capital funds. As a result, assessment of the conditions of facilities requires more than a physical inventory and a perusal of historical records of financial outlays. One should be more interested in the present economic worth of the various facilities and the opportunities for enhancing that worth through replacements and additions.

A second ramification of the durability-improved technology syndrome is the difficulty in forecasting future needs for beds and other facilities. Conceptually at least, one would like to determine, mathematically if possible, the relationship between a number of explanatory variables (such as population, age, and sex distributions, economic levels, and morbidity and mortality rates) and relevant dependent variables such as bed needs. Even when they cover short periods, such attempts at association are not always as successful as one would hope. Indeed, Feldstein and German have indicated that a simple time series projection of past utilization trends may be as reliable an approach as any (9). Presumably, long-run changes in treatment patterns and other technological changes will make present forecasts even less successful. Certainly, the bed is no longer a significant unit of measure in those areas of medicine where more and more procedures are performed on an ambulatory basis. A realistic view of our forecasting abilities, then, causes us to plan for facilities that are as flexible and adaptable to uncertainty as possible.

Population Changes

Population growth naturally affects the need for medical facilities and services. Uncertainties regarding future growth rates and distribution of the population form part of the forecasting problem discussed above. Population changes, especially qualitative ones, go beyond the matter of forecasting, however, and deserve attention on their own. To illustrate, the close tie between medical education and the provision of free hospital care has kept the level of medical services in the central cities of the United States higher than it would otherwise be. With increased government participation, however, patients who receive free care furnish a steadily declining fraction of all teaching material. This will affect decisions regarding the relationship between teaching and service, the location of facilities, and concern on the part of medical institutions for population shifts to and from the areas where they are located.

ASSESSING THE IMPACT OF HEALTH INVESTMENTS

The basic economic criterion for decisions as to health expenditure is the same criterion that guides businessmen in their decisions: the concept of return on investment.

The total investment in health can be viewed as the sum of a number of elements. As in business, spending on capital goods such as hospitals and durable equipment is classified as investment. In addition, current expenditures on health (supplies, payroll, and other items) can be viewed as an investment in the health of the population or indirectly as an investment in the goods and services which are expected to be produced by individuals in better health.

From the point of view of statistical measurement, the distinction between investing in *health* or in health *services* is important. An investment in health must measure its return in indices of health. Such indices are yet to be developed. Because of this, the negative aspect—reduction in morbidity and mortality—is commonly used. While this may indeed express health in terms of measurable characteristics, the problem of determining the return on the investment is complicated by the multiple causation mentioned earlier, which makes it impossible to attribute improvements in health (or reductions in morbidity and mortality) to the effect of the health services alone. To set a target of service is much simpler; service units such as bed-days of hospitalization, physician-hours of consultation, nurse-hours of patient care, or vaccinator time can be calculated relatively easily, and the return on investment in health services can be measured in terms of the units of service provided.

The pioneering work of Dublin and Lotka, *The Money Value of a Man,* dates back to the 1920's (10); in the subsequent forty years, students of the return on investment in health pursued the problem with increasing statistical virtuosity. The common method of such studies was to use statistics of morbidity and mortality as the basis for calculating the wages foregone (including, at times, an imputed wage for housewife services) because of avoidable illness or death. These earnings were then viewed as the positive return on investment in programs to prevent or cure the diseases causing absenteeism, disability, and death. Many of the studies also calculated the cost of treatment of the diseases and added this to the estimated return on health investment on the basis that prevention or early treatment means subsequent medical care costs foregone. By and large, however, this approach seems to have turned into a dead end, and by the 1960's had lost much of its earlier popularity as economists focused their attention on the more limited aspects of the problem involved in cost-benefit analysis.

This approach can be criticized in a number of ways. The existence of unemployment as a variable and unpredictable future quantity makes it impossible to obtain a valid present estimate of future wages lost. Also, calculations must be made for individual diseases, since the data on death and disability are available on this basis, with combined results depending on the aggregation of a large number of individual estimates which may introduce new errors. A general problem is the requirement that inputs and outputs be measured in comparable terms and that the quantitative association between them be known. In practice, the inputs are often most conveniently measured in such terms as man-days, bed-days, and dollars, whereas the outputs may be quite differently expressed as deaths or illness averted. Beyond this, the number of man-hours of effort required to avert a death is seldom clear; someone may venture to calculate the potential benefit of reducing heart disease to negligible proportions but he would be hard pressed to tell how this benefit could be achieved. Moreover, decisions do not often include the alternative of complete eradication; nor are they often made at a point when nothing whatsoever has previously been done about the problem. Instead, we are forced to contemplate the marginal effects to be expected from modifications of existing programs, and these marginal changes may be difficult to measure.

Among the more ambitious recent attempts are the economic valuations by disease category for health expenditures and productivity losses in the United States made by Dorothy Rice (11). A sample of her results is included as Table 7.6 for illustration. Economic studies have also been done in recent years on vocational rehabilitation programs, heart disease, cancer, stroke, and other problems (12). Most of these studies have been politically motivated and have been undertaken by government agencies with a budgetary stake in the results;

Table 7.6
Annual Economic Costs: Distribution of Direct Expenditures and Indirect Costs of
Morbidity and Mortality, by Selected Diagnosis, 1963

Diagnosis	Total	Direct Expenditures	Indirect Cost		
			Total	Mortality	Morbidity
Amount (Total)	$46,303,100	$22,530,000	$23,773,100	$2,731,000	$21,042,200
Percent (Total)	100.0	100.0	100.0	100.0	100.0
Neoplasms	5.6	5.7	5.6	17.7	4.0
Mental, psychoneurotic, and personality disorders	15.2	10.7	19.5	0.4	22.0
Diseases of nervous system and sense organs	7.0	6.3	7.7	11.0	7.2
Diseases of circulatory system	13.8	10.1	17.4	44.9	13.9
Diseases of respiratory system	10.6	7.0	13.9	5.1	15.0
Diseases of digestive system	11.9	18.5	5.7	4.5	5.8
Diseases of bones and organs of movement	5.7	6.3	5.2	0.2	5.8
Injuries	8.1	7.6	8.6	8.9	8.6
All other	21.9	28.0	16.4	7.4	17.8

SOURCE: Rice, Dorothy. "Estimating the Cost of Illness." *American Journal of Public Health* 57:437, 1967.

the results, therefore, have to be viewed with a modicum of skepticism. Other investigations have simply listed known consequences for qualitative appraisal without attempts at valuation, or have established indirect associations such as the historical relationship between mortality rates and hospital bed needs, or ratios of health personnel to population.

Some attempts have also been made to calculate the value of the goods and services produced by investment in health in the sense of production losses avoided by prevention or treatment of disease in the labor force. These studies have usually been very limited in nature, for only in exceptional circumstances can a clear and direct relationship between disease and economic activity be established. Malaria has been a favorite subject for such studies, since successful malaria programs are usually marked by a rapid and dramatic decrease in the incidence of the disease that can often be correlated successfully with statistics of agricultural production in single-crop cultivation (e.g., sugar cane, which depends heavily on manual labor with clear-cut seasonal requirements). The resulting estimates of economic loss from disease, however crude, have the advantage of being directly comparable in money terms with the anticipated return from alternative uses of the funds proposed to be invested in health.

Comparisons of the alternative return on investment (known in economics as "opportunity cost") provide a key measure of the economic desirability of different activities.

In contrast to the rough but economically important estimates of return to health investment when the target is either health or the gains in production attributable to health, the statistically more feasible and accurate calculation of returns in units of service, when the target is set in service terms, cannot be used for economic comparisons of the yield from investment. In addition, some classes of investment in health itself do not provide a calculable economic return: medical care of the aged, for example, responds to a moral rather than an economic imperative. As noted earlier, much of the demand for medical care services is related to the chronic and degenerative diseases of old age. In such cases, a true "cure" can hardly be said to exist and, as in the case of cancer, is often arbitrarily defined as survival for a given number of years. Palliation is the more likely product of medical care of many older people, and complete cure or rehabilitation in the sense of a return to productive economic life is rare. In other cases, such as vaccination against smallpox in a country where the disease is not known to exist, the money value of protection against the possible importation of the disease cannot be calculated even if the persons protected are employed workers with known rates of pay.

From the viewpoint of the health planner, the important issue is to find measures to reconcile the moral imperative to prevent and treat disease in cases where no economic return is apparent, with the estimated yield from investment in those areas of health activity where income foregone because of illness and death, and the cost of treatment avoided by preventive activities, can in fact be calculated. Neither economic nor moral criteria alone will suffice, and reconciliation of the two is usually a matter of political compromise at the decision-making level.

COST-BENEFIT AND COST-EFFECTIVENESS

Cost-Benefit Analysis in Health Planning

Since estimates of the economic return on investment in health are commonly related to individual diseases, the problem of aggregating the results into some measure of the return on investment in "total health" runs the risk of compounding errors. When the yield on investment in health (assuming that it can be estimated) is to be compared with the alternative yield from investing the same money in schools, roads, or factories, it is virtually impossible to arrive at a satisfactory calculation of "opportunity cost" because the outputs of the different activities are not commensurable (e.g., lives saved, graduates from secondary schools, miles of road, pairs of shoes). Even when the outputs are all expressed in money terms, cases exist in which an "educated guess" must be used when market prices are not available. Even then, available market price quotations for different goods and services may not necessarily reflect the value of the relative contribution of each activity to society; more likely, they reflect what consumers are disposed to pay at a given time and place. In addition, any major health planning decision may alter prices, wage levels, and other elements entering into the original calculation, if its impact is sufficiently great on the economy as a whole.

The problem of common measures of output is somewhat more manageable in the health sector even if some difficulty remains in comparing death deferred by organ transplant with sickness or death avoided by vaccination, health restored by chemotherapy of tuberculosis, or pain and anxiety relieved by active measures in terminal cancer. Many planning decisions, however, involve deciding among alternative ways to reach the same goal. Should x-rays or examination of sputum be made standard in tuberculosis case-finding? Should chemotherapy or house spraying with insecticide be the method of choice in a given malaria situation? In such comparisons, the benefits are clearly measurable in common units, and the decision will relate to the output (benefit) of the proposed methods and their relative cost. A useful technique in such cases is that known as cost-benefit analysis.

Cost-benefit analysis was first applied to estimates of the utility of public works about the middle of the nineteenth century, and it is still quite popular in that field. More recently, it has been extended to other areas of economic activity, including the planning of health services at the project level. The distinguishing characteristic of cost-benefit analysis is not the comparison of costs and benefits at a given moment, but rather the present comparison of a stream of anticipated future benefits and costs. To take the most common example encountered in practice, when a water or sewer system is installed in a community it is anticipated that the short-run investment of capital will bring about long-run returns over succeeding years. Yet before one investment project is chosen above another, it is necessary to anticipate those returns and compute the present value of the expected future benefit to compare with the present cost of the proposed investment and the present value of future operating costs.

This is done by means of the compound interest formula, which permits economists to calculate the "discounted present value" of future benefits and costs at any given rate of interest. In the conventional business calculation, the future value of a sum of money P invested at interest rate r for a period of t years is $P(1 + r)^t$. In numerical terms, $100 invested at present at 6 percent interest compounded annually will be worth $(1.06)^{10}$ after ten years, or $179. If it is anticipated that $179 will result at 6 percent interest after ten years, then the present value of that future benefit is held to be $100. It is also clear from the formula that, in order to have $179 at a higher rate of interest (e.g., 10 percent) at the end of ten years, a smaller initial investment is required, whereas at a lower rate of interest a higher initial investment is required.

This means that the present value of future benefits, other things being equal, is inversely related to the rate of interest. Common sense bears this out, for when the rate of interest is low (i.e., when capital is cheap) an investment promising given benefits is more attractive than when the rate of interest is high (i.e., when it costs more to obtain the capital that promises the same benefits). In practice, the interest rate does act as a principal determining factor when the attractiveness is measured by the relation between present costs and future benefits. Just as an individual may hesitate to purchase a house when mortgage interest rates are high, so a community may hesitate to undertake the construction of a water system or a hospital or other major public works under similar circumstances.

The question of the choice of interest rate for cost-benefit calculations is of particular interest to economists. It has not been solved satisfactorily and is still a matter of debate. At any given time, several rates of interest may be quoted in capital markets: the rates of interest on local and national government bonds will seldom be the same; higher rates will be charged for consumer credit or high-risk loans than for industrial working capital. Exactly as in the case of goods and services, it is not certain to what degree the market price of money (the rate of interest) reflects a social valuation of the future return from present investment, and to what degree a given rate of interest mainly reflects businessmen's and bankers' short-term expectations of the relative profitability of different kinds of investment and lending.

In terms of the priority-setting formula $P = f(M, I, V, C)$, cost-benefit analysis can be viewed as the examination of the C and V terms (perhaps, ideally, of all four terms) over time, with emphasis on the calculation of a present value for future reduction in M (evidently dependent on V) that can be compared with the investment term C. As in the priority formula, the numerical results must be subject to the same cautious interpretation, and the same reservations must be made with respect to the adequacy of the statistical indicators to provide a precise reflection of social valuations.

Finally, it should be noted that some future benefits of health services cannot be given a present value, since they cannot be identified until they occur. The long-run benefits accruing from a healthier population (ranging from higher potential productiveness to intangibles such as a more satisfying life) are mainly a matter of conjecture at present, and the effect of inputs as different from one another as health education of the public and basic scientific research is also hard to put in numerical terms.

Cost-Effectiveness Analysis in Budgeting

While the principal use of cost-benefit analysis is in long-run investment planning, the related concept of cost-effectiveness is often used in planning current activities. The emphasis in both long-run and general health planning is on the yield from investment in health; in short-run operational planning, particularly at the level of the local project or service unit, the general priorities and program choices are taken as given, and the focus is on efficient fulfilling of planned tasks. Cost-effectiveness analysis is simply a way of making budget decisions in order to maximize delivery of service and to minimize cost by making the best choice among alternative ways of reaching planned targets.

The budget is an essential instrument at the project or operating level because it provides a two-way flow of information for planning purposes. The budget request or submission from the project or service unit to the next higher authority (be it a local governing body or the next unit in a bureaucratic chain of command) embodies the ideas of the operating unit as to how it conceives its tasks and how it plans to go about them. The budget submission may be technically justified in every detail, or experience with the reviewing authority may lead to deliberate overestimates (in the hope that anticipated cuts will leave adequate resources for operation) or underestimates (based on a realistic assessment of the limited resources likely to be provided). The process of budget review and approval involves evaluation; it also serves to communicate the constraints on funding and human resources at the next higher level and the priority decisions made at that level for the allocation of funds and manpower to operating units.

Simplistic as it may sound, experience in a number of countries has shown that it is possible to plan activities that are not realized for lack of budgetary provision; it is also possible to maintain activities that are not included in current plans or that are scheduled by the planners for de-emphasis or termination, simply because a concurrent change from previous budgetary allocations is not made by the financial authorities.

Aside from its use as an instrument of financial accountability and control, the budget ideally should be the monetary expression of the activities embodied in the health services plan. The difficulties in achieving this goal are administrative rather than economic in nature. For example, common sense indicates that the budget should refer to the same time period as the plan. In point of fact, however, budgets are usually established on a yearly basis, and seldom more than one or two years ahead, while plans may be drawn up to cover five or ten year periods. Clearly, a ten-year plan should involve at least a gross estimate of the ten-year operating and investment budget. Similarly, if the annual budget is the real operating instrument of the health service, then the plan of activities must also have a yearly component corresponding to the budget year.

Some conflict also arises between the budget as the first step in an accounting process whose basic goal is the control over disbursement of funds, and the budget viewed as the grant of money that enables a series of planned program activities to be undertaken. From the viewpoint of accounting control, the budget clearly has to be broken down into items that are classified in the same way as expenditures (wages and salaries, drugs, medical supplies, office supplies, and so forth), even though any one of these categories of expenditure may be shared among a number of different planned activities. The salary of the director of a health service, for example, is attributable in part to direction of each activity the service undertakes.

The conventional budget for control of disbursement is referred to as a "line item budget" because each line in the budget relates to an item of expenditure, while budgets in which the line items are regrouped so as to show expenditures for different planned activities are commonly referred to as "program budgets," "activity budgets," or "performance budgets" (when the emphasis is on evaluation). The latest fashion in budgets is the planning-programming-budgeting system (abbreviated to PPBS) which was made general at the federal level in the United States in 1965 after successful experience in programming military activities. The PPBS combines the setting of planned priorities with the budgeting of the activities designed to achieve the plan targets. The basic criterion for choice of operating programs is a cost-effectiveness comparison (again introducing the V and C elements of the priority-setting formula).

As early as 1967, some students of public health administration in the United States had expressed their worry over the applicability of PPBS to health services. The Canadian government PPB manual of 1969 was explicit in its recognition of the limitations of the method in planning research support in particular (13). Despite its limitations, however, the approach is becoming increasingly popular and widespread.

CONCLUSION

Although this presentation of the economic considerations in health planning has necessarily been brief, it has led us into virtually every facet of health services. The importance of economic factors has been underscored, yet we have been forced repeatedly to point out difficulties of quantification and measurement, particularly with reference to physician care. We must finally agree with Fuchs:

> The practice of medicine is still more an art than a science. The intimate nature of the relationship between patient and doctor, the vital character of the services rendered, and the heavy responsibilities assumed by medical personnel suggest the dangers inherent in reducing health care to matters of balance sheets, or supply and demand curves. Economics has something to contribute to health problems, but it should proceed as the servant of health, not its master (8, p. 95).

The basic function of economics is to point out how to economize—how to get the greatest output per unit of input. This essentially managerial function at the local project or operating level requires the modern tools of operations research. At higher levels, the process of economizing involves comparing returns from alternative projects within the health sector, and deciding the relative priorities of health and other activities. For the health planner, economics is primarily a supporting service, providing grounds for decision at each level and searching for data to point up the complex relationships and issues that sometimes arise. While it may be easier for most health planners to master the mathematics required for operations research than it is to convert operations researchers into health specialists, it is often helpful to consult specialists in both fields as part of the decision-making process.

REFERENCES

1. Samuelson, P. W. *Economics.* Eighth ed. New York: McGraw-Hill, 1970.
2. Abel-Smith, B. *Paying for Health Services.* Public Health Papers No. 17. Geneva: World Health Organization, 1963.
3. Leontief, W. W. *Input-Output Economics.* New York: Oxford University Press, 1966.
4. Navarro, V. "Planning Personal Health Services: A Markovian Model." *Medical Care* 7:242-249, 1969.
5. Piel, G. "Technological Change in the Medical Economy." In: *Planning for Health: Report of the 1967 National Health Forum.* pp. 188-197. New York: National Health Council, 1967.
6. Klarman, H. E. "Economic Factors in Hospital Planning in Urban Areas." *Public Health Reports* 82:721-728, 1967.
7. Correa, H. "Health Planning." *Kyklos* 20:909-923, 1967.
8. Fuchs, V. R. "The Contribution of Health Services to the American Economy." *The Milbank Memorial Fund Quarterly* 44:No. 4, Part 2, pp. 65-111, October, 1966.
9. Feldstein, P. J. and German, J. J. "Predicting Hospital Utilization: An Evaluation of Three Approaches." *Inquiry* 2:13-36, 1965.
10. Dublin, L. E. and Lotka, A. J. *The Money Value of a Man.* Revised ed. New York: The Ronald Press Co., 1946.
11. Rice, D. P. "Estimating the Cost of Illness." *American Journal of Public Health* 57:424-440, 1967.
12. Klarman, H. E. "Present Status of Cost-Benefit Analysis in the Health Field." *American Journal of Public Health* 57:1948-1953, 1967.
13. Government of Canada. *Planning, Programming, Budgeting Guide.* Revised ed. Ottawa: Queen's Printer for Canada, 1969.

ADDITIONAL READINGS

Primary

Abel-Smith, B. *An International Study of Health Expenditure and Its Relevance for Health Planning.* Public Health Paper No. 32. Geneva: World Health Organization, 1967.

Results of a questionnaire survey, mainly concerned with the amount of national income and government budgets going for health. Unfortunately, this work is becoming dated, but it has not been repeated.

Feldstein, M. S. *Economic Analysis for Health Services Efficiency: Econometric Studies of the British National Health Service.* Amsterdam: North-Holland Publishing Co., 1967.

Econometric analysis principally concerned with the determinants of hospital bed utilization under the National Health Service.

Hobson, W., editor. *The Theory and Practice of Public Health.* Third edition. London: Oxford University Press, 1969.

Useful general text. Chapter 33 by J. H. F. Brotherston and G. D. Forwell, "Planning of Health Services and the Health Team," is of particular interest, while Chapter 34 by A. P. Ruderman, "Economic Aspects of Health Planning," contains an earlier version of some of the ideas expressed in the present chapter.

Kindleberger, C. P. *Economic Development.* New York: McGraw-Hill, 1958.

Useful general textbook on economic development. Written when massive development aid was still in vogue, but surprisingly timely in 1971.

Klarman, H. E. *The Economics of Health.* New York: Columbia University Press, 1965.

Helpful review of the general literature prior to 1965.

Klarman, H. E. and Jaszi, H. H. "Empirical Studies in Health Economics." *Proceedings of the Second Conference on the Economics of Health.* Baltimore: Johns Hopkins Press, 1970.

First anthology of the "new wave" of quantitative analysis of health economic problems.

Mushkin, S. J. "Toward a Definition of Health Economics." *Public Health Reports* 73:785-793, 1958.

Classic pioneering discussion.

Mushkin, S. J. "Health as an Investment." *Journal of Political Economy* 70:129-157, 1962.

Typifies the Chicago "human capital" approach.

Prest, A. R. and Turvey, R. "Cost-Benefit Analysis: A Survey." *The Economic Journal* 75:683-735, 1965.

Exhaustive review of the field of cost-benefit analysis, including a substantial section on health.

Rice, D. P. and Cooper, B. S. "The Economic Value of Human Life." *American Journal of Public Health* 57:1954-1966, 1967.

Good illustration of current computations in a classic field.

Taylor, C. E. and Hall, M.-F. "Health, Population, and Economic Development." *Science* 157:651-657, 1967.

Review of available literature and conceptualization of the interactions of health, population, and economic development.

Secondary

Division of Public Health Methods. "Economic Benefits from Public Health Services: Objectives, Methods, and Examples of Measurement." U.S.P.H.S. Publication No. 1178. Washington, D.C.: Government Printing Office, 1964.

Economics of Health and Medical Care. Proceedings of the Conference on the

Economics of Health and Medical Care, 1962. Ann Arbor: University of Michigan, 1964.

Evans, R. G. "Behavioral Cost Functions for Hospitals." *Canadian Journal of Economics* 4:198-215, 1971.

Frederiksen, H. "Dynamic Equilibrium of Economic and Demographic Transition." *Economic Development and Cultural Change* 14: 316-322, 1966.

Goldman, T. A., editor. *Cost-Effectiveness Analysis.* Washington Operations Research Council. New York: Frederick A. Praeger, 1967.

Linnenberg, C. C. "Economics in Program Planning for Health." *Public Health Reports* 81:1085-1091, 1966.

Rohrlich, G. F., editor. *Social Economics for the 1970's: Programs for Social Security, Health, and Manpower.* New York: The Dunellen Co., 1970.

Ruderman, A. P. Review of: Oznobina, N. M., editor. "Ocherki po sovremmenoy i zarubsezhnoy ekonomike." Vol. 1. Moscow: State Plan Publishing House, 1960. In: *American Economic Review* 217-218, March, 1962.

Tucker, M. "Utilization and Price Analysis: Prospects for Avoiding Higher Program Costs in Health Care." *American Journal of Public Health* 59:1226-1242, 1969.

Vergin, R. C. and Rogers, J. D. "An Algorithm and Computational Procedure for Locating Economic Facilities." *Management Science* 12:B240-B254, February, 1967.

Weisbrod, B. A. *Economics of Public Health.* Philadelphia: University of Pennsylvania Press, 1961.

8

The Demographic Base for Health Planning

MARGARET BRIGHT

Demography is the study of the size, territorial distribution, and composition of population. It is also, concerned with the components of population change—fertility, mortality, and migration—and with the changing characteristics of the population.

This chapter first describes certain features of population change that provide the demographic context within which planning takes place. Second, in the hope that health planners will become more frequent and knowledgeable users of demographic data, attention is given to common sources of these data and to some of their limitations and inaccuracies. Finally, mention is made of some specific uses which can be made of demographic data in health planning.

GENERAL DEMOGRAPHIC CONSIDERATIONS

Patterns of Population Growth

In developing countries the present rate of population growth is without historical precedent. Annual growth rates are of the magnitude of 2 to 3.5 percent. These rates, if continued, would result in a doubling of present population within a mere 25 to 35 years. Large declines in mortality have caused the acceleration of population growth in the developing countries, and in many countries will still be a factor in increasing growth rates. Growth rates will continue to be high even when death rates have leveled off, because birth rates remain high and in most developing countries have been resistant to change.

Even in the few developing countries where birth rates have declined, the birth rates so far exceed the death rates that large population increases continue. A case in point is Taiwan. In this country a decline in the death rate has been underway for some time, and the expectation of life at birth is now 65-70 years and approaching that of the developed countries. On the other hand, the birth rate, although declining from 41 to 29 per 1,000 since 1959, is still sufficiently above the death rate to produce large annual population increases. Thus, between 1958 and 1968, Taiwan's estimated population increased from 10.2 to 13.5 million.

In the already developed countries, the present potential of population increase is much less than in the developing countries, although there is considerable variation among developed countries. In most European countries, the annual rate of growth in recent years has been below 1 percent and in some countries below 0.5 percent. Rates for the USSR and for developed countries outside Europe are higher: USSR (1.0 percent), United States (1.0 percent), Japan (1.1 percent), Canada (1.7 percent), New Zealand (1.7 percent), and Australia (1.9 percent).

All developed countries have low death rates which may continue to decline slowly but not in sufficient magnitude to affect population growth appreciably in the near future. Fertility levels will thus be the main determinant of population growth, and since childbearing is to an increasing extent subject to control in these countries, population growth may be expected to fluctuate from time to time in response to changing conditions.

It is necessary to recognize, then, that the ability to make accurate projections of the future population in any instance depends on the ability to assess correctly what the future fertility behavior of the population in question will be. This is difficult at best. Short-term projections are likely to be better predictors than long-term projections. Indeed, there is no past performance to demonstrate accuracy of population projections over a long-term period. The present conventional practice in population projection is to prepare different population projections, based on different assumptions about future fertility levels, and to revise the projections at regular intervals. In the United States, for example, the total population was estimated at 205 million at midyear 1970, and the latest population projections for 1980 vary from 222.5 million to 237.8 million, depending on what assumptions about future fertility are used (1).

The effects of net immigration or net emigration on national growth have not been emphasized here, since in recent years neither has much affected the rate of population growth in either developed or developing countries. If immigration is permitted, however, its importance in national growth will be in inverse relationship to natural increase, i.e., the same volume of immigration will contribute more to population growth when birth rates are lower than when they are higher. At the present time, birth rates in the United States are low, and about one-fifth of the annual population growth of the United States is attributable to net immigration.

Age Structure

Since health needs are to a large extent age-connected, the age structure of a population is one of the more important features of its population composition to be considered in health planning. In general, the age structures of developing and developed countries are distinctly different. Developing countries characteristically have greater proportions of young and smaller proportions of old than do developed countries. They also have higher dependency burdens, i.e., higher ratios of persons in dependent ages to those in the productive ages.

How do countries come to have the kind of age structures they have? A fact not generally known is that the age structure of a population—the proportion of old or young—depends mainly on the birth rate and not on the death rate (2, pp. 47-58). Developed countries have a higher proportion of their population in the older ages because their birth rates have declined from higher levels and not primarily because death rates have declined in the older ages. Persons in older age groups are the survivors of the birth cohorts produced when birth rates were higher, and populations become older as members of earlier and larger birth cohorts advance in age. On the other hand, developing countries have higher proportions in the younger ages because their birth rates have remained high. Also, contrary to common sense notions, mortality declines may even contribute to making a population younger. This is the case where reductions in infant and childhood mortality have occurred and increased the ranks of the young. Thus, countries which have maintained high birth rates and have at the same time had large reductions in mortality at the beginning of life have the youngest populations of all.

Birth rates and the age structure of a population are related, therefore. Where birth rates are high, the young tend to comprise a larger share of the population. In turn, a young population will produce more births, for more young women will enter and survive the childbearing period. A young population is, therefore, one with great potential for population increase.

Implications of Population Growth and Age Structure for Health Planning

Typically, the developing countries have demographic characteristics which, in addition to social and economic conditions, reduce their options in health planning. With present rates of population growth, most such countries are faced with the problem of providing services to populations which will be doubling within a period of 20 to 35 years. Will they find it possible to provide the same type and volume of health services to such extended numbers? Is it possible to expand present services under the pressure of increased numbers? Will it be necessary to institute further priorities in health planning with the result that some services will be emphasized and others not, some segments of the population provided for and others not? Children predominate in these countries, and should health services for children predominate at the expense of services aimed at improving the health status of those in the economically productive age groups? Are increases in mortality, rather than decreases in mortality, a distinct possibility in some countries (3)? Given the rate of population growth and the unfavorable structure (i.e., high dependency ratio), what priority should be given to health as opposed to other needs such as education, welfare, economic development programs, and other public needs?

Recently, many developing countries have established national family planning programs, usually in conjunction with health programs, in the hope of slowing birth rates and their population growth. Health planners in these countries should not, however, be overly optimistic about the consequences of these programs in easing the constraints on planning for health services in the several years ahead. With possibly a few exceptions, these programs have not yet had any effect on the birth rates and population growth. Even in Taiwan, where possibly the most successful family planning program has been undertaken, the potential for population increase has been shown to be very great. It has been calculated, for example, that even under drastic reductions in fertility—i.e., if fertility declined so that the two-child family (half its present size) became the average at once for all new families in the future—Taiwan's population would still continue to grow for another 60 years, at which time it would level off at 22 million, or about 60 percent above its present population level (4). Of course, no evidence indicates that any such substantial decline in fertility is in sight.

The case of India is a dramatic one, since present fertility levels are much higher than in Taiwan, and the national family planning program to date has not been successful in reducing the birth rate. In 1970, India's estimated population was around 555.2 million, and under present levels of fertility would grow to 899.6 million by 1985 and to 1.5 billion by the year 2000, intervals of a mere 15 and 30 years. Even if the two-child family became the average at once, the population would still grow to 724.8 million in 1985 and 888.2 million by the year 2000 (5). Such an assumption for India is, of course, ridiculous for prediction purposes, but the figures do illustrate that even under the most successful reduction in fertility, India's population growth in the future would still be enormous. Because of her age structure, India's potential for population growth is still great, no matter what reduction in fertility is achieved.

Thus, while health planners in countries with high fertility levels and age structures conducive to rapid population growth should be aware that family planning programs will not ease the burdens in health planning for many years into the future, they will be ill-advised to ignore the importance of attempting to reduce fertility. The longer the interval before the reduction in fertility begins, the more distant the time when the rate of population growth begins to level off. Farsighted health planning will call for reasonable allocation of resources between the prevention of births and the nurturing and saving of lives.

Developed countries, on the other hand, have social and economic as well as demographic characteristics which provide far greater options in health planning than exist in the developing countries. Their greater resources, theoretically at least, may be allocated to providing a greater range of health services to all segments of the population. Thus, as the proportion of older persons has increased, more resources have gone to providing health services for those with chronic diseases, a luxury which few of the developing countries have yet been able to afford. Services for the chronically ill are enormously costly, however, and medical advances and institutional innovations for sustaining the well-being and life of the chronically ill are only in process of development and less often yield the dramatic results which similar resources applied to the health needs of younger populations do. Thus, partly at least as a consequence of the age structure of their population and the generally larger proportions of old people, developed countries face the problem of determining how resources for health shall be allocated among different age segments of the population.

A final point is that health planners will need to take into account the consequences of fluctuations in the birth rate in order to plan for how many people there will be in the future and how many in particular age groups. Already, ample evidence from among the developed countries shows that even where contraceptive practice is widely diffused throughout the population, birth rates on occasion fluctuate upward and downward. Marriage and child-spacing patterns, as well as changes in family size preference, vary in response to a variety of social and economic conditions and may cause birth rates to fluctuate within rather broad limits. Most developed countries experienced "baby booms" after World War II; in some countries, notably the United States, Canada, Australia, and New Zealand, rises in the birth rate were sustained for a long enough time to affect greatly the size of the total population, their age structure, and the potential for future growth.

There is, therefore, no way of knowing what the unborn portion of the population at some future date will be. For the immediate future, the number of women in the childbearing ages can be estimated, but the number of children to whom they will give birth cannot. Probably no one anticipated the fluctuation in the number of live births that took place in the United States after World War II. Just prior to the war (1940), the number was 2.3 million. It rose to 3.7 million in 1947, to a maximum of 4.3 million in 1957, and declined again to 3.5 million by 1968. There is now much uncertainty about the future annual number of births. Large increases in the number of persons in the childbearing ages (survivors of the "baby boom" years) suggest increases in the number of births for future years. The number of births has been increasing since 1968, but the future number is problematic. It depends upon marriage and childbearing patterns of those now entering their reproductive years.

Fluctuations in the size of birth cohorts create problems for planning which are different from those which derive from consistent increases or declines in the number of births. Under consistent declines, demands for particular services will be less with each successive cohort; under consistent increases, services will be in greater demand. When, however, the size of birth cohorts fluctuates greatly, resources and personnel needed for services may be alternately inadequate and overabundant. Rises in the number of births, for example, call for additional maternal and child health services. By the time they have been provided for, and often at considerable investment in buildings, equipment, and the training of personnel, the need may have diminished. Meanwhile, services needed for other age segments, such as school health services, may have been curtailed, but are now in short supply as the births of earlier periods swell the ranks of the school age population.

Theoretically at least, the greatest impact of fluctuations in the size of cohorts may be felt as survivors move into older age groups. Here the prevalence of chronic diseases is high, the cost of providing services great, and the organization of services most complex. Thus, in the United States, consequences of fluctuations in births may be more acute in the next century than in the present one.

Geographic Distribution of the Population

In the developing countries, high proportions of the population generally live in rural areas deficient in modern medical and sanitary facilities. The physical remoteness of the rural population poses serious problems for extending even minimum health services and facilities. Many health planners question the efficiency of using scarce personnel and resources for the small achievements which efforts in such cases would bring, yet there will be pressures to equalize the geographic availability of health services to all segments of the population.

The rapid growth of population in cities of the developing countries undoubtedly contributes to the neglect and delay in providing health services in rural areas. In many of the developing countries, cities are growing at a much more rapid rate than the rural hinterland. In several Latin American countries, for example, recent population growth has been twice as great in cities as in rural areas, and the most rapid growth has been in the largest cities. Latin American countries tend to have larger proportions of their population in cities than do those in Africa and Asia, and the pace at which urbanization has occurred exceeds that of most developed countries when they were urbanizing. The pace of urbanization most likely will also accelerate considerably in Asia and Africa.

The developed countries are more urbanized than the developing ones, but the former are not without problems in planning for an equitable distribution of health services to all localities. In the United States, for example, the provision of health services is probably most acute for that one-third of the population widely dispersed throughout the nonmetropolitan areas of the country. The majority of nonmetropolitan areas are losing population or have little potential for maintenance of their present levels of population, and many have little opportunity for attracting health and medical services for a population that is predominantly young and/or old. Within the metropolitan areas, the problem of provision of services is being altered by the changing distribution of the population between the central cities and suburbs. Suburbs around central cities now contain more than one-half of the population of the SMSA's (Standard Metropolitan Statistical Areas), and 16.3 of the 17.2 million increase between 1960 and 1969 was in the suburbs. Thus, demands to provide increased services for the suburban populations are heavy, but demands are also heavy for the maintenance of services within central cities to increasing numbers with special health problems: children, the aged, nonwhites, and the poor.

In the past, public health professionals have traditionally limited their purview of demography to changes in mortality. Analysis of mortality changes represented one means of assessing their achievements. Increasingly, however, health planners must take account of other demographic changes as well. They may from time to time benefit by the assistance of demographers. However, the relevance of population changes for health planning will probably be best attended to if health planners themselves make some attempt to understand in a general way how populations change. The foregoing discussion was an attempt to assist in this direction.

SOURCES OF DEMOGRAPHIC DATA

Demographic data derive from several sources. They are collected both by a canvass of the population and from record systems (6).

The Population Canvass

Two types of population canvass have evolved for obtaining information on the size and characteristics of the population: the population census and the sample survey.

The *population census* is the older method. Although early censuses were taken in China and the Roman Empire, in various European cities and states in the sixteenth and seventeenth centuries, in certain of the French and British colonies in colonial America, and in French Canada, the first continuous series of reliable reports on population was that of Sweden. Here, however, the system of house-to-house enumeration was soon replaced by a continuous accounting system. Periodic censuses began in the United States in 1790 and in England and Wales in 1801. Between 1855 and 1865, complete census enumerations were carried out in 24 countries and the number rose to 49 in the years 1925-34. The increase in the number of sovereign nations in the period following World War II, together with the encouragement and technical assistance provided by the United Nations, has greatly stimulated census-taking. By 1964, over 200 countries, sovereign and nonsovereign, had undertaken population censuses, some for the first or second time only.

The *sample survey* is a more recent innovation, following the development of sampling theory. The sample survey is presently the main source of demographic data in some of the newly-formed African nations, where scarcity of resources and personnel and other factors present awesome obstacles to a complete population canvass and where vital registration systems are virtually nonexistent.

Sampling in conjunction with the decennial census was first employed in the United States in 1940 and has since been greatly extended. In 1960 and 1970, a total count of the population was made on only five items (age, sex, race, relationship to head of household, and marital status). The remaining data were obtained on a sampling basis.

Governments sometimes conduct periodic sample surveys to obtain demographic data in addition to those data obtained from their regular population censuses and registration systems. Cases in point are the National Sample Survey in India and the Current Population Survey in the United States. Special sample surveys restricted to certain population groups are also undertaken by governmental and other agencies. For example, much of what is known about the changes and variations in the fertility of American women since World War II has been derived from information obtained in sample surveys. The advantages of the sample survey are timeliness, economy, and quality. It cannot, however, replace the census in supplying demographic data for small areas.

Population censuses in different countries vary in the information collected and the tabulations published, although the United Nations has encouraged the collection of certain types of data and certain basic tabulations. The United Nations itself publishes in the *Demographic Yearbook* the distributions of population by age and sex available from population censuses of various countries. Recently, where sample surveys have been used in lieu of the total population canvass, the United Nations has published the distribution of population by age and sex estimated from these surveys.

The best source of the basic demographic data available from population censuses is the subject-matter index which appears at the end of *Demographic Yearbook,* published annually. Here are given the types of data tabulations published, the year in which the data appeared in the *Yearbook,* and the time coverage on the item or tabulation under consideration.

Also, introductory remarks at the beginning of each *Demographic Yearbook* are extremely useful in providing an understanding of definitions used in census taking. Each table showing either frequencies or rates has footnotes which describe the departure from usual procedures in the case of particular countries.

For these reasons, it is recommended that the *Yearbook* be consulted in advance of the published census reports of individual countries.

Record Systems

Three major types of record systems providing demographic data are the vital registration system, the population register, and administrative records of government agencies.

Vital registration systems have been established in many countries for the purpose of the legal recording of births, deaths, marriages, and divorces. The first such national system was begun in England and Wales in 1837; that of the United States was among the last of the highly developed countries. In the United States, the first mortality statistics from registration data (including only 40 percent of the United States population) were published in 1899 and the first birth statistics (including 90 percent of the population) were published in 1915. Not until 1933 was the last state admitted to the registration system for births and deaths, and several states still are not included in the registration system for marriages and divorces. Evolving a vital registration system has been an enormous task in the United States, not only because of the size of the country, but also because of the federal system.

Probably at least one-half of the world's population still lives in areas where the registration of births and deaths does not occur or is so incomplete that reliable crude birth rates and death rates cannot be calculated. Records of vital events are needed for many purposes, personal and administrative as well as for demographic analyses. But the establishment of complete registration of vital statistics requires an extensive administrative apparatus and a thorough re-education of the public.

The United Nations and its specialized agencies as well as the international organizations which preceded them have all devoted much effort to the improvement of vital statistics. They have specified definitions to distinguish all vital events. They have specified types of information which should appear on certificates. They have given technical assistance to the establishment and improvement of registration systems in various countries. Even so, availability of reliable statistics on vital events improves slowly.

In some countries, registration is compulsory only for births and deaths; in others for only part of the population (e.g., "European nonindigenous" population). In other countries no national provision exists for compulsory registration, and municipal or state ordinances do not cover all geographic areas. Still other countries have registration areas which comprise only part of the country, the remainder being excluded because of inaccessibility or other conditions. Vital statistics coverage is particularly incomplete for Africa, having been confined largely to European populations and including only partial statistics or estimates for the indigenous segments. Similarly, coverage is uneven and statistics incomplete and unreliable for much of Asia and parts of Latin America.

The best published single source of data on vital statistics for countries as a whole is the *Demographic Yearbook*. On the basis of information obtained from various sources, the United Nations classifies the reliability of vital statistics data from various countries into three categories: (C) those stated to be relatively "complete," i.e., representing at least 90 percent coverage of the events occurring each year; (U) those stated to be "unreliable," i.e., less than 90 percent coverage; and (. . .) those concerning which no specific information is available.

As with population census data, it is well to consult the tables in the *Demographic Yearbook* before referring to the official reports of individual countries to get some notion of the reliability of the data for the country in question. The tables in the *Yearbook* also provide numerous footnotes which are useful for evaluating definitions used for determining population coverage, and for ascertaining whether tabulation is by date of occurrence or of registration. Such detail may not be provided in official reports of governments, yet it is necessary for evaluating the usefulness of the vital statistics and for determining comparability among countries.

The *Yearbook* has not yet published mortality statistics for subdivisions within countries, but on occasion has provided birth statistics according to whether mothers were residents of urban or rural areas. When vital statistics data for local areas are needed, the *Yearbook* may provide information about coverage and reliability which will determine whether such data exist for different localities and if they are worth seeking out in other sources.

In Taiwan and a number of European countries, a continuous *population register* is maintained to serve many legal and administrative functions. Such registers are important sources of demographic information, possibly providing data equivalent to those obtained from population censuses and a registration of vital events. One advantage of the population register is that in the calculation of vital rates (e.g., birth and death rates), the data for both the numerator (i.e., births, deaths) and the denominator (population) are from the same source. In most countries, the two types of data are compiled under different systems of collection. Another advantage of the registration system is that it may be used as a source of information on internal migration. One problem of population estimation for intercensal years in local areas is that the extent of in-migration and out-migration is unknown and must be estimated with data other than that on migration.

The problems of maintaining population registers is in many respects not unlike that of maintaining vital registration systems. Procedures must be defined and followed on a continuous basis, government functionaries and the public must be educated, and data must be processed at various levels of government. Continuing studies are needed to evaluate the accuracy of the demographic data.

Various *administrative record systems* from both governmental and private agencies also serve as sources of demographic data. In the United States, the Bureau of Immigration and Naturalization is the only source of data on the number of immigrants and emigrants. The Department of Defense is the source of data on the number of persons in the armed forces both in the United States and overseas. Both agencies regularly make these data available to the Bureau of the Census for the preparation of population estimates in intercensal years. Data on school enrollment are sometimes used for estimating migration in making intercensal population estimates in local areas.

Another of the more comprehensive governmental record systems is that dealing with individuals covered by various social security programs, of which those under Medicare and Medicaid are recent additions in the United States. Data from such sources are in some instances useful when the interest is in special populations.

ERRORS IN DEMOGRAPHIC DATA

This section is intended to make health planners aware of the more common types of deficiencies and limitations of these data. Here we emphasize the limitations of data found in a wide range of circumstances.

Type of Errors

The simplest and sometimes hardest errors to detect are those of *omission or inflation of numbers.* Omissions (usually more frequent than inflations) are more common in some biological and social subgroups than in others. Babies and young children are frequently underreported in censuses and surveys and sometimes those of one sex, usually females, more than the other. In the United States, nonwhites (especially young adult males) are more frequently underreported than whites; in certain countries, the indigenous populations are more often underreported than other sections of the population.

A second type of error is *placing people in the wrong subgroups.* These errors can occur during the collection of data or at a later stage in the data processing. A common type of such error is age inaccuracy. In some cases, people simply do not know their age and no improvement in the system of data collection will yield accurate age information. Often, however, errors of this type are systematic rather than random ones. For example, people tend to show "digit-preference" in reporting age, i.e., ages ending in zero or five.

A third type of error commonly encountered in census enumerations are those which result from *biased measurements of time.* A substantial body of evidence indicates that the longer the interval of time between the event and the time of the census, the more likely the event will be forgotten and not reported. For example, older women are more likely to underreport the number of children they have ever borne, especially if the children died in early childhood. Also, this error is greater among women who have had a large number of children, indicating that both memory and mental arithmetic ability may be factors.

The above types of errors occur also in the data on vital events obtained from registration systems. As indicated earlier, the registration system may not cover all areas of the country and all segments of the population within it. Omission will probably be less frequent when the birth or death occurs in a hospital than when it does not. Completeness may vary with the event, i.e., birth registration may be more accurate than death registration, even when both sets of data are collected under the same system. Any information about personal characteristics which appears on the certificate may be incorrect—age, sex, occupation, marital status, nationality or ethnic background, and so forth.

Vital events, also, seem susceptible to certain types of errors in classification. Live births may be incorrectly registered as fetal deaths, or as infant deaths. Births may be classified incorrectly according to parity. Vital events may also be registered at the wrong place or time. They may be registered at the place of occurrence rather than at the place of residence. Many events are recorded as taking place at the time they are recorded rather than at the time they occurred.

Cause of death statistics, which are of great importance from the public health point of view, are unfortunately among the poorest data supplied by the vital statistics system. The validity of cause of death is dependent upon the quality of medical diagnoses. The percentage of deaths medically certified varies greatly among countries; moreover, even when medically certified, the knowledge upon which the medical certification is based varies. Even though medical certification may yield fairly reliable statistics for the major broad groups of causes of death, improvement is still needed both in specificity and in accuracy.

The *Demographic Yearbook* publishes the number of deaths by cause and cause-specific death rates for countries in each of its issues. It also indicates the percentage of deaths which are medically certified. The cause of death tabulation is according to the "Classification of the Abbreviated List of 50 Causes for Tabulation of Mortality of the International Statistical Classification of Diseases, Injuries, and Causes of Death." Cause-specific rates are not computed when at least 25 percent of the reported deaths are reported as due to senility, ill-defined and unknown causes (B-45). A cursory glance at the size of this group serves as a rule of thumb barometer for a first evaluation of the quality of cause of death statistics.

Assessment of Accuracy in Demographic Data

A number of rule of thumb procedures may be applied initially in making assessments about the accuracy of demographic data. First, a general knowledge of the circumstances of collection and processing is always valuable. All too often consumers of published demographic data do not bother to read the explanations and footnotes which accompany published demographic data. Previously we have referred to the utility of the United Nations *Demographic Yearbook* in supplying definitions of terms, footnotes explaining the data used, and an evaluation of the accuracy of the data published. Second, bizarre and unusual findings—data which depart from expectation—should be viewed with skepticism and carefully checked. Third, if more than one source exists for the same or similar data, consistency checks between series of data may be undertaken. Fourth, the source of error is sometimes easier to locate in detailed tabulations. For example, age reporting may be more deficient in some age groups than others.

Comparative checks used in assessing the quality of demographic data may be external or internal checks. *External checks* are those in which records obtained from separate collection systems (or from different operations of the same system) are compared with one another. *Internal checks* refer to the comparison of various data obtained in one collection process.

The simplest type of *external check* is the comparison of data from two different collection systems, e.g., data from a census and a registration system. A case in point would be the comparison of the number of children enumerated in a census as 0 to 9 years, compared with the number of births recorded in the vital statistics in the 10 years prior to the census with allowance for attrition by mortality in the interval. Any great discrepancy would indicate further assessment before either set of data was used.

One method now widely used for estimating errors in the enumeration of a population, or segments of it, is the "survival method" or the "reverse survival method." For example, the size of the same age cohort is compared at two successive census dates (i.e., those 5 to 9 years in 1960 and those 15 to 19 in 1970), with account taken of the attrition from mortality which would occur in the interval between censuses. Large discrepancies indicate differences between the two censuses in the accuracy of enumeration of persons in specific age groups.

Record linkage studies provide external checks for assessing the accuracy of certain types of data. Examples include age and diagnoses entered on hospital records compared to those entered on death certificates. These procedures are time-consuming but may in certain instances justify the effort. For example, preference for coding of the cause of death on the death certificate may be allotted to the cause which precipitates the death. Other diseases present in the individual at the time of death may escape tabulation. These, however, may be of special concern for those interested in the prevalence of certain diseases or for those interested in certain health programs.

Internal checks of the data have been used more commonly in evaluating demographic data because the discrepancies in a set of data often become apparent to the consumer in the course of his use of it and because they require recourse only to data easily and already available. Such comparisons will not provide clues as to whether a population is undercounted or overcounted. They do, however, allow for more accurate estimation of distributions and rates. For example, one may question why the number of infants under one year is less than the number between one year and two years, if there appears to be no reason to expect that infant mortality has increased or birth rates have declined.

In many cases, internal checks are based upon comparisons with the accumulated experience from many populations. For example, we know that the sex ratio (males per 100 females) at birth varies within a very narrow range in those countries with reliable birth registration data. If in a birth series which we examine the sex ratio is exceptionally high, we might suspect that female births are underreported.

SPECIFIC DEMOGRAPHIC DATA NEEDED FOR HEALTH PLANNING

A serious gap exists between the quantitative information about populations necessary for all kinds of social and economic planning and the amount and quality of data actually available. Several reports have now been prepared by the United Nations outlining the types of demographic data needed for different types of planning (7, 8).

Studies of Health Levels

Health planning requires indicators for evaluating health conditions among different segments of the population. Various measures of mortality have commonly been used for this purpose. The demographic data required for the simplest of these measures are as shown below.

Measure	*Demographic Data Required*
1. Crude *death* rate	Total deaths in year; total population at midyear
2. Age-specific *death* rate	Deaths tabulated by age; population tabulated by age
3. Age-sex specific *death* rate	Deaths tabulated by age and sex; population tabulated by age and sex
4. Age-sex-cause specific *death* rate	Deaths tabulated by age, sex, cause; population tabulated by age and sex
5. Infant mortality rate	Deaths under one year of age; live births during year

As indicated above, reliable data for even these simple measures will not always be available for many national populations. They will, of course, be even more deficient if the interest is in rates for particular areas of a country or for different subgroups of the population. Where population data are available for denominators, death registration data may be missing or of poor quality for numerators. Or, as in even a country such as the United States, the death data may be available on an annual basis for different jurisdictions (e.g., countries, cities), but during the intercensal years the population data will either be unavailable or of doubtful quality owing to poor methods of population estimation. The methodology for population estimation for local areas is as yet poorly developed even in the developed countries.

It would be optimistic to assume that data collected from routine procedures, such as a population census or a vital registration system, will ever exist in the detail needed by health planners. Such data are costly to collect, and innovations in data collection systems tend to be infrequent. Health planners will need to recognize that, even in the most developed countries, either they make use of the limited data available, or they be prepared for costly expenditures for special surveys to obtain the data needed.

Other indicators of the health conditions in the population are morbidity and disability prevalence rates. Data on morbidity and disability obtained by sample survey can be used in conjunction with census data to determine morbidity and disability rates in different segments of the population. Such data are available in the United States National Health Survey and sometimes from studies done in local areas. Wherever possible, local area surveys should be taken around the time of the population census, for at that time the population "at risk" is most accurately known.

Studies of the Availability of Health Services

In planning health services, the extent of match between services and population requires information about the geographic distribution of both. Gross measures for national populations, e.g., number of hospital beds or number of physicians per 1,000 population, have limited use, for they conceal differences in distribution of both services and population. Such measures are needed for smaller geographic areas. If information about services (numerator data) can be coded to the same geographic base as population (denominator data), such measures can be obtained for geographic units which make sense for health planning purposes. Such procedures depend heavily upon the employment of modern techniques of data processing. Eventually, when information in one data system (e.g., birth records) are linked to that of another (e.g., infant mortality records) through standardized geographic coding, it will be possible to identify areas where particular types of health programs (e.g., pre- and postnatal clinics) need to be concentrated.

Studies of Projected Needs for Health Services and Facilities

Estimates of the future population are crucial for projecting the need for future services and facilities. Historically, demographers have shown little daring with respect to the preparation of population projections for local areas. Recently, however, the United States Bureau of the Census has developed a method for use in local area population projection (9, 10) and a handbook on the subject is in preparation. In addition, the need for such projections and certain underlying principles to be considered in undertaking them has been outlined in a report of the United Nations (8). Several papers prepared for the World Population Conference in Belgrade in 1965 also considered the problem of projections for smaller areas than an entire country (11, pp. 6-9, 61-65, 91-96).

The United Nations has recommended separate projections for the urban and rural population sectors, since this distinction is useful in many types of planning. Also, separate projections should be made for the principal cities of a country and for certain administrative or economic regions involved in national development plans. The United Nations has recommended that projections of the population be prepared for not more than 20 to 25 years into the future. Alternative sets of projections should be prepared to include not only what appears to be most likely in terms of past experience but also plausible deviations from the past.

The "component method," or variations of it (10), is usually suggested as the method most suitable for making local area projections. At the base year, a distribution of the population by sex and by age (single years preferably; quinquennial age groups alternatively) is required. The number of males and females in each age group at the base date is taken as a basis for estimating the number of survivors in successively higher age groups at successive future dates. The size of each future generation of births is estimated by applying projected fertility rates to the number of women in the childbearing age groups. Estimated net additions or subtractions through migration should also be taken into account. Thus, the preparation of the projections requires separate projections of mortality, fertility, and net-migration.

REFERENCES

1. Bureau of the Census. "Projections of the Population of the United States, by Age and Sex (Interim Revisions), 1970 to 2020." *Current Population Reports.* Series P-25, No. 448. Washington, D.C.: Government Printing Office, 1970.
2. Freedman, R., editor. *Population: The Vital Revolution.* Garden City: Doubleday & Co., 1964.
3. Davis, D. "The Climax of Population Growth: Past and Future Perspective." *California Medicine* 133:33-39, 1970.

4. Avery, R. "Taiwan: Implications of Fertility at Replacement Levels." *Studies in Family Planning.* The Population Council, No. 59: 1-4, November, 1970.
5. Population Reference Bureau, Inc. "India: Ready or Not, Here They Come." *Population Bulletin* 26:5, 1970.
6. Hauser, P. M. and Duncan, O. D. *The Study of Population.* Chicago: University of Chicago Press, 1959.
7. United Nations. *National Programmes of Analysis of Population Census Data as an Aid to Planning and Policy-Making.* ST/SOA/Series A/36. New York: United Nations, 1964.
8. United Nations. *General Principles for National Programmes of Population Projects as Aids to Development Planning.* ST/SOA/Series A/38. New York: United Nations, 1965.
9. Bureau of the Census. "Methods of Population Estimation: Part I. Illustrative Procedure of the Census Bureau's Component Method II." *Current Population Reports.* Series P-25, No. 339. Washington, D.C.: Government Printing Office, 1966.
10. Bureau of the Census. "Illustrative Projections of the Population of States." *Current Population Reports.* Series P-25, No. 326. Washington, D.C.: Government Printing Office, 1966.
11. United Nations. *Proceedings of the World Population Conference, Belgrade, 30 August to 10 September 1965.* Vol. III, E/CONF. 41/4. New York: United Nations, 1967.

ADDITIONAL READINGS*

Primary

Barclay, George W. *Techniques of Population Analysis.* New York: John Wiley and Sons, 1958.
  A clear, systematic exposition of basic demographic procedures: computation of rates and ratios, standardization, life table construction, estimation, forecasting, etc. Many of the examples are drawn from the developing world. Although one of the earlier works, this is still a good basic reference.
Berry, Brian J. L. and Horton, Frank E. *Geographic Perspectives on Urban Systems.* Englewood Cliffs, New Jersey: Prentice-Hall, Inc., 1970.
  A comprehensive presentation of current theory and method in the study of population distribution and human settlement patterns. Integrating a wide selection of readings and text, the authors focus upon those worldwide processes bringing about a spatial redistribution of population into organized urban systems. The theory and some examples are drawn from both the developed and developing world; the discussion of urban structure relates primarily to the United States.
Bogue, Donald A. *Principles of Demography.* New York: John Wiley and Sons, 1969.

* Prepared by Jeanne S. Newman, Ph.D.

Both a comprehensive text and a reference work, covering the entire field of population study. The text is clear and readable, emphasizing research findings, principles, and implications, rather than techniques of analysis; readers wishing to develop operational skills should also obtain one of the manuals of demographic procedure listed in this bibliography. The many tables represent an inventory of basic worldwide data as of about 1965.

Bureau of the Census. *The Methods and Materials of Demography* (2 vols.), by Henry S. Shryock and Jacob S. Siegel. Washington, D.C.: Government Printing Office, 1971.

A systematic presentation of the methods currently used by technicians and research workers in demographic analysis. Data availability and analytical methods for statistically underdeveloped areas are emphasized. Materials of the United States are also covered in detail.

United Nations Department of Economic and Social Affairs. *The Concept of a Stable Population: Application to the Study of Populations of Countries with Incomplete Demographic Statistics.* Population Studies, No. 30, Series A. New York: United Nations, 1968.

Demographers rely heavily upon Lotke's stable population model for estimating and forecasting. Under conditions of relatively constant or slowly falling fertility the model may be used to estimate certain population parameters even when data are incomplete. The model is discussed and its application illustrated in this work.

United Nations Population Branch. *Manuals on Methods of Estimating Population.* New York: United Nations, 1952-

Manual I. Methods of Estimating Total Population for Current Dates. Population Studies, No. 1, Series A, 1952.

Manual II. Methods of Appraisal of Quality of Basic Data for Population Estimates. Population Studies, No. 23, Series A, 1956.

Manual III. Methods for Population Projection by Sex and Age. Population Studies, No. 25, Series A, 1956.

Manual IV. Methods of Estimating Basic Demographic Measures for Incomplete Data. Population Studies, No. 42, Series A, 1967.

Manual V. Methods of Analyzing Census Data on Economic Activities of the Population. Population Studies, No. 43, Series A, 1969.

Manual VI. Methods of Measuring Internal Migration. Population Studies, No. 47, Series A, 1970.

The above series of demographic manuals constitutes a useful guide to demographic procedures, and is an important reference for those who wish to develop operational skills in demographic analysis.

Model life tables, based on the concept of age patterns of mortality, have become indispensable tools in demographic analysis, particularly in those cases where data are incomplete or unreliable. Three systems are currently in use. The earliest and probably still the most widely used is that developed by the United Nations, although many demographers have adopted the system of Coale and Demeny. The Brass system has not yet been as widely used as either of the other two, but forms the basis of an estimating model in use at the London School of Economics. Many countries, of course, also publish national life tables.

Carrier, Norman and Hobcraft, John. *Demographic Estimation for Developing Societies.* London: The Population Investigating Committee, London School of Economics, 1971.

Coale, Ansley J. and Demeny, Paul. *Regional Model Life Tables and Stable Populations.* Princeton: Princeton University Press, 1966.

United Nations Population Branch. *Age and Sex Patterns of Mortality. Model Life Tables for Underdeveloped Countries.* Population Studies, No. 22, Series A. New York: United Nations, 1955.

U.S. National Center for Health Statistics. *Vital Statistics of the United States 1967.* Volume 2. *Mortality.* Part A, Section 5, Life Tables. Washington, D.C.: Government Printing Office, 1969.

Secondary

Demographic Materials and Methods

Bogue, Donald J., editor. *Rapid Feedback for Family Planning Improvement. Family Planning Research and Evaluation Manuals.* (In series) No. 1- . Chicago: University of Chicago, Community and Family Study Center, 1971- .

Bureau of the Census. *Census of Population and Housing, 1970.* (In series) Washington, D.C.: Government Printing Office, 1970- .

Bureau of the Census. *Census Use Study.* (In series) Report No. 1- . Washington, D.C.: Government Printing Office, 1970- .

Bureau of the Census. *Current Population Reports.*
Series P-20 Population Characteristics
Series P-23 Special Studies (formerly Technical Studies)
Series P-25 Population Estimates and Projections
Series P-26 Federal-State Cooperative Program for Population Estimates
Series P-27 Farm Population
Series P-28 Special Censuses
Series P-60 Consumer Income
Series P-65 Consumer Buying Indicators
Washington, D.C.: Government Printing Office.

Bureau of the Census. *International Population Statistics Reports.* Series P-96 Demographic Reports for Foreign Countries (Panama, Chile, Tunisia, Peru).

Morrison, P. A. *Demographic Information for Cities: A Manual for Estimating and Projecting Local Population Characteristics.* Santa Monica: Rand Corporation, June 1971.

Reinke, William A., Taylor, Carl E., and Immerwahr, George E. "Nomograms for Simplified Demographic Calculations." *Public Health Reports* 84:431- 444, 1969.

United Nations. *Demographic Yearbook.* New York: United Nations.

Population Trends and Components of Change

Arriaga, Eduardo E. *Mortality Decline and Its Demographic Effects in Latin America.* Monograph Series, 6. Berkeley: University of California, Institute of International Studies, 1970.

Bourgeois-Pichat, Jean and Taleb, Si-Ahmed. "Un taux d'accroissement nul pour les paysen voie de developpement en l'an 2000. Reve ou réalite?" *Population* (Paris) 25:957-973, September-October, 1970.

Frejka, Tomas. "Reflections on the Demographic Conditions Needed to Establish a U.S. Stationary Population Growth." *Population Studies* 22:379-397, 1968.

Friedman, John. "The Strategy of Deliberate Urbanization." *Journal of the American Institute of Planners* 34:364-373, 1968.

Johnson, E. A. J. *The Organization of Space in Developing Countries.* Cambridge, Massachusetts: Harvard University Press, 1970.

Preston, Samuel H. "Empirical Analysis of the Contribution of Age Composition to Population Growth." *Demography* 7:417-432, 1970.

Rodwin, Lloyd. *Nations and Cities. A Comparison of Strategies for Urban Growth.* Boston: Houghton Mifflin Co., 1970.

Simmons, James W. "Changing Residence in the City: A Review of Intraurban Mobility." *Geographical Review* 58:622-651, 1968.

United Nations Department of Economic and Social Affairs. *The Aging of Populations and Its Economic and Social Implications.* Population Studies, No. 26, Series A. New York: United Nations, 1956.

United Nations Department of Economic and Social Affairs. *Demographic Aspects of Manpower. Report I. Sex and Age Patterns of Participation in Economic Activity.* Population Studies, No. 33, Series A. New York: United Nations, 1961.

United Nations Department of Economic and Social Affairs. *Planning of Metropolitan Areas and New Towns.* New York: United Nations, 1967.

United Nations Department of Economic and Social Affairs. "Urbanization: Development Policies and Planning." *International Social Development Review.* No. 1. New York: United Nations, 1968.

United Nations Department of Economic and Social Affairs. *Growth of the World's Urban and Rural Population, 1920-2000.* Population Studies, No. 44, Series A. New York: United Nations, 1969.

9

Assessment of Personal Health Problems: An Epidemiologic Approach

M. ALFRED HAYNES

SCOPE AND PURPOSE OF ASSESSMENT

Assessment of personal and environmental health problems is one of the initial steps in health planning. This chapter deals only with personal health problems. These include the disease problems of illness, impairment, and death; problems related to the delivery of health care such as availability, accessibility, and acceptability of services; and problems of effectiveness and efficiency. One is concerned with identifying the *nature* of the problems, their *magnitude, severity,* and *distribution,* and *trends.* In attempting to assess problems, health planners will ask several fundamental questions: What are the real problems? How frequently do they occur? How serious are they? How are the problems distributed? Are they increasing or decreasing?

Assessment of health problems is not an exact science. What the health expert considers a problem may not be perceived as such by the layman, and vice versa. Planning, therefore, often requires compromise between conflicting points of view. The greater the congruence between the assessment of the expert and that of the community, the greater the chance of implementing an effective program.

Assessment implies comparison. Unfortunately, no well-defined absolute standards exist for either health or disease. In actual practice, one makes comparisons with some reference population. One may compare the infant mortality rate of the nonwhite population with that of the white population of the United States. A rate in the nonwhite population twice that of the white may suggest a problem in infant care. Trends in both populations may be considered and one will note that for many years the rate declined faster in the white population. The specific nature of the problem is further identified to be primarily the diseases of the respiratory and digestive systems, and some of these conditions may be more severe than others in that they constitute a greater threat to life. Other comparisons are frequently made on the basis of age, sex, economic status, geographic location, or time of occurrence. In order for the comparison to be valid, it may be necessary to adjust for certain variables, such as age and sex, when two or more populations are compared.

One reason for assessing health problems is to provide the planner with a rational basis for setting priorities in the allocation of resources. There are never enough resources available to solve all recognized problems, and the planner must decide on attacking those problems which will yield the greatest results using resources that can reasonably be mobilized. This chapter deals with the epidemiological basis for making these decisions, although it does not imply that such criteria are the only ones to be used, since political considerations often outweigh epidemiological ones.

Epidemiology has been defined as the study of the distribution and determinants of disease frequency in man (1). Its importance for effective health planning should be, but unfortunately is not always, self-evident. Health planners often become preoccupied with sophisticated planning methods that are useless without good epidemiologic data. The link between epidemiology, planning, and effective action is as important today as it was when Dr. John Snow analyzed the distribution of cases, and then removed the pump handle from the contaminated well, to control a cholera epidemic in London.

Having decided on the problems to be tackled, initial assessment will aid in defining program objectives and repeated assessment will provide a logical basis for making modifications. The same procedures are necessary to measure the effectiveness of health programs. Many health programs fall short of being effective because the objectives are not clearly defined—and the objectives are not clearly defined because the problems are not clearly identified. The whole object of health planning is to improve the health status of the population more effectively and efficiently than would have occurred by chance alone. Assessment at various points in time will also help to determine if planning makes any difference.

In some countries, the health problems are so great that some administrators consider it unnecessary to plan. Almost anything that one does may appear to be worthwhile. These countries, however, are also the ones with the most limited resources, and this is what makes planning critical. Planning began to be popular in the United States only when it became clear that the demand for health care was rapidly exceeding what was possible with current resources. On this basis, good planning always serves a useful purpose.

SOURCES AND RELIABILITY OF DATA

In the assessment of problems, the health planner is dependent upon the quantity and quality of data available. In some countries, the paucity of data is disturbing; in others, the amount is well-nigh overwhelming. Reliability of the data will depend upon the state of sophistication of the public health and vital registration system of the country or the information system of a particular program. It will also depend on the data in question. Variations in the reliability may depend on the method of collection, the location, or the type of illness. For example, data obtained from the United States Health Interview Survey do not always coincide with those obtained from the Health Examination Survey (2-4). International sources may present an additional problem due to the delay in collecting data from several countries. Differences in the method of classification, even within a country, may complicate analysis and interpretation.

Six major types of data should be noted.

1. Routine vital statistics are compiled by national, state, or local governments. These data are disease-oriented and do not give a well-rounded view of the health problems of a local area. They also fail to consider morbidity. In less-developed countries, underreporting tends to detract from their usefulness, particularly for regions of any great distance from the capital cities. Misclassification of causes of death is frequent in countries where doctors are scarce.

2. Routine morbidity statistics of a quality adequate for health planning are rare. In most countries only communicable diseases are routinely reported, and generally even these are grossly and variably underreported.

3. When health care is organized into a comprehensive program serving a well-defined population (such as the Indian Health Service of the United States Department of Health, Education and Welfare), it is possible to obtain more comprehensive program data depending upon the sophistication of the information system. Such data should define the population, provide a health profile, give estimates of utilization, costs, and resources in manpower and facilities, and also include the usual clinical records. These types of data are service-oriented and may help to assess not only disease problems but also problems in the delivery of health care. In the United States, this type of information is now being developed in a more sophisticated manner. In countries such as the USSR and Sweden, comprehensive health data systems have been available for many years. As countries develop national health services, the opportunities for effective data gathering increase.

4. Data from specific programs may be published as either research or service reports (5-9). In the United States, several such reports have come from programs such as the Health Insurance Plan of Greater New York or Kaiser-Permanente. The study of capitation programs can provide useful comparisons for fee for service programs. Before applying such data in planning for a different population, however, careful consideration has to be given to certain variables. Utilization rates may vary in a low income group from those observed in a middle income group. Hospitalization rates under a capitation program will differ from rates in a fee for service setting. The difference between

utilization in one clinic as compared with another may be largely due to personal factors rather than to a program itself. National tuberculosis control or similar specific programs provide extensive data on single diseases. Data from specific hospitals or public health centers and clinics are difficult to evaluate or use, as the population base is rarely known. If all hospitals or other facilities are under one system, however, their records may be of somewhat more value to the planner.

5. Even with the above types of data, it is often necessary to use current surveys of both providers and consumers. Data from providers tend to be disease-oriented, while information from consumers tends to be oriented toward problems in community service. In carrying out such special surveys, consideration must be given to proper sampling techniques, taking into account, for example, specialty of physicians, age, or socioeconomic level of consumers. Consumer surveys are essential in countries with multiple sources of medical care, particularly when a large sector is supported by private payments. The costs of data from surveys are generally high in comparison with routine data sources, and partly for this reason, poor countries should consider "one shot" surveys rather than continuing ones.

6. A whole block of epidemiologic data frequently neglected in health planning is measurement of the *effectiveness* of various types of treatment and prevention. As a case in point, health planners should know comparative cost-effectiveness ratios for water supply programs, general sanitation programs, rehydration programs, and immunization programs, in control of diarrheal disease.

United States

The greatest source of data in the United States is the National Center for Health Statistics. The Center publishes annual volumes on mortality, natality, marriage, and divorce (*Vital Statistics in the United States*). It also publishes monthly and cumulative data on births, marriages, divorces, deaths, and infant deaths. In addition, several series deal with statistics other than those included in the monthly and annual reports. The more important among these are given below.

Series 10. Data from the Health Interview Survey. Statistics on illness, accidental injuries, disability, and other topics based on data collected in a continuing national household interview survey.

Series 11. Data from the Health Examination Survey. (1) Estimates of the medically defined prevalence of specific diseases in the United States and the distribution of the population with respect to physical, physiological, and psychological characteristics. (2) Analyses of relationships among the various measurements from national samples of the population.

Series 12. Data from the Institutional Population Survey. Statistics relating to the health characteristics of persons in institutions.

Series 20. Data on Mortality. (1) Various statistics on mortality other than those included in annual or monthly reports: specific analysis by cause of death, age, and other demographic variables. (2) Geographic and time series analyses.

Series 22. Data from National Natality and Mortality Surveys. Statistics on characteristics of births and deaths not available from the vital records. Based on sample surveys stemming from these records and dealing with such things as mortality by socioeconomic class.

Annual and special reports of the various state and local health departments provide important health statistics on local areas and may be more specific indicators of local problems, especially in the case of mortality data. Morbidity data based on a well-defined population are not commonly available, although some cities may conduct their own health surveys. *Special diagnostic and screening surveys* have been done for single or multiple diseases. The usefulness of the data may depend upon the bias of the population studied. *Special registries,* such as those for cancer and tuberculosis, may provide reliable data on specific problems, depending on their completeness. *Hospital in-patient data* may be used in some cases; they have their own bias, however, and in many cases the population denominator is unknown. *Records of physicians' practices* and *health insurance records* may also be valuable sources of data, if one is cautious about their inherent bias and limitations.

In the case of morbidity data, one may simply have to use the data available, although it may not be truly representative of an area. A decision whether or not to use regional data in the absence of local data will depend upon specific circumstances. The planner often has to decide whether to conduct a special survey (at a cost) or plan without facts (which may also be costly).

International

Other Developed Countries

Most other developed countries have sources of data similar to, or better than, those in the United States, excluding the special information compiled by the National Center for Health Statistics. The British National Health Service has a unique, and underexploited, potential for generating much valuable data on various health problems, local and national. The health system of the USSR generates a wealth of data to aid in its own evaluation and future planning. Although the Russian data *is* utilized in health planning, its collection led one Russian Minister of Health to complain of the amount of professional time spent in recordkeeping. As planners we must always balance the cost of data with its value. Most countries with monolithic health systems have better potential for securing health planning data from official records than countries with pluralistic systems.

Developing Countries

In the developing countries, the range of possibilities is wide. At one extreme are those countries which have not even conducted a census and which have poorly developed public health systems. In these countries, information on the precise magnitude of the problems may simply not be available, but the problems may be so great and so obvious as to justify planning without facts. Malnutrition may be seen everywhere. No one knows how many children die of measles, but everyone knows that there are too many. Epidemics of smallpox are common. Any attempt to assess the problems rather than to "get on with the job" may be met with impatience. Furthermore, economic resources may not permit a detailed analysis of problems. In these countries, estimates of even the crude death rate, not to mention morbidity rates, may be unreliable.

In other, slightly more developed countries, however, public health and vital registration systems may be well organized for at least parts of the population, such as the urban areas. In such cases, one may use data available from local health departments. Where national data are compiled from information submitted by subdivisions, the national data clearly cannot be more reliable than the primary sources. Extrapolations may be made from cities to rural areas based on "epidemiological judgment" and on the few sporadic surveys that may have been or can be carried out.

International Comparative Data

The most important sources of comparative international data are the publications of the World Health Organization, specifically the *World Health Statistics Annual.* This report carries information on estimated population, births, deaths, and infant deaths for selected countries. Deaths according to cause are also published by sex and age. Much of the data is compiled from a questionnaire sent to the reporting countries. The annual *Reports of the Director of the Pan American Health Organization* provide useful information on health conditions in the Americas, as do special reports such as that of Puffer and Griffith (10).

Regardless of the country, one never seems to have all the data desired for a full assessment of problems. Planners must reconcile themselves, therefore, to the fact that good planning is essentially the art of making the wisest decisions on the basis of the best available information.

NATURE OF HEALTH PROBLEMS

Much of health planning deals with disease entities or groups of diseases. A universal classification of diseases is thus very useful, since it allows agreement in identifying the problems. To serve its purpose in health planning, a classification of diseases should have a limited number of categories which encompass the entire range of illness. The *International Classification of Diseases (ICD)* seems most generally used for this purpose and will be used in other sections of this chapter. Unfortunately, the classification is more appropriate for an anatomist than a health planner. Hopefully, a classification based on types of treatment or prevention will be developed and move into more general use. The 17 major categories of the *ICD*, which are used for both mortality and morbidity, are listed below, along with their code numbers as of the eighth revision.

I.	Infective and Parasitic Diseases	000-136
II.	Neoplasms	140-239
III.	Endocrine, Nutritional and Metabolic Diseases	240-279
IV.	Diseases of the Blood and Blood-Forming Organs	280-289
V.	Mental Disorders	290-315
VI.	Diseases of the Nervous System and Sense Organs	320-389
VII.	Diseases of the Circulatory System	390-458
VIII.	Diseases of the Respiratory System	460-519
IX.	Diseases of the Digestive System	520-577
X.	Diseases of the Genitourinary System	580-629
XI.	Complications of Pregnancy, Childbirth and the Puerperium	630-678
XII.	Diseases of the Skin and Subcutaneous Tissue	680-709
XIII.	Diseases of the Musculoskeletal System and Connective Tissue	710-738
XIV.	Congenital Anomalies	740-759
XV.	Certain Causes of Perinatal Morbidity and Mortality	760-779
XVI.	Symptoms, Senility and Ill-Defined Conditions	780-796
XVII.	Accidents, Poisonings, and Violence (External Cause and Nature of Injury)	E800-E999 and N800-N999

The United States Division of Indian Health uses the *ICD* classification in planning and lists the more important advantages as follows:

1. It is comprehensive; all diseases and conditions are included.
2. Diseases are grouped according to similar etiology; thus, diseases vulnerable to the same methods of attack are considered under the same problems.
3. The current magnitude and changes in magnitude of the problem are for the most part measurable from available statistics.
4. Program packages for attacking the problems are more easily designed because of disease similarity within the problems.
5. Performance budgeting is facilitated; expenditure for any disease is readily assignable to a health problem.
6. Health problems of lower magnitude in the study population than the same health problems in the reference populations are included so that resource expenditures for required health maintenance activities are accounted for.
7. Cost-benefit analysis can be made not only with health problems but

among health problems, in order to provide proper direction for program emphasis (11).·

Unfortunately, no similar international classification exists for other types of health problems related to the delivery of health care. A patient goes to the clinic at 9:00 a.m. for an appointment, waits until 12:00 to see a doctor who tells her that she is in the wrong place. She goes to the other clinic and waits until 2:00 p.m., but there are still many people ahead of her and she has to leave to meet her children who get out of school at 2:30 p.m. This patient has a very real problem which is common throughout the United States but which has not been systematically classified and coded. The problems related to the accessibility of care may be due to the location of health facilities, difficulty with transportation, or economic barriers which make care inaccessible. If the nature of these problems can be nationally or internationally classified and coded, it will be a great step forward for health planners.

MAGNITUDE OF HEALTH PROBLEMS

Some problems occur more frequently than others, as causes of either death or illness. Mortality rates for major causes of death in the United States and Peru are given in Table 9.1, with category numbers from the *ICD*. Heart disease, cancer, and stroke account for almost two-thirds of the deaths in the United States, an assessment which justified the development of the Regional Medical Programs. If a successful attack can be made upon these major killers in the United States, it will have a major impact on the mortality rate. Heart disease, cancer, and stroke are of relatively less concern in many other countries, such as Peru, where diseases of the respiratory and digestive systems are primary causes of mortality. Clearly, the priorities for health planners in Peru differ from those for planners in the United States.

Unlike death, illness has duration, and this forms the basis for two classifications—acute and chronic. Other important measures are the incidence (occurrence of new cases over a given unit of time) and the prevalence (total number of cases, new and old, at one point in time). Table 9.2 provides data from the United States National Health Survey on the incidence, percentage of distribution, and the number per 100 persons per year of certain acute conditions. The importance of respiratory conditions and injuries is clear. The analysis can be taken further to show that upper respiratory conditions account for the greatest proportion of all respiratory conditions and that among respiratory conditions the common cold has the highest incidence.

In the same manner, prevalence of chronic conditions and impairments is

Table 9.1
Five Leading Causes of Death, United States of America and Peru (1967)

U.S.A.

Cause of Death*	Number of Deaths	Rate per 100,000 Population
Diseases of the heart (410-443)	720,892	364.3
Malignant neoplasms, etc. (140-205)	310,983	157.2
Vascular lesions affecting the central nervous system (330-334)	202,184	102.2
Accidents (E800-E962)	113,169	57.2
Influenza and Pneumonia (480-483, 490-493)	56,892	28.8

Peru

Influenza and Pneumonia (480-483, 490-493)	16,620	134.2
Certain diseases of early infancy (760-776)	10,505	84.8
Gastritis, enteritis, etc. (543, 571, 572)	6,138	49.6
Accidents (E800-E962)	5,291	42.7
Bronchitis (500-502)	4,745	38.3

SOURCE: *Health Conditions in the Americas, 1965-1968.* Scientific Publication No. 207. p. 95. Washington, D.C.: Pan American Health Organization, 1970.
* According to Seventh Revision, *International Classification of Diseases.*

given in Table 9.3. Heart conditions, arthritis and rheumatism, mental and nervous conditions, and certain types of impairments are the most prevalent.

SEVERITY OF HEALTH PROBLEMS

So far, we have considered examples of the nature and magnitude of various health problems. Clearly, given the same magnitude, pneumonia would represent a more serious problem than the common cold. It is useful to have objective measures of the severity of an illness, and there is need for an acceptable technique for combining the days of activity lost due to morbidity and the future years of activity lost due to preretirement mortality.

For acute illnesses, the United States National Health Survey uses rates of restricted activity, bed disability, and work loss or school loss. Respiratory illnesses account for not only the highest incidence among acute conditions but result in the highest rates of restricted activity, bed disability, or loss from work and school. Limitation in activity due to chronic conditions is graded into

Table 9.2
Incidence of Acute Conditions, Percent Distribution, and Number of Acute Conditions per
100 Persons per Year by Condition Group, United States, 1968

Condition Group	Incidence of Acute Conditions in Thousands	Percent Distribution	Number of Acute Conditions/ 100 Persons/Year
ALL ACUTE CONDITIONS	399,095	100.0	204.3
Infective and parasitic diseases	41,592	10.4	21.3
Respiratory conditions	238,475	59.8	122.0
Digestive system conditions	19,390	4.9	9.9
Injuries	51,620	12.9	26.4
All other acute conditions	48,017	12.0	24.6

SOURCE: National Center for Health Statistics. *Current Estimates from the Health Interview Survey, United States–1968.* U.S.P.H.S. Publication No. 1000, Series 10, No. 60. Washington, D.C.: Government Printing Office, 1970.

Table 9.3
Average Number and Percent Distribution of Persons Reported as Limited in Activity
for Seven Most Frequent Causes of Activity Limitation,
United States, July, 1963-June, 1965

Rank	Condition	Average Number of Persons in Thousands	Percent
1	Heart conditions	3,619	16.0
2	Arthritis and rheumatism	3,481	15.4
3.5	Mental and nervous conditions	1,767	7.8
3.5	Impairments of back or spine	1,769	7.8
5	Hypertension without heart involvement	1,369	6.1
6	Impairment of lower extremities and hips	1,325	5.9
7	Visual impairments	1,285	5.7

SOURCE: National Center for Health Statistics. *Chronic Conditions Causing Activity Limitation, United States–July, 1963-June, 1965.* U.S.P.H.S. Publication No. 1000, Series 10, No. 51. Washington, D.C.: Government Printing Office, 1969.

categories by the National Health Survey: (1) no limitation of activity, (2) limitation but not in major activity, (3) limitation in amount or kind of major activity, (4) unable to carry out major activity (such as school or work). Such a breakdown reveals that heart conditions account not only for the largest number of cases but also for the greatest severity of limitation.

Objective measures have not been developed for problems related to the delivery of health care and there is often wide divergence between provider and consumer with respect to characterizing severity. One common area of contention is the definition of emergency services. The physician tends to define an emergency as a life-threatening event. The consumer is likely to include many other events which he considers worthy of urgent attention.

DISTRIBUTION OF HEALTH PROBLEMS

Age

Major health problems are not evenly distributed throughout the population. Heart disease and cancer are not leading causes of death in all age groups. Knowledge of the relative importance of health problems at various ages provides a firmer basis on which to plan for target populations. Although 40 percent of a given population may be in the pediatric age group, only a small percentage of the health problems may be concentrated there. The age group over 65 may require a much larger share of the resources than would be justified merely on the basis of numbers.

Age is a factor in the accessibility of health care because older people often have greater problems in getting to their source of care than do younger people. Persons of working age may find it inconvenient or expensive in terms of hours of work lost in order to seek care during the working day. In this respect, care may be inaccessible to them.

Consideration of age adds another dimension to the assessment because the condition which kills or debilitates early in life may be weighted more heavily than one which kills or debilitates near the end of the normal life span. There are, of course, other views, which tend to attach greater significance to economic productivity. We prefer to take the approach that life is inherently valuable and do not weigh the productive years more heavily than others.

In Table 9.4, we show the death rates from malignant neoplasms and from accidents at various ages in the United States for the year 1966. To measure the relative impact of death from the two conditions, one could measure the person-years lost as a result of death from each cause by multiplying the rates at specific ages by the difference between that age and the life expectancy at that age. For example, using Table 9.4, it is seen that the death rate for malignant neoplasms in the under-one-year age group is 5.6 per 100,000; for accidents, it is 84.5 per 100,000. Assuming that the life expectancy at that age is 70, and that if the person had not died from that cause he would have lived, on the average, the remaining 69 years, then the number of person-years lost due to malignant neoplasms is 5.6×69. Likewise, the number of person-years lost due to accidents is 84.5×69. On this basis, programs designed to reduce accidents

Table 9.4
Death Rates from Malignant Neoplasms and Accidents by Age,
United States, 1966

Age	Malignant Neoplasms (Rate per 100,000)	Accidents (Rate per 100,000)
Under 1 year	5.6	84.5
1-4	8.3	33.4
5-14	6.4	19.8
15-24	8.4	67.1
25-34	18.3	51.9
35-44	61.1	47.9
45-54	180.1	55.6
55-64	406.7	67.3
65-74	756.6	92.5
75-84	1098.7	199.2
85 years and over	1493.7	591.9
Total	155.1	58.0

SOURCE: National Center for Health Statistics. *Monthly Vital Statistics Report* 16: No. 12 Supplement. Washington, D.C.: Department of Health, Education and Welfare, March 12, 1968.

would have a higher priority for this age group than programs to reduce neoplasms.

A more delicate problem arises when the number of person-years is approximately the same but the number of persons differs significantly. The question is posed in the following form: If resources are limited, which is the better plan, one which will save 10 lives for an average of 10 more years, or one which will save 5 lives for an average of 20 more years? This dilemma is more theoretical than real. The question is hardly ever answered on purely statistical grounds.

Sex

At all ages, women in the United States have a lower death rate than men, but women have a higher rate of morbidity from chronic conditions. Similar differences are also noted in other countries. The death rate from cancer of the lung is almost seven times as high for men as for women, whereas diabetes is a more frequent cause of death among women. Mortality and morbidity data based on sex are easily available from the sources quoted above. Women seem to make more use of health services than do men. The reasons seem to be both social and pyschological, as well as the fact that women find it more convenient than men to receive services during the day.

Race

Differences in morbidity and mortality associated with race are striking in the United States. When appropriate adjustments are made for age, the nonwhite population has higher rates for most major causes of death. Table 9.5 illustrates this point.

The disease hypertension is twice as frequent among nonwhites as it is among whites. Although the proportion of the population with one or more chronic diseases or impairments is greater for the white population than for the nonwhite, a smaller proportion of white persons report limitations affecting their major activity (12). This illustrates the smaller magnitude but greater severity of problems reported by nonwhites. The morbidity and mortality rates of the white population may in many cases be assumed to be a reasonable goal for the total population, and the existing gap between the races may be a measure of deficiencies which currently exist in health programs.

Table 9.5
Age-Adjusted Death Rates for Specified Causes, by Color, United States, 1966

Causes of Death	White (Rate per 100,000)	Nonwhite (Rate per 100,000)
ALL CAUSES	709.2	1,051.1
Major cardiovascular-renal diseases	368.0	502.2
Malignant neoplasms	125.9	152.7
Accidents	53.0	75.8
Influenza and pneumonia (except pneumonia of newborn)	21.2	43.3
Diabetes mellitus	12.7	24.8
Cirrhosis of liver	12.1	20.4
Tuberculosis	2.6	10.8

SOURCE: National Center for Health Statistics. *Monthly Vital Statistics Report* 16: No. 12 Supplement. Washington, D.C.: Department of Health, Education and Welfare, March 12, 1968.

Income

Although we do not know very much about the relationship of poverty and disease, we do know that a greater prevalence of illness exists among the poor (13, 14). The power to purchase care is perhaps the single most important factor in the distribution and utilization of health services in the United States. This situation has great relevance for urban health planning, as income differentials within many of our cities are quite marked. The present policy in the United States tends to favor efforts aimed at the elimination of these disparities and the achievement of a higher standard of health care for all.

Geographic Distribution

Geographic differences may refer to differences between census tracts within a city, rural-urban-suburban differences, or differences among states or countries (15). Inner city health problems are different from those of suburbia both in kind and in degree. It would be unwise to plan as if these differences did not exist. Differences among geographic areas in both mortality and morbidity levels are often related to differences in race and income. The differences are also related to the variability of health services due to a maldistribution of health manpower and other resources.

Interrelationship of Factors

Although variables are listed separately above, they are not necessarily to be considered singly. Data are often available in combination and in this form can be more valuable. For example, Table 9.6 portrays suicide rates for the United States for 1959-1961 by color, sex, marital status, and age. It shows that suicide as a health problem tends to increase with age, is more frequent among males than females, is more frequent at all ages among the divorced than the married, and is more frequent for both marital states among the white than the nonwhite.

TRENDS

Knowledge of current trends is useful for planning and evaluation. One is able to determine which problems are increasing and which are decreasing. It may also be evident that despite a large expenditure of funds, some problems persist to an embarrassing degree. The farther back the observations go, the greater the confidence one can place in the trends. Where changes are observed, they may be due to increase or decrease in the frequency of disease or death, changes in the method of classification, changes in accuracy of reporting, improved diagnosis, or a combination of these and other factors. Sometimes the factors causing the change can be easily identified, such as a new revision of the *ICD*. In most cases, the causes are not so clear-cut. Trends are often used to show an association between factors without necessarily establishing a causal relationship. Proper interpretation of the trends is as important as observation of the trends. Wrong conclusions may lead to an investment of funds in a futile program.

Table 9.6

Suicide Rates, by Color, Sex, Marital Status, and Age, United States, 1959-1961 (3-Year Average)

Marital Status and Age	WHITE			NONWHITE		
	Both Sexes	Male	Female	Both Sexes	Male	Female
	Rates per 100,000 Population					
Married						
15 – 19 years	3.6	8.3	2.4	*2.3	*4.5	*1.8
30 – 34 years	8.5	12.0	5.3	6.8	11.1	3.3
45 – 49 years	17.0	25.1	8.6	6.7	10.7	2.5
60 – 64 years	21.9	32.9	8.6	8.5	12.6	*2.9
75 – 79 years	26.1	37.1	6.0	8.9	12.1	*1.3
85 + years	33.0	43.1	*3.3	*2.1	*2.7	–
Divorced						
15 – 19 years	*12.3	*6.8	*13.8	–	–	–
30 – 34 years	47.9	77.6	27.1	*12.0	*22.5	*6.6
45 – 49 years	56.9	107.0	22.5	15.6	34.1	*4.1
60 – 64 years	64.9	118.8	21.7	*22.3	*36.3	*9.7
75 – 79 years	78.0	125.9	*26.7	*17.7	*30.7	–
85 + years	*60.4	*101.8	*16.6	–	–	–

*Age-specific rates based on fewer than 20 deaths.

NOTE: Only a portion of the original table is shown.

SOURCE: National Center for Health Statistics. *Suicide in the United States, 1950-1964.* U.S.P.H.S. Publication No. 1000, Series 20, No. 5. Washington, D.C.: Government Printing Office, 1967.

PRIORITIES

Factors which influence the assignment of priorities are both quantitative and qualitative and are not always developed in a logical manner. This chapter deals primarily with the epidemiological factors which influence these decisions; even within this area, the criteria are not easily quantifiable. Problems arise with the attempts to combine the effects of morbidity and mortality and to give appropriate weight to each. Planning groups have used different indices for ranking problems quantitatively. For example, the Division of Indian Health has devised a Health Problem Index which combines a number of factors as follows (11, p. 10):

$$Q = MDP + (274LA/N) + (91B/N)$$

where

    M = Health problem ratio (Indian rate/U.S. rate)
    D = Crude Indian mortality rate per 100,000
    P = (65 − average age at death)/50
        (1.0 when average age at death is less than 15
        or 0.01 when average age at death is greater than 65)
    L = Length of hospital stay ratio (Indian/non-Indian)
    A = Total number of in-patient days
    B = Total number of out-patient days
    N = Population
    274 = Conversion constant = 100,000/365
    91 = Conversion constant = (100,000/365) × (1/3)

The Q value is weighted for amenability to treatment and lost production potential, quite apart from the level of unemployment in the population. In-patient visits are rated three times as heavily as out-patient visits. These features may make this index unacceptable to some planners. It has proved useful to others and, in any event, does allow a ranking of health problems on a uniform basis.

The Latin American Institute includes four factors in an index of priorities (16):

$$MIV/C$$

where

    M = Magnitude (number of deaths)
    I = Importance (deaths rated by age of occurrence)
    V = Vulnerability of the disease to attack
    C = Costs

Age is used as an indicator of importance or significance. Vulnerability is a measure of the susceptibility of conditions to therapeutic and/or preventive measures and is based either on experience of health services or special studies. For example, malaria is rated 1 (or very vulnerable) and tumors 0.10 (least vulnerable). Cost is the cost of avoiding a death. The index is oriented toward mortality; hence, it would be more valuable in a country where death rates are high from preventable causes than in a country where morbidity is a more sensitive indicator of health problems.

In the absence of detailed information, certain rates have often been used as indices of the general health of a country. The most common of these are the infant mortality rate, the crude mortality rate, and the life expectancy at birth. These rates are usually compared with the rates for some country which is known to have an excellent standard of health, or they may also be used to compare the same country at different times. The infant mortality rate of 114 per thousand in Chile (1964) may be compared with 14.2 per thousand in Sweden, or the rate for Sweden in 1964 may be compared with the rate in 1960. A great deal is currently made in the United States of the fact that this country now ranks fourteenth with respect to infant mortality. The comparison of crude mortality rates fails to give proper weight to age and other structural differences in the population. In general, these health indices do not provide enough specific information to form the basis for planning. Obviously, many health problems exist in a community where the life expectancy at birth is only 45; this information, however, does not in itself provide sufficient grounds for the selection of alternatives.

The whole question of health indices has recently been reviewed in an excellent monograph of the National Center for Health Statistics (17). The same series of the National Center includes a monograph on another index of health, which includes time lost due to death and time lost due to illness during a calendar year (18). The index has a value between 0 and 1 and increases as the population becomes healthier. Like other summary statistics, it gives a general impression but cannot be as useful as a more detailed consideration of the various components which are summarized in the single figure. This index is not useful for setting priorities or defining objectives, but may be useful in evaluation.

In recent years, it has become increasingly evident that assessment from the experts' point of view is not enough if one is to assure a concerted attack on the problems. Providers and consumers who have "lived with the problems" may have a different assessment; sometimes the differences are semantic. In such cases, the expert must recognize the semantic barriers and use language which will more effectively communicate. In other cases, differences with respect to priorities may be strong. What the expert considers serious and of high priority the community may consider trivial. For example, a health expert may decide that dental care for children is a more pressing need than providing dentures, but the older and more vocal population may have accepted the development of dental caries as natural and may fail to cooperate unless some recognition is given to their own need for fillings, extractions, and dentures. Compromises may be necessary. The important point is that even expert planning cannot lead to effective action unless substantial agreement on the nature and relative importance of the problems is reached.

EVALUATION

The initial assessment of health problems is the first step in evaluation. It forms the baseline for the measurement of performance within a given plan of action. Specific objectives can be defined and change measured only after assessment. Hopefully, the results of planned change will be greater quantitatively and qualitatively than those which occur by chance alone. This change may be in mortality, morbidity, or both. Elimination of disease problems may or may not be associated with changes in level of satisfaction with the delivery of health care. This requires measurement of process as well as end results, and involves the difficult task of demonstrating cause and effect among complex and interdependent variables. The same measures should be used for evaluation and for the initial assessment and, therefore, agreement on measures must be reached at an early stage in planning. One cannot overestimate the value of a clear understanding and a cooperative working relationship between those who plan and those who evaluate.

REFERENCES

1. MacMahon, Brian, Pugh, Thomas F., and Ipsen, Johannes. *Epidemiologic Methods.* Boston: Little, Brown and Company, 1960.
2. Woolsey, T. I., Lawrence, P. S., and Bolamuth, E. "An Evaluation of Chronic Disease Prevalence Data from the Health Interview Survey." *American Journal of Public Health* 52:1631-1637, 1962.
3. Simmons, R. and Bryant, E. "An Evaluation of Hospitalization Data from the Health Interview Survey." *American Journal of Public Health* 52:1638-1647, 1962.
4. Sanders, B. S. "Have Morbidity Surveys Been Oversold?" *American Journal of Public Health* 52:1648-1659, 1962.
5. Shapiro, S., Williams, J. J., Yerby, A. S., Densen, P. M., and Rosner, H. "Patterns of Medical Use by the Indigent Aged under Two Systems of Medical Care." *American Journal of Public Health* 57:784-790, 1967.
6. Shapiro, S., Weinblatt, E., Frank, C. W., and Sager, R. V. "Incidence of

Coronary Heart Disease in a Population Insured for Medical Care (HIP)." *American Journal of Public Health* 59:Suppl.:1-101, 1969.

7. Cook, W. H. "Kaiser-Permanente Program. Experience with a Comprehensive Prepaid Medical Plan and Its Implication for Future Medical Practice." *Journal of the Kansas Medical Society* 70:379-383, 1969.

8. Williams, J. J., Trussell, R. E., and Elinson, J. "A Survey of Family Medical Care under Three Types of Health Insurance." *Journal of Chronic Diseases* 17:879-884, 1964.

9. Densen, P. M. *Prepaid Medical Care and Hospital Utilization.* Hospital Monograph Series No. 3. Chicago: American Hospital Association, 1958.

10. Puffer, R. R. and Griffith, G. W. *Patterns of Urban Mortality.* Scientific Publication No. 151. Washington, D.C.: Pan American Health Organization, 1967.

11. *The Principles of Program Packaging in the Division of Indian Health.* Silver Spring, Maryland: U.S. Public Health Service, Bureau of Medical Services, 1966.

12. National Center for Health Statistics. *Chronic Conditions and Activity Limitations.* U.S.P.H.S. Publication No. 1000, Series 10, No. 17. Washington, D.C.: Government Printing Office, 1965.

13. National Center for Health Statistics. *Medical Care, Health Status, and Family Income.* U.S.P.H.S. Publication No. 1000, Series 10, No. 9. Washington, D.C.: Government Printing Office, 1964.

14. National Center for Health Statistics. *Selected Health Characteristics by Occupation.* U.S.P.H.S. Publication No. 1000, Series 10, No. 21. Washington, D.C.: Government Printing Office, 1965.

15. National Center for Health Statistics. *Health Characteristics by Geographic Regions, Large Metropolitan Areas and Other Places of Residence, United States, July 1962-June 1965.* U.S.P.H.S. Publication No. 1000, Series 10, No. 36. Washington, D.C.: Government Printing Office, 1967.

16. Ahumada, J., *et al. Health Planning: Problems of Concept and Method.* Scientific Publication No. 111. Washington, D.C.: Pan American Health Organization, 1965.

17. National Center for Health Statistics. *Conceptual Problems in Developing an Index of Health.* U.S.P.H.S. Publication No. 1000, Series 2, No. 17. Washington, D.C.: Government Printing Office, 1966.

18. National Center for Health Statistics. *An Index of Health–Mathematical Models.* U.S.P.H.S. Publication No. 1000, Series 2, No. 5. Washington, D.C.: Government Printing Office, 1965.

ADDITIONAL READINGS

Primary

Berg, R. L., Browning, F. E., Hill, J. G., and Wenkert, W. "Assessing the Health Care Needs of the Aged." *Health Services Research* 5:36-59, 1970.
The article reports on findings of a sample survey of the health care needs of the aged population in Monroe County, New York, living at home and in health care institutions. Sampling problems are discussed, as well as the

correlation of physical and mental disability with demographic and socioeconomic factors.

Kisch, A. I., Kovner, J. W., Harris, L. J., and Kline, G. "A New Proxy Measure for Health Status." *Health Services Research* 4:223-230, 1969.

This article describes a new proxy measure for health status developed as part of a study to quantify determinants of demand for health care. The health status of approximately 2,000 individuals in two sample populations was to be assessed, and results of two pretests of the proxy measure are presented.

Meltzer, J. W. and Hochstim, J. R. "Reliability and Validity of Survey Data on Physical Health." *Public Health Reports* 85:1075-1086, 1970.

This paper evaluates survey data on physical health from two points of view: (1) how consistently do people answer questions about their health when a survey is repeated after a short interval and (2) how closely does the information collected by survey agree with that obtained from clinical records? Results show that chronic conditions were reported more reliably than other types of complaints, and negative answers more reliably than affirmative.

"Methodological Issues in Health Statistics." *Milbank Memorial Fund Quarterly* 48:Suppl., October, 1970.

This supplement includes papers presented at the American Public Health Association Conference during a special memorial session honoring Mortimer Spiegelman, a former staff statistician for the APHA.

Stewart, G. T. "Epidemiological Approach to the Assessment of Health." *Lancet* 2:115-119, July 18, 1970.

The author describes some basic concepts of epidemiology and the main principles underlying Joseph Lister's research into the causes of disease. He explains how these concepts and principles are applicable to the assessment of health problems.

Wylie, C. M. "The Definition and Measurement of Health and Disease." *Public Health Reports* 85:100-104, 1970.

The author analyzes current problems in defining and measuring health and disease and suggests ways to reach clearer definitions of these concepts.

Secondary

Bradfield, R. B. and Coltrin, D. "Some Characteristics of the Health and Nutrition Status of California Negroes." *American Journal of Clinical Nutrition* 23:420-426, 1970.

Buck, Alfred A., Sasaki, T. T., and Anderson, R. I. *Health and Disease in Four Peruvian Villages.* Baltimore: Johns Hopkins Press, 1968.

Densen, P. M., Jones, E. W., Bass, H. E., *et al.* "A Survey of Respiratory Disease among New York City Postal and Transit Workers. I. Prevalence of Symptoms." *Environmental Research* 1:265-286, 1967.

Densen, P. M., Jones, E. W., Bass, H. E., *et al.* "A Survey of Respiratory Disease among New York City Postal and Transit Workers. II. Ventilatory Function Test Results." *Environmental Research* 2:277-296, 1969.

Densen, P. M., Ullman, D. B., Jones, E. W., and Vandow, J. E. "Childhood Characteristics as Indicators of Adult Health Status. Relation of School

Records to Selective Service Classification." *Public Health Reports* 85:981-996, 1970.

Donabedian, Avedis. *Medical Care Appraisal.* Volume II of *A Guide to Medical Care Administration.* New York: American Public Health Association, 1969.

Haber, L. D. "The Epidemiology of Disability: The Measurement of Functional Capacity Limitations." *Social Security Survey of the Disabled.* Report No. 10. Washington, D.C.: Social Security Administration, July, 1970.

Kane, R. L. "Determination of Health Care Priorities and Expectations among Rural Consumers." *Health Services Research* 4:142-151, 1969.

Kerr, M. and Trantow, D. J. "Defining, Measuring, and Assessing the Quality of Health Services." *Public Health Reports* 84:415-424, 1969.

National Center for Health Statistics. *Facts of Life and Death.* U.S.P.H.S. Publication No. 6000. Revised edition. Washington, D.C.: Government Printing Office, 1967-1968.

Sullivan, D. F. "Disability Components for an Index of Health." *Vital and Health Statistics,* Series 2, No. 42. Washington, D.C.: Department of Health, Education, and Welfare, Health Services and Mental Health Administration, July, 1971.

10

Health Manpower Planning

TIMOTHY D. BAKER

What is health manpower planning? Very simply, it is the process of trying to make sure that we shall have enough health workers to meet, but not exceed, the future *effective economic demand* for their services—that is, to fulfill perceived needs that are backed by willingness and ability to pay.

The importance of health manpower planning should be self-evident, but, throughout the world, decaying water systems, unmanned health centers, and empty hospitals stand as monuments to dismally inadequate manpower planning. The urgency of health manpower planning should be equally clear, because of the long lag time in training health professionals. Hospitals can be built in months; it takes a decade to train a doctor.

The details of health manpower planning are extremely complex, as pointed out in Butter's excellent review of health manpower (1). Problems vary from country to country. To understand the principles, a framework for analysis is necessary. The analytic framework presented here will certainly not remove all complexities from the planning process. It has proved useful, however, in practical tests in countries as varied as Taiwan, Turkey, Peru, and Nigeria, where cooperative manpower studies have been conducted under the auspices of the Department of International Health of Johns Hopkins University (2-5).

The analytic framework has seven parts:

1. *Supply analysis:* measuring the current supply of all types of health workers in some detail.

2. *Projection of supply:* projecting the supply of health workers forward to target dates 10 to 20 years in the future, with anticipated additions of new graduates and estimated subtractions for death, migration, retirement, and change of profession.

3. *Demand analysis:* evaluating the effective economic demand for health services from both the private and public sector.

4. *Projection of demand:* projecting the effective economic demand forward to the 10 to 20 year target dates.

Revised with permission of the publisher from: Baker, T. D. "Dynamics of Health Manpower Planning." *Medical Care* 4:205-211, 1966.

5. *Productivity:* estimating the average number of services per health worker per unit of time.

6. *Will future supply match demand? Recommendations to effect a balance:* comparing the projected supply with the projected demand and recommending necessary adjustments to effect a balance.

7. *Constraints:* describing the limiting factors inherent in any recommendations made.

Supply can be brought into balance with demand by either (1) increasing supply (S′) or (2) increasing productivity (Figure 10.1). Increase in productivity is limited by standards of acceptable quality. On an economic basis, total services may be increased at the same cost by increasing the units of service per health worker, or by substituting less expensive health workers. This sounds quite simple, and as a concept it is. Complexities arise in practice, however, as will be discussed below.

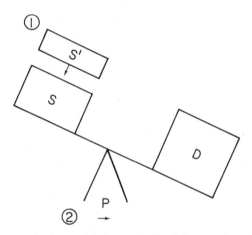

Fig. 10.1 Supply-demand balance on the fulcrum of productivity.

SUPPLY ANALYSIS

Categories of Health Workers

The first step in supply analysis is to decide who to count. Of course, doctors, nurses, dentists, technicians, and pharmacists should be included. Midwives, herbalists, and similar categories should be counted in countries where they are numerically important. Groups such as health educators may be included for the sake of completeness. Sanitation workers with special training should probably be counted. It is not generally considered necessary to count *untrained* persons who happen to be working for medical institutions. Most ambulance drivers, hospital maids, and hospital clerks should not be counted as they are a part of larger general manpower pools.

Definition of categories of health workers is the next step in analysis of supply. Just what will be included under the term "doctor"—should osteopaths, licentiates, grade-B graduates be included? How about chiropractors, herbalists, curanderos? Although definitions will vary from country to country, a useful guiding principle is to have one group of doctors comprising all persons licensed to practice modern, scientific medicine. This is not to say that the herbalists and curanderos should not be counted. Such groups may be important, but only should be studied separately.

In measuring supply, overclassification of health professions into many subgroups is confusing. For each class of health worker, three groups—professional, assistant, and aide level—should be adequate for most general health manpower planning. Usually, a definition based on years of training is most useful in determining these groupings.

Table 10.1 classifies health workers by length of training, income, and type of practice. Health professionals are included in both the high and medium income groups. Specific tasks often show considerable overlap between the groups. Supervision is not included in Table 10.1 because in most cases there will be supervision within groups as well as across professional lines.

The importance of measuring the various specialty groups varies from country to country. In any case, information on numbers of teachers in the health professions will be useful for measuring capacity for expansion of schools.

Sources of Supply Information

Information on the current supply of health workers varies from country to country and profession to profession as to source and accuracy. Obviously, most professional health workers come from the country's training institutions. A count of the past graduates, corrected for migration, deaths, and retirement from the profession, will give the potential number of professionals available. This source is only as reliable as the estimates of deaths, retirements, and migration, however, and these figures are hard to get. Also, health workers in subprofessional categories often have not been formally trained in educational institutions, but have merely taken an examination or, in some cases, simply applied for and received a license.

This leads us to the second source of data on current supply, namely the licensing institution. This institution, if its basic registration is complete, can serve as a good source of the maximum numbers of legal practitioners in a given country. This source of data is often out of date, however, as most licensing agencies lack adequate methods for removing those who leave the licensing area, die, or stop practicing.

Table 10.1

Health Workers by Income and Type of Practice

Type of Practice	High Income, Long Education (12 Years Basic + 6-13 Years Professional)	Medium Income, Medium Education (10-12 Years Basic + 2-5 Years Professional)	Low Income, Short Education (6-12 Years Basic + 0-2 Years Professional)
Unsupervised independent general clinical practice	Physician (GP)	Assistant medical officer, licentiate, behdar, health officer (Gondar), feldsher, nurse	Dresser
Hospital or group practice	GP and specialist: e.g., surgeon, pathologist, radiologist, physiatrist, orthopedist	Nurses (general duty and specialist), surgical technician, laboratory technician, X-ray technician, physical therapist, etc.	Nurses' aide, practical nurse, dresser, laboratory assistant
Antenatal, delivery, and postnatal care	Physician-obstetrician	Midwife	Auxiliary midwife, dai
Drug compounding and dispensing	Pharmacologist	Pharmacist	Dispenser, compounder
Mental health	Psychiatrist	Psychiatric nurse, psychiatric technician	Psychiatric aide
Dental practice	Dentist	Dental hygienist	Dental aide
Public health	Health officer (M.D.)	Health visitor, public health nurse, health educator	Home health aide, etc.
Environmental sanitation	Sanitary engineer	Sanitarian	Malaria assistant, sanitary inspector, etc.
Average cost of training:	X	1/3 - 1/2 X	1/10 - 1/5 X
Average earnings per year:	Y*	1/5 - 1/2 Y	1/10 - 1/5 Y

*Including consideration of private practice as well as government salary.

SOURCE: Baker, T. "Paramedical Paradoxes--Challenges and Opportunity." In: G. Wolstenholme and M. O'Connor, editors. *Teamwork for World Health*. CIBA Foundation Symposium, p. 130. London: J. & A. Churchill, 1971.

Professional registries, which are maintained in many countries, are a third source of data. Registries maintained by an annual, biennial, or triennial registration system give a fairly up to date estimate of the total number of active practitioners. In many countries, however, this system misses practitioners who are working in government institutions, for government institutions do not require registration. Combining government payrolls with the registry of private physicians makes estimates of total manpower possible, but name checks are required to prevent double counting of professionals with more than one job.

In countries lacking a general registration, one often finds a special registration for permission to use narcotics. Since essentially every physician in private practice will require narcotics at one time or another in his practice, this is a reasonably good source of information, *if* the regulations are enforced. The same problem of enforcement exists with lists of health workers paying the professional taxes required in some countries. A *laissez faire* governmental policy toward licensure and registration enforcement will lead to highly inaccurate data from official sources.

Professional societies will occasionally have an accurate roster of all members of the profession, and in some cases even will include those who are not members of the society. This is more usually found in developed countries.

Census data may prove useful if the general census mechanism in the country under study is worthy of confidence. The major drawbacks of a general census are that it is usually out of date and that census enumerators accept the statements of informants without verification. Thus, many unqualified practitioners may be listed as qualified professionals.

Pharmaceutical companies occasionally have accurate and up to date lists of private practitioners. Our experience, however, has been that these lists are far from complete and frequently the companies are reluctant to release their lists.

The last and undoubtedly most accurate method of determining the current supply of health workers in the country is to conduct a special survey. Unfortunately, this method is both time-consuming and expensive. If a country has no good source of information on numbers and distribution of professionals, however, a survey could be the starting point for an effective registration system. Such a system is a necessity for logical health planning in any country of the world today.

Characteristics of Health Workers

In addition to the total number in each class of health professional, distribution by age, sex, educational background, income, type of practice, specialization, productivity, and geographic location are crucial factors.

Knowledge of age composition is essential for making predictions of change in supply. For example, in Taiwan we found almost five times as many doctors of age 35 to 44 as age 25 to 34 (2). Authorities were unaware of this dangerous gap in physician manpower, which would not have manifested itself until 1985, when it would have been too late to institute corrective measures. The sex distribution of health professionals is particularly important in countries where women have a very different working pattern from men. Educational background is especially useful in defining categories of health workers and in comparing contributions of different training institutes to the various sectors of the health industries.

Income level is important for all projections, and attempts to change the supply will require adequate information on the costs of these changes. Reluctance of professionals, especially in the private sector, to disclose their incomes hinders the determination of income levels. In many cases, disclosure of real income would bring major penalties in the form of increased taxes. In Taiwan, we had to approach the problem indirectly (2). We found the average monthly expenditure for physician services (from 66,000 persons in the random sample), multiplied this average by the total island population, and divided the product by the number of physicians practicing in Taiwan. Thus, we calculated the *average* physician income.

Another significant attribute of the health worker is his type of practice, i.e., the number of hours he works and for whom (in private, for the state, for a commercial concern, for a voluntary agency, or for a combination of these). If an adequate method of defining specialists exists, numbers of specialists can sometimes be of value.

Some knowledge of productivity—the number of patients seen by the average practitioner per unit of time—is essential (6). (Of greater value would be the number "helped," but such information is virtually unobtainable.) Information on variation in productivity from region to region and from sector to sector is also useful. Where productivity falls below acceptable norms, supply can be effectively increased without adding a single person merely by increasing productivity.

In order to measure the importance of immigration of health professionals, the number of native-born and native-trained workers is needed. Knowledge of geographic distribution is necessary because a country may have an adequate over-all number of health workers so poorly distributed that corrective action is indicated. Finally, special studies of professional and student attitudes on rural practice, migration, retirement, and so forth can be very worthwhile.

PROJECTION OF SUPPLY

Losses

Change of supply may be divided into losses and increases. Losses are primarily by death, retirement, and migration.

Losses from Death

Theoretically, the most accurate method of age-specific professional death rate determination is to divide all registered deaths of professionals for each age group by the population of professionals in each age group. If the professional group is small, we must use a period longer than a year. Where professional associations keep accurate records of memberships and deaths and where all professionals are counted in their statistics, these records offer an alternative source of data for direct calculation of professional death rate. The use of official registration data and professional association data may be combined to secure a more accurate determination of professional deaths (6). This method has the drawback of being time-consuming if separate classes of health professionals are not distinguished on the death certificates. Where accurate information is not readily available, this direct calculation of professional mortality for manpower studies is not justified.

The second alternative is the use of age-specific death rates for the general population, assuming that the physician death rates equal the general death rates. The weakness of this method is that the assumption is a bad one, for physician age-specific death rates are uniformly lower than the general population age-specific death rates. In studies as widely separated in time as 1925 and 1951, and as widely separated in space as United States and Japan, lower mortality for physicians has been demonstrated.

The third alternative, applying a correction factor to the general mortality rates, follows logically from the above observation that physicians have more favorable rates than the general population. Since in reality the losses by death before the age of retirement represent a small part of the losses of the total health manpower pool, use of a general death rate with whatever approximate correction seems appropriate is strongly recommended.

Losses from Retirement

Retirement is usually the greatest source of loss to the profession. Age of retirement varies from country to country. In India, where the retirement system was designed for the British Colonial Service, retirement was compulsory at age 55. In other countries, the age of official retirement is 65 or even 70. In private practice, in which usually one does not retire but "fades away," median retirement age is a matter of judgment. Some private physicians will work beyond this median age while others will retire earlier and the "fading away" is assumed to be a gradual process continuing over a period of 10 years or so.

In some countries, losses by change of occupation are very significant. In most of Latin America, where the medical degree is as much a mark of an educated man as it is the key to a professional career, many physicians do not practice medicine. Determination of these losses may be made by surveys of one or more cohorts of graduates of professional schools. In some countries, many physicians are reported to leave the practice of medicine because they are unable to make a living in medicine—evidence of defective health manpower planning. Special cases of change in profession, such as Taiwanese midwives going into nursing, also occur. One change of "profession" of particular significance for the female health worker is marriage. One must carefully examine the working pattern of women to see if marriage causes an interruption to work, and to see if children represent a temporary interruption, or if they keep the mother out of work for their preschool years or even for the rest of her life. Studies of this kind are particularly important in examining the nursing profession, as they give a basis for planning retraining of women who re-enter the labor market.

Losses by Migration

The last major source of losses to the profession is migration. This is a well-recognized phenomenon and for some countries represents a considerable loss. Migration takes place for training and for future work, and in practice it is very hard to separate the two. If a professional from a developing country undertakes a 10-year course in a highly specialized field that has no application to the problems of his own country, he is essentially as much of a loss to his profession as the professional who actually migrates. Furthermore, regional or state manpower planning is difficult in countries with appreciable interstate or interregional migration.

Increases

Increases in supply are primarily from new graduates. Obviously, training schools are a major source of new health professionals, but it is not enough merely to take the number of graduates from each school for the past 10 years and average them. Evaluation of the plans and proposals of educational authorities in the various health professions gives a better estimate of the increase by new graduates than statistical projection of past performance. Increase of health professionals by immigration is extremely rare in most developing countries. The creation of a new group of professionals occasionally occurs when one class of professionals is upgraded in status by governmental decree.

Availability of Applicants

Four basic factors determine a country's potential for increasing its number of trained health professionals. The first is the "raw material," that is, qualified applicants. Training institutions should be able to give the annual number of qualified applicants for admission each year. Correction should be made for multiple applications when several training institutions exist. In estimating the number of future applicants, the demands of other sectors of the nation's economy for trained manpower must be taken into consideration. Generally, in relation to the number of openings, medical schools will have a higher number of qualified applicants than the other health professional schools.

Educational Plant Capacity

The second determinant of potential for increased supply is the educational plant capacity, that is, the number of students who can be taught in existing teaching facilities. For clinical fields such as nursing and medicine, this also implies the availability of *suitable* "teaching" hospital beds, as well as the classroom facilities normally associated with educational institutions. In addition to the study of the existing facilities, both the feasibility of new construction and methods of extending the present facilities should be reviewed, so that more students can be handled by using more efficient teaching methods.

Availability of Funds

The third factor determining potential for increase is capital: the funds available for expanding training facilities and paying for the recurring costs of training and education.

Availability of Teachers

The fourth determinant in the health manpower field is the availability of teachers; because of the long time lag in preparing a teacher, it is also probably the most important. Reviews of existing resources of qualified teachers are needed, as are determinations as to whether salary and prestige are adequate to attract the teachers needed to expand training facilities. As in the problem of limitation of educational plant capacity, existing numbers of teachers can be extended by converting some part-time faculty to full-time. This must be planned with extreme care, however, as exclusively full-time teaching staffs involve some hazards.

DEMAND ANALYSIS

Many different methods exist for determining the demand for health workers. In clinical medicine, if one disease has many remedies, one assumes that none of these remedies is really adequate. Such is the case in demand analysis for health workers.

Basic Biological Need

Determination of the basic biological need is based on: (1) determining the level of mortality and morbidity of a country; (2) estimating the time of health professionals needed to care for each type of case representing the various types of morbidity and mortality; (3) multiplying the time per case by the estimated annual number of cases to get the total professional hours *needed;* (4) determining the average hours worked per year by the professionals; and (5) dividing total hours *needed* by hours per professional to determine total required supply of health professionals to meet basic biological needs. The best known document on this method is the report by Lee and Jones (8).

Although this approach has the seductive appeal of seeming to be the most scientific appraisal, for many practical reasons it is unworkable. First, no country in the world has sufficiently detailed and accurate morbidity and mortality statistics to give the exact figures needed for this type of estimate. Second, no measure of health professional time required by any given level of morbidity or mortality can be accurate when health problems have many alternative solutions that require entirely different types of health manpower. For example, should one equate the morbidity from diarrhea with a sanitary engineer's time to design a water supply system, or with the services of the nurse and doctor in the rehydration clinic? Practically speaking, this problem has no answer. Third, and most important, even if one could calculate the "need," this is no measure of public "demand" for the services of health professionals. Unused health clinics in areas of high health need stand as examples of this, as do physicians unable to earn a living in the larger cities of underdeveloped countries (where there are crying "needs" for medical attention which the people cannot afford to express in terms of "effective economic demand").

The Status Quo

The most common approach to health manpower analysis is the normative approach, where existing professional-to-population ratios are enshrined as norms. This *status quo* approach, despite its many theoretical drawbacks, is the basis of many past estimates of demand for the various types of health workers. Examples of this method are the otherwise excellent reports *Physicians for a Growing Nation* (9) and *Nurses for a Growing Nation* (10). The major flaw in this method is that it fails either to determine the suitability of present ratios or to account for changes in demand due to changed demographic character of the population. Closely akin to the status quo approach is the "Parkinsonian" modification which says in effect: "Our doctors and nurses are busy now, therefore we need more." This was the method used in early efforts to set standards for public health nurse staffing in the United States. Some communities had a ratio of public health nurses to population of 1 to 10,000. In the opinion of authorities, the nurses were overworked, so the ratio was changed to 1 to 5,000.

Comparative Method

The comparative method takes the ratios for other countries, and reasons that the country under study has effective economic demand for at least as many health workers as in the reference country. The flaw in this method lies in the fact that very few countries are truly comparable.

Expert opinion is often used for estimation of demand for health workers. Indeed, in some instances, this is probably the best estimate available, particularly in fields that employ small numbers of health workers for which there is no real public demand, such as health educators, sanitary engineers, and other highly specialized personnel.

The Russian System

In Russia, where essentially all medical care is given by government personnel, estimation of demand for doctors has been based on observed norms of practice. On the average, one out-patient doctor sees five patients an hour, works 5.5 hours a day, 240 days a year, and, theoretically, handles about 6,600 visits in a year. Total visits per 1,000 population are observed and doctors are "allocated" on the basis of total population. Similar methods are used for allocation of medical specialists, nurses, and feldshers. The Russian system is said to work satisfactorily in practice, but it is complex and exacting. The Russian Minister of Health recently complained that Russian doctors spent half their time on paperwork. Apparently, the full extent of demand in Russia has not yet been measured, for the most recent publication proposes increasing the doctor/population ratio from 1/610 to approximately 1/350 (11).

Effective Economic Demand

In countries where the private sector offers an appreciable source of financing for health services, an entirely different approach must be used: measurement of effective economic demand. This is best determined by a random sample survey of patterns of demand for health services throughout the country to be studied. Demand should be quantified by basic demographic attributes of the population, thus giving a basis for predicting change of demand as the age pattern changes and the population becomes better educated, more urban, and wealthier.

In the public sector, the number of budgeted vacancies may be used as an index of unmet demand.

In countries with both private and public payment for medical care a mixed method of analysis of demand is appropriate. Indeed, since no perfect method for measuring demand exists, one should utilize elements of all relevant methods and arrive at a composite judgment on the current demand for medical services.

PROJECTION OF DEMAND

Population Increase

The primary factor affecting change of demand in countries with slight to moderate manpower shortages is population increase—the more people, the more doctors and nurses demanded, assuming economic growth at least keeps pace with population growth. Very few countries have large unmet effective economic demands. More often they have a supply of doctors and nurses in keeping with the countries' ability to pay for them.

Economic Development

In countries with severe health manpower shortages, economic development may also play a major role in increasing demand. Increased per capita income will result in increased demands for medical care in virtually all the developing countries of the world. High income groups demand more medical care at the present time. Logically, therefore, as the present low income groups increase their real per capita income, they will be able to afford and demand more medical services.

Improved Education

Formerly, improved education was believed to result in increased demand for medical care. This is certainly not true for all health professions and is probably a minor factor in causing change of demand in many countries. Although one would expect a decrease of demand for herbalists and untrained physicians as the general level of education improves, one may not assume that the increase in the demand for modern medical practitioners will be more than just compensatory. Since increase in income and increase in education are often closely correlated, multivariate analysis may be useful to separate the effects of these two changes on demand for medical services. This procedure is seldom justified in a health manpower survey because of the small effect that increased education has on increased demand.

Change of Supply

Another determinant of change in demand which should be considered is the available supply of health workers. Effective economic demand for a physician does not exist in a village where physicians are unkown or unavailable. However, a new road which would make a physician available to the people in the village would definitely change their demand for physician services.

Age Distribution and Population Redistribution

As part of the general population increase, changes in the age structure of the population exert a special effect. If a population gains higher percentages of older people and of small children, demand for medical services will increase, because these groups universally require more medical attention. Another effect of population increase is population redistribution. As populations shift from rural to urban areas, the demand pattern of the country will change.

Unpredictable Factors

Whereas the previous changes of demand may be predicted with some degree of accuracy, the following factors, which may be very important in changing the pattern of demand, are virtually unpredictable. These include changes in disease patterns, technological advances, and social and organizational change.

Measles has changed markedly in the past years in many countries from an extremely severe disease with high morbidity and mortality to a far milder condition. Leprosy is thought to have changed considerably during man's experience with it. New diseases may be introduced where they did not exist previously, completely distorting the picture of demand for medical care.

In addition to disease pattern changes, technological changes affect health manpower demand. Certainly the demand for radiologists would never have been predicted before the discovery of x-ray. The discovery of antibiotics has changed the health service demand picture considerably, probably more from the standpoint of shifts within the health professions than from shifts of total demand. For example, the discovery of isoniazid and PAS has very definitely reduced the number of chest physicians and tuberculosis hospital nurses required and has increased the demand for public health nurses to carry out home care programs.

Social changes are also very significant in altering demand for health workers. As village women become less satisfied with the unqualified, unsafe, untrained midwife and shift to the trained midwife and health center, demand for midwives clearly changes. On a larger scale, as a country changes the balance of financing of medical care from the public sector to the private sector, obvious changes in demand may result.

Modifications in the organization of health services will influence both the available supply of health workers and demand. For example, as health ministries "ruralize" their health services, more demand may develop. Changes in administrative policies now in existence could have marked effects on the demand for medical care. For example, in some clinics only the first 20 patients in line are admitted each day. The people know this and know that they must suppress demands for medical care since it is not available under the present organizational system.

Demand for *salaried* health professionals is less directly related to economic and demographic change than to government health budgets. (Of course, government budgets are directly tied to a nation's economy.)

In summary, many factors influence demand for health services. Some of these factors are measurable; others are more in the realm of prediction and guesswork. Health manpower studies should include all available methods of analysis to predict the effect of these factors on future demand for health workers.

PRODUCTIVITY

Measurement of productivity in the health sector is a special and complex problem. In most instances, individuals of different professional background and capability jointly supply services of widely different natures. The simplest example is a solo practitioner dentist who restricts his practice to filling teeth. In this case, his productivity would be the number of teeth filled per hour, per day, per month, or per year—that is, the number of procedures over a given unit of time. In general, a relatively longer time period is more appropriate, in order to include losses from vacation, time spent in continuing education, administration, and other deviations from normal activities. The most complex example is a hospital staff offering a range of services from brief patient visits to complex surgical procedures and including personnel from janitors to cardiac surgeons. Measuring the productivity of a hospital complex or its individual members calls for modern methods of industrial engineering, systems analysis, and detailed time and motion studies.

After careful measurement of the time actually required for given procedures, and the nonproductive administrative time which must be allocated to these procedures, equivalency units may be established. For example, one surgical procedure may equal ten out-patient visits, or one medical in-patient day may equal five out-patient visits.

The problem of measurement of productivity is further complicated by the differing levels of salary of the various members in a complex medical organization. It may well be that a more highly trained, and better paid, technician may be more productive even in terms of salaries than a less qualified and less well paid worker. However, major economies usually can be realized as functions are transferred from high salary to low salary workers, because the main costs in the health industry are for services rather than goods. This principle is based on the assumption that productivity does not decrease at the same rates as salary.

Examples from dentistry show the magnitude of increases in productivity that may be expected from use of auxiliaries and aides. An American Dental Association survey showed that each additional full-time auxiliary working with a practicing dentist increased the dentist's productivity by approximately 30 percent (12, 13). A United States Navy study showed that each middle-level dental technician could boost the productivity of a dentist well over 50 percent (14).

There are limits to this principle; otherwise, we would have the janitor performing all health sector functions. Downward delegation of functions is limited by (1) quality of care expressed as end-results of services, (2) acceptability to consumers, and (3) perhaps most important, acceptability to the professionals who set standards for care. Physicians in developing countries often state that nothing but physician care is good enough for their people, when, in fact, only a small portion of the people have the benefit of any modern medical services at all (15).

WILL SUPPLY MATCH DEMAND? RECOMMENDATIONS TO EFFECT A BALANCE

A most important concept in health manpower planning is "start where you are." Grandiose and visionary schemes to correct the nation's health manpower problems by completely redesigning the system have little value. As mentioned earlier, the process of changing a country's health manpower status involves a great time lag.

After one has estimated the future demand and the future supply for periods 10 and 20 years in the future, a trial balance should be analyzed. For most professions in most countries, this trial balance will reveal future potential shortages. In many cases the trial balances will show more marked shortages in the rural areas. In a few cases, one might predict surpluses of certain categories of health workers, in respect to the effective economic demand (for example, herbalists in Taiwan).

Types of Action

Increased Personnel
To avert predicted shortages, three general types of action may be undertaken. The first is direct. This involves increasing enrollments in the training institutions and possibly increasing the number of training institutions. To make such recommendations, obviously one must know if there are adequate numbers of qualified applicants to fill the institutions, adequate teachers, and adequate funds to support the increased training programs. Possibly, government subsidies will have to be provided for the students and for the training institutions. To prevent losses of professionals in short supply, migration laws may have to be made more strict.

Substitution

The second general way to avert shortages is to substitute the auxiliary for the nurse or the nurse for the doctor. Such changes imply changes in training programs to fit professionals better for their new roles. If, for example, a nurse is to act as a physician in rural clinics, she should be trained in elements of diagnosis and treatment rather than merely in bedside nursing. Such changes also call for new patterns of supervision and quality control. If the qualtiy of medical care is not to deteriorate markedly when lower level personnel are substituted for higher level personnel, good supervision is essential.

Increased Productivity

The third type of solution to the shortage problem is based on increasing productivity of physicians by offering inducements for more efficient and effective practice. Regular refresher training may increase the effectiveness of the health worker. Group practice may result in increased output. Good supervision may also help to increase the productivity of health workers.

Special Measures

In addition to over-all personnel shortages, distribution is often unbalanced. For example, securing physicians for rural practice is often a major problem. This problem calls for suitable orientation in the medical schools. It also may call for reserving places in the medical schools for candidates from rural villages. It may, if the people's representatives so decide, call for increased salaries for rural posts.

ALTERNATIVES AND CONSTRAINTS IN POLICY DECISIONS

Since all these recommendations have social and economic costs, the ultimate policy decisions will not be in the hands of the health manpower planner, but rather at higher levels of government. These policy decisions will involve such issues as: equal distribution of care regardless of ability to pay *versus* better care for the more productive members of society; equal rural-urban distribution of medical personnel *versus* the efficiencies of group and hosptial practice; the hazards of restrictive migration policies for health workers; the pros and cons of governmental support for education; implications of changes in retirement age; the extent of governmental support of medical care; and types of governmental control that may be exercised on the health industry.

While the manpower planner cannot make these decisions himself, he must pose clear and detailed alternatives for implementing programs to alleviate shortages. At the same time he should describe the various constraints in initiating new training programs or new systems to increase productivity. These constraints fall into the categories listed below.

Constraints

Educational

How many applicants with the desired prerequisites would be available? Are the educational prerequisites appropriate for the types of training programs recommended? Are the training programs appropriate for the jobs to be filled?

Social

Would assistant doctors be acceptable in all communities? Are there limitations to the employment of males in certain health professional roles? For females? Is upward mobility of prime concern (e.g., does the opportunity exist for dressers to become medical assistants, or for medical assistants to become doctors)? Do regional or tribal prejudices block free job mobility of health workers? Does the social level of certain health professions thwart recruitment of qualified applicants?

Economic

What are the total costs of training adequate numbers of a given type of health professional? More important, what are the total earnings in the profession? (For instance, what would be the total annual cost for education and maintenance of replacing all short-trained nurses by university graduates?) Are the short-term education costs and the long-term maintenance costs in keeping with the nation's ability to pay? (Some health professionals are clearly unable to accept the fact that most countries cannot afford to meet all health manpower *needs.*)

Political

Are there imperial decrees that "a medical college shall be established?" What are the political pressures toward centralization or decentralization? Does the existing tax structure favor national, state, or locally financed training institutions? How strongly (in deed, not word) is the nation committed to equal medical care for all?

Administrative

Are health workers hired by one major employer or many? Are positions now filled by unqualified persons? Is staffing adequate enough to permit supervision? Are present employment rolls "padded?"

Professional

Will existing professionals refuse to work with assistants? Are there professional practice laws that bar the use of new types of health workers? Would these laws be difficult to change? How restrictive are present licensing or certification laws? Change can often be instituted more easily through the training of new graduates than through persuasion or re-education of established practitioners. For example, new dentists can be trained to utilize assistants more successfully than established dentists can be persuaded to change their current habits of practice.

To return to our initial questions, we trust that the importance of health manpower planning has been established and the process clarified. The additional readings noted below cover the topic in even greater detail.

REFERENCES

1. Butter, I. "Health Manpower Research: A Survey." *Inquiry* 4: 5-41, 1967.
2. Baker, Timothy and Perlman, Mark. *Health Manpower in a Developing Economy.* Baltimore: Johns Hopkins Press, 1967.
3. Taylor, Carl, Dirican, Rahmi, and Deuschle, Kurt. *Health Manpower Planning in Turkey.* Baltimore: Johns Hopkins Press, 1968.
4. Hall, Thomas. *Health Manpower in Peru.* Baltimore: Johns Hopkins Press, 1969.
5. National Manpower Board of Nigeria. *Health Manpower Survey 1965.* Lagos, Nigeria: Federal Ministry of Economic Development, 1969.
6. Ciocco, A. and Altman, I. "The Patient Load of Physicians in Private Practice." *Public Health Reports* 58:1329-1351, 1943.
7. Dickinson, F. and Martin, L. *Physician Mortality, 1949-1951.* Bulletin 103, Bureau of Medical Economic Research. Chicago: American Medical Association, 1956.
8. Lee, Roger I. and Jones, Lewis W. *The Fundamentals of Good Medical Care.* Chicago: University of Chicago Press, 1933.
9. Bane, G. *Physicians for a Growing America.* Report of the Surgeon General's Consultant Group on Medical Education. U.S.P.H.S. Publication No. 709. Washington, D.C.: Government Printing Office, 1959.
10. National League for Nursing. *Nurses for a Growing Nation.* New York: National League for Nursing, 1957.
11. Rozenfel'd, I. I. *Planning and Allocation of Medical Personnel in Public Health Services.* Translated from Russian and published for the National Science Foundation, Washington, D.C. Jerusalem: Israel Program for Scientific Translations, 1963.
12. American Dental Association. Bureau of Economic Research and Statistics. "Survey of Dentist Opinion, 1964." *Journal of the American Dental Association* 70: February, March, April, May, and June, and 71: July and September, 1965.
13. American Dental Association. *Reports of Offices and Councils. Section on Dental Education.* Chicago: American Dental Association, 1965.
14. American Dental Association. *Reports of Offices and Councils. Section on Dental Education,* pp. 37-47. Chicago: American Dental Association, 1965. Cited by: Cassidy, J. E. "Maryland Dental Manpower Projection." Doctoral thesis, Johns Hopkins University, Baltimore, Maryland, 1968.
15. Baker, T. "Paramedical Paradoxes—Challenges and Opportunity." In: G. Wolstenholme and M. O'Connor, editors. *Teamwork for World Health.* CIBA Foundation Symposium, pp. 129-141. London: J. & A. Churchill, 1971.

ADDITIONAL READINGS

Primary

Baker, T. D., Cassidy, J. E., Galkin, J. D., *et al. Projection of Maryland's Health Manpower Needs through the 1980's.* Baltimore: Maryland Council for Higher Education, 1968.
> Extensive source for methods of estimating future demand and supply of doctors, dentists, and nurses in one state.

Baker, T. D. and Perlman, M. *Health Manpower in a Developing Economy.* Baltimore: Johns Hopkins Press, 1968.
> Source of useful concepts and techniques for projecting manpower supply and demand in developing countries. The importance of private practice in Taiwan makes the study relevant for American health manpower planners. The multivariate analysis of demand has great potential as a research technique.

Butter, I. "Health Manpower Research. A Survey." *Inquiry* 4:5-41, 1967.
> Thorough review of major works in the field, primarily in the United States, up to the time of publication.

Bryant, J. *Health in the Developing World.* Ithaca: Cornell University Press, 1969.
> A notable, although uneven, analysis of the obstacles to the provision of adequate health care on a nationwide basis, with examples drawn from Latin America, Africa, and Southeast Asia. Particular attention is given to manpower needs and training.

Fein, Rashi. *The Doctor Shortage, An Economic Diagnosis.* Washington, D.C.: The Brookings Institute, 1967.
> Excellent study of physician manpower in the United States.

Fendall, N. R. E. "The Auxiliary in Medicine." *Israel Journal of Medical Sciences* 4:614-628, 1968.
> Excellent review of problems of training, supervision, and utilization of auxiliaries in the delivery of preventive and curative health services.

Hall, Thomas L. *Health Manpower in Peru.* Baltimore: Johns Hopkins Press, 1969.
> Of particular interest for Latin American governmental health agencies. Presents the concept of "rationalized demand:" disaggregation of demand by parts of the health sector; projection; and reaggregation.

Health Manpower Source Book Series. U.S.P.H.S. Publication No. 263, Sections 1-21. Washington, D.C.: Government Printing Office, 1952-1970.
> A series of official documents on United States health manpower. Early sections covered physicians, nurses, medical social workers, medical record librarians, dentists, dental hygienists, pharmacists, sanitarians, and medical specialists. The current section (21) deals with allied health professionals.

National Center for Health Statistics. *Health Resources Statistics, 1969.* U.S.P.H.S. Publication No. 1509. Washington, D.C.: Government Printing Office, 1970.
> A basic document for United States health manpower planners: data on most health professions and training institutions, including 230 pages on health manpower.

Study on Health Manpower and Medical Education in Columbia. Volumes 1 and 2. Washington, D.C.: Pan American Health Organization, 1967.

Extensive study in Columbia to determine both the incidence of disease
and the demand for medical care.

Taylor, Carl, Dirican, Rahmi, and Deuschle, Kurt. *Health Manpower Planning in
Turkey.* Baltimore: Johns Hopkins Press, 1968.
Stresses the distribution of manpower within the country, which is a major
problem in Turkey. Presents the concept of "technically feasible demand
(politically and administratively)."

Secondary

Acton, J. P. and Levine, R. A. *State Health Manpower Planning: A Policy
Overview.* R-724-RC. Santa Monica, California: Rand Corporation,
December, 1971.

Badgely, R. F., Last, J. M., and Paredes, R. "Review Article: *Health Manpower
in a Developing Economy, Health Manpower Planning in Turkey,* and
Health Manpower in Peru." Milbank Memorial Fund Quarterly 48:203-237,
No. 2, Part 1, April, 1970.

Butter, I. and Grenzke, J. "Training and Utilization of Foreign Medical
Graduates in the United States." *Journal of Medical Education* 45:607-617,
1970.

Butter, I. and Schaffner, R. "Foreign Medical Graduates and Equal Access to
Medical Care." *Medical Care* 9:136-143, 1971.

Carlson, C. L. and Athelstan, G. T. "The Physician's Assistant. Versions and
Diversions of a Promising Concept." *Journal of the American Medical
Association* 214:1855-1861, 1970.

Fahns, I. F., Choi, T., Barchas, K., and Zakariasen, P. "Indicators of Need for
Health Care Personnel: The Concept of Need, Alternative Measures
Employed to Determine Need, and a Suggested Model." *Medical Care*
9:144-151, 1971.

Forgotson, E. H. and Forgotson, J. "Innovations and Experiments in Uses of
Health Manpower: A Study of Selected Programs and Problems in the
United Kingdom and the Soviet Union." *Medical Care* 8:3-14, 1970.

Hiestand, D. L. "Health Services Research II: Research into Manpower for
Health Service." *Milbank Memorial Fund Quarterly* 44:146-179, No. 4,
Part 2, October, 1966.

Hyde, H. Van Zile, editor. *Manpower for the World's Health.* Evanston, Illinois:
Association of American Medical Colleges, 1966.

National Advisory Commission on Health Manpower. *Report.* Vol. 1.
Washington, D.C.: Government Printing Office, 1967.

National Health Forum. *Health Manpower: Adapting in the Seventies.* New
York: National Health Council, 1971.

Schaefer, M. and Hilleboe, H. E. "The Health Manpower Crisis: Cause or
Symptom?" *American Journal of Public Health* 57:6-14, 1967.

Shuman, L. J., Young, J. P., and Naddor, E. "Manpower Mix for Health
Services: A Prescriptive Regional Planning Model." *Health Services
Research* 6:103-119, 1971.

Sidel, V. W. "Feldshers and 'Feldsherism' in the USSR." *The New England
Journal of Medicine* 278:987-992, 1968.

Silver, H. K. and Hecker, J. A. "The Pediatric Nurse Practitioner and the Child
Health Associate: New Types of Health Professionals." *Journal of Medical
Education* 45:171-176, 1970.

11

Physical Facilities

PHILIP D. BONNET AND A. PETER RUDERMAN

This chapter outlines those characteristics of existing facilities which are useful for identifying the starting point and the background for planning. Since society is dynamic and in a continuing state of change, time perspective is important. In addition, all inventories of health facilities need to be regularly updated. We should recognize that facilities are instrumental means and not ends in themselves. In most countries until quite recently, more attention has been given to facilities planning than to any other part of health services. This should not be allowed to distort one's perspective about their importance. Facilities tend to be highly visible, organized, and expensive; they are also major sources of documented information. Thus, they tend to be regarded as more manageable and more important than other parts of health services.

Facilities are necessary for the provision of health services but in themselves are not sufficient. Thus, it is important to define as clearly as possible their appropriate roles and functions in the total arrangement of health services. This is complicated by the fact that many (although not all) health facilities have a "residential" function in addition to their health service functions of prevention, diagnosis, treatment, and rehabilitation. Although identification of that residential function and its components separately is desirable, it is neither easy nor always possible.

From the point of view of investment planning, physical facilities clearly represent a capital item. In planning physical facilities, however, it is important to take into account that the physical plant *by itself* is not a producing unit. The output of health care facilities is patient care, and this requires personnel and consumable supplies as well as capital. In a number of developing countries—although not only in such countries—construction of physical facilities independent of considerations of staffing and operation has meant that expensive capital resources were wasted because appropriate personnel to staff them were unavailable. In other cases, failure to make adequate budgetary provision for operating expenses resulted in similar waste, even when the facilities might have been put into full operation by recruiting personnel available in the labor market and by purchasing supplies available in commodity markets.

Because of the many historical influences on the development of health service facilities, types of facilities for personal health services are quite diverse—not to mention various other types of facilities relating to prevention and to environmental health. Except for acknowledging the existence of those other types of facilities, this chapter will deal only with facilities where health services are provided to individuals.

CLASSIFICATION OF FACILITIES

No single classification system for facilities exists. The trend is steadily toward the adoption of a system developed by refinement and combination of those used most widely for separate categories such as hospitals, clinics, and nursing homes.

Objectives and Levels of Care

One such combined classification, based on the objectives of facilities and levels of care, is as follows:

I. Facilities for care of ambulatory patients
    A. Physicians', dentists', or other practitioners' offices
        1. Solo
        2. Associated group
        3. Organized group
    B. Hospital clinics—general or special
    C. Health department clinics
    D. Industrial clinics
    E. School clinics
    F. Other clinics
    G. Rehabilitation centers
    H. Neighborhood service centers
    I. Community mental health centers
II. Facilities for emergency services
    A. First aid stations
    B. Emergency service units
        1. Community-based
        2. Hospital-based
III. Facilities for patients requiring residential care (in-patient)
    A. Short-term general hospitals
    B. Short-term special hospitals
    C. Chronic disease and long-term hospitals
    D. Acute psychiatric hospitals
    E. General hospital sections of psychiatric communities
    F. Rehabilitation hospitals
    G. Extended care facilities
    H. Nursing homes

   1. Skilled
   2. Intermediate
 I. Infirmaries
   1. Schools and colleges
   2. Sections of homes for the aged and homes for children
IV. Facilities for organized home care services
  A. Comprehensive
   1. Community-based
   2. Hospital-based
  B. Visiting nurse agencies
V. Facilities for supporting services
  A. Pharmacies
  B. Clinical laboratories
  C. Dental laboratories
  D. Radiology services
  E. Ambulance stations
  F. Prosthesis and appliance fitters and makers
  G. Opticians
VI. Supply services
  A. Manufacturers and distributors of drugs
  B. Manufacturers and distributors of medical and dental supplies and equipment
  C. Publishers of health services literature

The concept of differing levels of care for bed patients is a rather recent development, although the old large Nightingale Ward contained some of its features in that the sickest person was often placed close to the nurses' station. As improvement occurred, the patient's bed was moved farther and farther from the nurses' station. Varying levels of care for bed patients have been designated "progressive patient care." Originally, three levels of care were described: intensive, intermediate, and minimal. In practice, only two have been widely adopted: intensive care and general care.

Although progressive patient care suggests the movement of a single patient through all three stages, experience has shown that many patients require only one level of care during their hospital stay. Even so, adopting the concept of different levels of care has some advantages: (1) conservation and better utilization of highly skilled and experienced manpower, especially nurses; (2) improvement in the quality and appropriateness of care of patients; and (3) greater availability of technical equipment and technical support services for the patient needing them.

Consideration of the levels of care to be provided has a major influence on design and layout of physical facilities. Precautions must be taken to avoid the creation of inflexible compartmented levels of care which may result in problems of low occupancy because the number of beds in each category does not match the variations in demand for each level of care. Estimates of the number of intensive care beds in a general hospital vary, but are of the order of magnitude of 5 to 10 percent of the total number of beds.

Facilities for all desired levels of care need not be combined in a single physical plant. Very often, the cost of construction of a truly flexible hospital with convertible units has proved prohibitive. As an alternative, patients may be transferred from one institution to another for different levels of bed care (e.g., general hospital to convalescent hospital or nursing home) with lower over-all capital cost. Since the anticipated lifetime of hospitals is fairly long, and methods of treatment can change, the ratio between active treatment space and bed space may no longer prove ideal five or ten years after construction has been completed. In this case, investment in hostels or other nearby accommodation facilities for patients who go to the hospital for day rehabilitation programs, radioisotope treatment, minor surgery, and so forth may prove economical. In urban areas of sufficient population density, an investment in specialized transportation equipment (e.g., buses with ramps for wheelchairs) may increase the output of a treatment or rehabilitation service at lower cost than the provision of additional beds. When a given capital sum is available for facilities, devoting the money to expanding facilities for treatment of out-patients may prove more efficient than providing additional beds. The decision will depend on a realistic assessment of the health care needs of the community as a whole and cannot be based on consideration of the hospital in isolation from the total system.

Ownership or Sponsorship

Other classifications of facilities relate to ownership or sponsorship. For purposes of planning, these considerations are somewhat secondary to the functional classification. Nevertheless, broad classifications by function may conceal important internal differences. Whole facilities cannot be regarded as providing a homogeneous pool of services equally available to all individuals interchangeably in accordance with need or demand. Important differences occur on the basis of biology—age and sex—and technology—urology and ophthalmology. Present data tend to portray facilities on an over-all basis, without clear indication of the extent to which their component services are interchangeably available to all. Some degree of specialization which limits interchangeability and universal availability exists in almost all health service facilities, especially those with a residential component.

DIMENSIONS IN PLANNING

Size of Facilities

One major dimension in facilities planning is size, which can be measured in several different ways.

I. Capacity
   A. Number of practitioners
   B. Number of sessions
   C. Number of beds
II. Utilization
   A. Number of patient visits by clinical function (medicine, surgery, obstetrics, pediatrics, and so forth)
   B. Number of services
   C. Number of admissions or discharges
   D. Number of patient days
   E. Average census
   F. Percentage of occupancy
   G. Average length of stay
   H. Rate of turnover (admission per bed per year)
   I. Turnover interval (average time from discharge of a patient to the admission of another patient)
   J. Waiting lists and waiting time
III. Economic magnitude
   A. Annual operating expenditures
   B. Capital invested

For planning purposes, size of facilities must be balanced with distribution. A larger facility tends to be stronger and more effective and to have lower unit costs because of economies of scale. Economists disagree about the most efficient size for any given type of hospital. Some have suggested 100 beds, and others have suggested 1,000 (1); still others feel that the U-shaped cost curve sometimes found in manufacturing industry does not exist at all for the hospital. Most important to remember, real or theoretical economies of operation alone cannot be used as the basis for determining size; political pressures, fund-raising possibilities, and the desires of the community make themselves felt even when hospital planners may not wish to take them fully into account. The advantages of larger size, furthermore, must be weighed against limited number and reduced accessibility and against the tendency for larger facilities to undertake a wider range of services with resulting higher costs. In any event, the aggregate capacity of all facilities inevitably must bear some reasonable relationship to the demands, needs, and numbers of people to be served.

Size of the Population

Certain rough criteria have developed for the general hospital needs of a population in an intermediate or advanced country. The estimated requirements range from three to six short-term beds per 1,000 population. When total hospital beds (including psychiatric, chronic disease, tuberculosis, and geriatric beds) are considered, the figures range from 11 to 16 beds per 1,000 population. The minimum technically efficient size for a hospital with the necessary basic services (such as operating rooms, clinical laboratory, radiology services, and delivery service) is considered by some to be 100 beds and by others 150 beds (2). Thus, the smallest population for a "complete" general hospital using these criteria would be 1,000 beds x 1,000/3 population = 33,300. Obviously, in some sparsely settled areas, strict application of these criteria would make reasonable availability impossible without special transport arrangements.

For smaller areas, a rule of thumb used in Canada by the Task Force on the Cost of Health Services is that no community with fewer than 5,000 or 6,000 people in the service area can keep three doctors fully employed, and that three doctors plus supporting staff represent the minimum team to provide any community with continuously available health care (3, pp. 293-294). Assuming that more difficult cases should be referred elsewhere, a minimum community hospital of 30 beds could be justified where travel time to another facility was more than 1.5 hours. In general, no hospital with fewer than 75 to 100 acute treatment beds should be considered unless travel time made it imperative. In planning the distribution of such facilities, incidentally, another important factor is the "portability" of different classes of cases. Thus, a small number of specially trained personnel in special coronary care facilities is considered important even for the smallest hospitals (or, at the least, two beds for a joint coronary-intensive care unit with two specially trained nurses), even though heart surgery would require a minimum market area of 500,000 population and a major hospital center.

Geographical Distribution

Distribution of facilities is usually related to the concept of service or catchment areas, which is dependent upon population density, the transportation network, and considerations of travel time or distance. Service areas may be defined either from the provider point of view or the consumer (population) point of view. In either case, a spontaneous regionalized arrangement develops; it may be formal, but usually has some aspects of both points of view.

Because of the increasing variety and levels of service being identified, no single regional pattern has so far evolved which is easily applicable to the full range of health services. As a result, many facilities, differing by level of service or by special function, serve several catchment areas. In the widely proposed three-tiered regionalization of hospitals, with peripheral hospitals, intermediate hospitals, and a medical center hospital, these levels are not mutually exclusive. The medical center hospital incorporates the levels of care for the other two types in addition to its superspecialty, educational, and research functions, thereby having a smaller catchment area for its peripheral hospital (basic) functions, a somewhat larger area for its intermediate (secondary) functions, and the largest area (the whole region) for its special (tertiary) functions. In regions such as metropolitan areas, where more than one medical center hospital and substantial numbers of other types of hospitals exist, the definition of catchment areas and the resolution of the many border problems between formal jurisdictions become complex indeed.

In spite of the difficulties, continuing efforts are being made to identify and define appropriate catchment areas or populations of primary responsibility for each facility. In advanced countries, this is being attempted by redefining the functions and responsibilities of existing institutions and appropriately filling in any gaps which are identified. In developing countries, the reverse tends to be true. As new facilities are established, attempts are made to relate them to the needs identified for specific areas or populations defined in advance.

Time Trends

It is very important to bring the inventories of facilities and services—as well as the measures of need and demand—up to date at least at 12 month invervals. People move in or out of an area; they grow older; they have more or fewer babies. The facilities available change from time to time. The availability of manpower changes. As infectious diseases are controlled by sanitary measures, fewer hospital beds may be needed. As new treatments are developed, out-patient care may be preferable to bed care. For all these reasons, documenting the changes in available services, in their utilization, and in identified needs of the people to be served is an essential part of effective planning. As changes are identified, the plan should be appropriately modified.

Design

Consideration of building layouts and design details are outside the scope of this chapter. In any plan, however, attention must be given to the question of standards, both minimum and maximum. Most countries have guidelines with respect to acceptable minimum standards, although they vary to some extent with climatic conditions of the area, local customs, available building materials, sanitation and safety regulations, and concern for providing convenient access to people with disabilities and impairments. Beyond these basic requirements are those relating to the level, range, and variety of services needed to support the specific objectives of the facilities.

A general hospital is one of the more complex types of buildings in existence because of the mixture of scientific, technological, and personal needs; because of the need to provide for future expansion; and because of the complex interaction and sequencing of services to patients. With the steady rise in labor costs, the increasing number of special skills needed, and the high proportion of labor in operating costs, the design of health facilities should be expected to incorporate increasing numbers and types of labor-saving features in countries such as the United States. In planning labor-saving features, the capital cost and the rate of interest must be taken into account. Not all labor-saving devices are also cost-saving; in countries such as Canada where capital is more expensive and skilled labor more available, different decisions would often be indicated. One attempt to stimulate rational decision-making in this area was made by the Task Force on the Cost of Health Services in Canada in 1969, when it proposed an incentive plan for hospitals that permitted substantial retention of savings by hospitals when the savings were in fact realizable and could first amortize the cost of the capital investment (3, pp. 78-79). An incentive plan along these lines was adopted by the Ontario Hospital Services Commission in 1970, but did not elicit uniform response from different hospital administrators and boards, and was (by the end of 1971) producing results in only a few hospitals.

Financing

The amount and form of financing—tax appropriations, philanthropy, or mortgage loans—have a powerful influence on the quantity and quality of health services facilities, since the providers of the funds either explicitly or implicitly establish the conditions to be met in obtaining the funds. The conditions vary among countries and rarely are all facilities financed from a single source. In many cases, a combination of all three sources is used. A serious deficiency in nearly all provisions of capital for facilities is the scarcity of funds for modernization and for replacement of outmoded facilities. A plan for facilities should recognize the problem of obsolescence and make some appropriate provision for it.

The importance of the interest rate in making capital investment plans should be emphasized. Private mortgages involve interest rates that vary with the state of the general capital markets of a country. Governments, too, must often borrow, and the rate of interest paid to holders of government bonds will also vary with financial circumstances. Furthermore, money raised by taxation may indirectly affect the supply of loanable funds. The key role played by interest rates is discussed in connection with cost-benefit and cost-effectiveness analysis (see Chapter Seven).

REFERENCES

1. Bridgman, R. F. "Integration of the Organisation of Medical Care into Health and Town Planning." *World Hospitals* 3:50-53, 1967.
2. Carr, W. J. and Feldstein, P. J. "The Relationship of Cost to Hospital Size." *Inquiry* 4:45-65, 1967.
3. *Task Force Reports on the Cost of Health Services in Canada.* Vol. 2. "Hospital Services." Ottawa: Minister of National Health and Welfare, 1969.

ADDITIONAL READINGS

Primary

American Hospital Association. *Classification of Health Care Institutions.* Revised edition. Chicago: American Hospital Association, 1968.
> The definitions which distinguish hospitals from nursing homes, and nursing homes from residential homes, are spelled out in this report.

Bridgman, R. F. "Integration of the Organisation of Medical Care into Health and Town Planning." *World Hospitals* 3:50-53, 1967.
> This article is a convincing plea for the full integration of town planning with health planning and full cooperation among the planners. It includes an interesting historical perspective on the location of health care facilities.

Carr, W. J. and Feldstein, P. J. "The Relationship of Cost to Hospital Size." *Inquiry* 4:45-65, 1967.
> A report of a regression analysis involving 3,147 general hospitals in the United States. Average cost per day declined initially with increase in size but rose again as the complexity of provided services increased.

Division of Hospital and Medical Facilities. *Procedures for Areawide Health Facility Planning—A Guide for Planning Agencies.* U.S.P.H.S. Publication No. 930-B-3. Washington, D.C.: Government Printing Office, 1963.
> This manual describes policies and procedures for guiding the development of general hospitals in specific geographic areas.

Hudenburg, Roy. *Planning the Community Hospital.* New York: McGraw-Hill Book Company, 1967.
> A good description of hospital functions and the methods which are generally helpful in solving the problems of planning a new hospital. It recognizes the accelerating changes which are revolutionizing hospital architecture.

Joint Committee of the American Hospital Association and Public Health Service. *Areawide Planning of Facilities for Long-Term Treatment and Care.* U.S.P.H.S. Publication No. 930-B-1. Washington, D.C.: Government Printing Office, 1963.
> This manual describes policies and procedures for guiding the development of facilities for nursing homes, rehabilitation centers, chronic disease hospitals, and home care. Emphasis is placed on emerging patterns of service such as day care, community mental health centers, and affiliations among facilities.

Reed, Louis S. and Hollingsworth, Helen. *How Many General Hospital Beds are Needed?* U.S.P.H.S. Publication No. 309. Washington, D.C.: Government Printing Office, 1953.
> A definitive review of the several different methods and bases used to determine the need of populations of areas for hospital beds.

Task Force Reports on the Cost of Health Services in Canada. Volume 2. "Hospital Services." Ottawa: Minister of National Health and Welfare, 1969.
> A comprehensive review of hospital services in Canada from the standpoints of utilization, operational efficiency, personnel costs, bed needs, and distribution of facilities.

Wheeler, E. Todd. *Hospital Design and Function.* New York: McGraw-Hill Book Company, 1964.
> This book by an experienced hospital architect reviews the functions and staffing of individual hospital departments and considers the interrelations

among departments. Emphasis is placed on alternative solutions to a given problem.

Secondary

Clibbon, S. and Sachs, M. L. "Like Spaces vs. Bailiwick Approaches to the Design of Health Care Facilities." *Health Services Research* 5:172-186, 1970.

Coe, Rodney M., editor. *Planned Change in the Hospital: Case Studies of Organizational Innovations.* New York: Frederik Praeger, 1970.

Drosness, D. L. and Roach, C. I. "A State-Wide Information System for Health Facility Planning." *Proceedings of the Second Annual Conference on Applications of EDP Systems for State and Local Governments.* New York: New York University, 1966.

Klarman, H. E. "Some Technical Problems in Areawide Planning for Hospital Care." *Journal of Chronic Diseases* 17:735-747, 1964.

McNerney, Walter J. and Reidel, Donald C. *Regionalization and Rural Health Care. An Experiment in Three Communities.* Ann Arbor: University of Michigan Press, 1962.

Weeks, J. and Best, G. "Design Strategy for Flexible Health Sciences Facilities." *Health Services Research* 5:263-284, 1970.

Weeks, Lewis E. and Griffith, John R., eds. *Progressive Patient Care: An Anthology.* Ann Arbor: University of Michigan, Bureau of Hospital Administration, 1964.

Wheeler, E. Todd. *Hospital Modernization and Expansion.* New York: McGraw-Hill Book Company, 1971.

12

Health Care Systems and Financing

PHILIP D. BONNET AND A. PETER RUDERMAN

Use of the word "system" in connection with health services is relatively new, although the concept is not. It implies an identifiable array of interrelated and interacting components. At present, to draw a blueprint of the whole health service system is impossible because of its complexity and magnitude. In one way or another, health services involve all aspects of human existence, and to define the entire system would require a description of the whole human world. For this reason, what is here called a system should be understood as only a part of the larger whole.

The resources with which planning is concerned include both financing and the existing network of values, concepts, ideas, and institutional forms involved in the provision of health services. Each country has a unique historical, cultural, and political tradition, and has evolved a somewhat different pattern of health service arrangements. Although the problems are substantially the same everywhere, the emphasis, quantity and mixture of resources, and specific arrangements all differ. In general, where the decision-making with respect to allocation of resources is centralized and unified, the resulting system is more formal and identifiable. Where the decision-making is more diffuse and pluralistic, a less formal system results. Neither approach guarantees higher quality or greater economy, but it is widely believed that whenever resources are scarce a more equitable system is likely to result from coordinated, even if not fully centralized, decision-making.

Three basic aspects of health care systems should be recognized: (1) the state of knowledge and art; (2) the arrangements for providing care, i.e., the organizational arrangements among the providers—both people and facilities; and (3) the arrangements for paying for care. Comprehensive health planning may apply to any of the forms separately or, more usually, to a combination of the three, since they are not, after all, independent of one another.

HEALTH CARE SYSTEMS BASED ON THE STATE OF THE ART

Throughout recorded history mankind has attempted to deal in one way or another with problems of sickness, injury, and health. Individuals have been set apart as especially able, knowledgeable, or responsible for such problems—medicine men, witch doctors, healing priests, physicians. The three general types of systems developed by human society have usually been called primitive medicine, folk medicine, and scientific medicine. Primitive medicine invokes magical rites and rituals to solicit the aid of friendly spirits or to fend off unfriendly ones. Folk medicine relies on the use of herbs, unguents, and heat and cold, the benefits of which (actual or believed) have been learned by experience and handed down to succeeding generations. Scientific medicine utilizes the knowledge and technical apparatus developed through conscious testing, measurement, and controlled experiments. None of these has wholly replaced the others. Today, all three systems operate in different proportions in different parts of the world. One unstated premise in comprehensive health planning is that the objective should be to increase scientific and rational medicine and to reduce the domain of primitive and folk medicines—a premise which deserves some explicit examination in a more appropriate context.

Further examination of health care systems and financing in this chapter will deal only with those aspects based on scientific-rational methods. It concerns itself primarily with those personal health services which by circumstance are required to be provided to one individual at a time, not with major environmental services provided to areas or populations.

HEALTH CARE SYSTEMS BASED ON SPONSORSHIP AND ORGANIZATIONS

Two commonly recognized systems are the private sector and the public sector. Rarely does either exist in pure form. Everywhere, health services involve some mix of private and public effort, although in widely varying proportions. Even in the USSR, which has one of the larger public sectors, a small private sector continues to function.

Private Sector Health Services

Private medical care services are organized and sponsored in many ways, but they are all substantially influenced by the traditional physician-patient relationship, which assumes a confidential personal relationship between a doctor and a patient. Concern for confidence, confidentiality, privacy, and a continuing personal relationship persists in spite of increasing technical and professional specialization and growing numbers of persons other than physicians who help provide medical care.

Principal forms of provision of services in the private sector are the following: *Individual practitioners,* who arrange for their own independent offices, choose their own locations, and seek to develop a practice by becoming known as "good doctors." Advertising for patients is contrary to professional ethics.

Practitioners associated in informal groups, who choose a location in the same building as other practitioners and who may share waiting rooms and other facilities, but who maintain separate medical and financial records. Such geographical proximity promotes referrals, increases convenience to patients, and facilitates coverage during vacations, holidays, nights off, and attendance at medical meetings.

Organized practitioner groups, in which several physicians enter into a partnership and share the use and expense of the same office facilities and the same supporting services (e.g., medical records, nursing, receptionist, and laboratories). One requirement of an organized group practice is that revenue is pooled and, after payment of all expenses, distributed to all members according to some agreed formula. Practitioners may be employed individually by an organization sponsored by a group of consumers, such as a labor union or neighborhood group; in such cases, the practitioners may be paid a salary or on the basis of a fee per time period, per service, or per capita. It is more common, however, for practitioners to create an organized group, such as a partnership, which in turn contracts with the organization representing the consumers. Nevertheless, as of 1970, the largest number of organized practitioner groups in the United States were sponsored by physicians and did not undertake formal contractual obligations toward groups of consumers.

Industrial clinics, which undertake a limited range of service to handle emergencies and injuries at work, to minimize occupational hazards, and in some plants to conduct periodic examinations of employees for early detection of disease and maintenance of health.

Philanthropic (nonprofit) organizations, which primarily provide buildings (e.g., hospitals, convalescent and nursing homes) and those supporting services needed to create suitable conditions for the disabled sick to receive care from physicians. Many of these organizations were church-related or church-influenced at the time of their founding. Over the years, however, church support has declined relative to the whole. Now, 37 percent of general hospitals in the United States have no identification with any church denomination and are voluntarily sponsored by public-spirited citizens and community leaders (1).

Quasi-private organizations (or public authorities), which are public in legal form but in operating autonomy and dependence on revenue from services performed act more like private organizations.

Business organizations, which in legal form are typically American profit-making enterprises and which are usually limited to hospitals, nursing homes, and supply services, if practitioner partnerships are excluded. Limitations in the supply of capital and the low or absent prospects of a dependable return on invested capital have restricted the number of hospitals in this form.

Public Sector Health Services

Traditionally, in addition to public health services, the public sector has been called upon by society to fill gaps in the provision of personal health services for the disadvantaged, to protect society from those who are regarded as "dangerous" (e.g., isolation of individuals with contagious diseases or commitment of the mentally ill), and to provide for special groups (e.g., the military, merchant seamen, American Indians on reservations, and in some countries civil servants and the police).

The principal form of organization in the public sector is the government department or agency in which practitioners are almost always salaried or volunteer their services, expenditures are tied to budgeted appropriations, and all revenues are put into the general treasury without being directly applied to expenditures. Practitioners may be paid for part-time service on some basis other than salary, but only very rarely on a fee for service basis.

Since 1960, the limitations of municipal tax resources, the rigidities imposed by municipal bureaucracy on purchasing, on obtaining new employees, and on arranging for repairs and maintenance of buildings, and the difficulties of operating a hospital beset by frequent emergencies on the basis of a line item budget, have resulted in a deterioration of many municipal hospital services. As a result, serious consideration has been given to the transformation of some municipal hospitals into public authorities with substantial financial and managerial autonomy. In the case of New York City in 1970, a new public service corporation has been created to operate the municipal hospitals.

Public Health Services in the United States

The distribution of functions and responsibilities among the various levels of government in the United States is more or less as follows:

Local and municipal governments may provide general care clinics, general hospitals, emergency services, and immunization clinics. In very few instances, mostly large metropolitan cities, they provide institutions for the care of tuberculosis and some mental, chronic, and geriatric problems.

County governments are similar to municipal governments, although they are less likely to provide general services and more likely to provide long-term institutional services, such as mental hospitals, chronic disease hospitals, and tuberculosis hospitals.

Hospital districts are special jurisdictions created by state legislation for taxing purposes. They may be a group of counties or townships assembled to establish a special tax base to raise capital for hospital construction or occasionally to meet operating deficits. Once the facilities are built, they are usually operated by a board of trustees with fiscal autonomy (as in a private, nonprofit organization). This form is used most often for general hospital purposes, although occasionally it is applied to other activities.

State governments have generally limited their activities to providing services for mental health, tuberculosis, crippled children, and retired militiamen. Where individuals could not pay for care because of severity and duration of an illness and its cost, the state has been invoked to distribute the burden as widely as possible through taxes. In some instances, because of population dispersion and limited local resources, the state has provided general hospitals, most notably in the narrow coal valleys of Pennsylvania.

The *national government* up to 1945 limited its role to providing care for the military, veterans, American Indians, residents of the District of Columbia, merchant seamen, lepers, and drug addicts. Since 1945, the federal government has been increasingly involved in many aspects of health services, including hospital construction, biomedical research, health manpower development, financial support for special services, and programs in which costs are usually shared with individual states. The prevailing philosophy has been that each state was responsible for the health and well-being of its citizens. The federal role was limited to guiding, providing financial assistance, and setting standards. With the passage of Title XVIII of the Social Security Amendments of 1965—the Medicare Act—a partial compulsory national health insurance program was established under a social insurance plan, limiting the beneficiaries to persons 65 years of age and older but financed primarily by a payroll tax during the working years.

Special government agencies in the United States are involved in financing and assuring availability of medical care. Examples include the Social Security Administration, the Children's Bureau of the Social and Rehabilitation Service, and State Workmen's Compensation Commissions. The report *Federal Role in Health*, published by the Senate Committee on Government Operations in 1970, revealed the myriad ways in which the federal government has become involved in health matters (2).

Comprehensive Health Services

Comprehensive organizations for providing a complete range of services rarely occur. Those institutions which most nearly approximate such an organization are the medical services of the armed forces and prepaid group practices such as the Kaiser-Permanente Plan. In both instances, prevention is emphasized and most attention is given to acute illnesses. Both institutions involve a relatively young, healthy population and problems of chronic illness, geriatrics, and prolonged disability are underrepresented. In addition, they are neither heavily involved with training physicians and nurses nor deeply engaged in research.

Choice of a System

The advantages and disadvantages of each form of sponsorship and organization are not well understood. Experience indicates that public forms tend to be rigid in the United States and, although formally accountable, not very responsive. Private forms tend to be flexible, not formally accountable to the public without special legislation, variable in their responsiveness, and innovative. Many exceptions to these generalizations might be cited.

The problem for the planner is not so much that of selecting from among possible private and public forms of health care as of selecting the elements that will make the prevailing system responsive and efficient. Basic changes in sponsorship and organization, such as the absorption of friendly societies and mutual insurance groups into a social insurance system or the conversion of a social insurance system into a national health service providing direct benefits, are infrequent and usually result from political pressures rather than the choices of planners unless they are made in the immediate aftermath of revolution. Nevertheless, in any situation, the minimum requirements should be the same: (1) maintenance of standards of competence and safety; (2) minimum levels of accessibility and availability; (3) stability and dependability; and (4) responsiveness to new needs, demands, and opportunities.

The health services planner is generally not free to choose among the variety of possible forms, except in the rare case where no comprehensive health care system exists and the initial planning is being undertaken. Most commonly, the planner is in the employ of a ministry of health, a social security system, a regional hospital council, or some similar body and must work within the constraints already established. Experience has shown that, whatever the official system, as long as adequate facilities are made available and basic remuneration, conditions of work, and status rewards are considered satisfactory by the health workers, good health care can be provided.

HEALTH CARE SYSTEMS BASED ON FINANCING ARRANGEMENTS

In recent years, making a full range of services available to the total population has relied primarily on the development of financing mechanisms; even in financing arrangements, however, true comprehensiveness has not yet been achieved because of the problem, common to all arrangements, of insufficient resources of all types—manpower, facilities, and money.

Possible patterns of finance rely on either private or public sources of funds. Private sources of money include: (1) direct payments to the provider by the patient or user of services; (2) indirect payments to the provider through pooled funds and risk-sharing (insurance); (3) philanthropy; (4) industrial expenditures; and (5) lotteries.

Public sources include: (1) tax appropriations for direct provision of services; (2) tax appropriations for subsidy payments; (3) tax appropriations for purchase of services for the general population or a special segment of the population; (4) collection and disbursement of social insurance contributions by public authorities; and (5) lotteries.

Patterns or systems of financing involve questions of how fiscal resources are to be channeled and distributed to accomplish the health services objectives. Some patterns are more appropriate to one type of health service than to others. For example, most environmental services, being collective in nature, require collective financing, which is usually government or public financing. Personal health services, being individual in nature, sometimes have an element of coinsurance of personal payment even in countries providing comprehensive public programs. In many countries, the best-financed and most creative part of the medical care system is to be found under the aegis of social security or health insurance. The distinction must be made, however, between those countries whose public health funds are disbursed primarily as payment for services rendered in the private sector and those whose public health funds are used to operate hospitals and out-patient clinics and to provide direct service benefits.

Special Aspects of Financing

Payments to Providers

Resources can flow to the providers of health care through a variety of channels. The most direct route is from the patient (or his family) to the hospital and the physician. More commonly, funds are collected from many or all members of the community (persons covered by Social Security, taxpayers in general, or all residents able to pay) and flow through a financial intermediary such as an insurance organization, a prepayment organization such as Blue Cross, a social insurance fund, or a national health service to the institutions and/or individuals providing care.

Methods of paying providers of health service differ, too. The most widespread method is probably a fee for each specific item of service (fee for service). Other methods of payment to individuals include capitation based on the number of individuals in a calendar period, time-related payment based on the number of clinic sessions of specified duration, and salary. Each entails a different set of incentives and disincentives. Other methods of payment to institutions include retroactive cost determination and prospective budgeting, each of which involves a contract to provide services to patients (service benefits) rather than merely dollars to credit toward charges for services (indemnity benefits).

Sources of Revenue

When the method of financing has not been predetermined by past history or political considerations, the planner, in choosing among available methods, should consider ability to pay. The once-familiar argument that the burden of health care should rest most heavily on those directly benefited has been shifted in most of the world in favor of a concept of the citizen's (or resident's) right to health care. Financing health care through a single flat rate of insurance contribution or premium clearly bears most heavily on the poor. Financing health care by a retail sales tax is similarly regressive except when the basic necessities of life are exempted or the tax is levied on dispensable items (e.g., tobacco or alcohol) or on luxury goods. While real property taxes have been used to finance health care in few cases, the tendency is to rely increasingly on the general revenues of government. These funds, in a growing number of countries, tend to come from direct (income) taxes rather than indirect (sales or turnover) taxes; thus, they tend to be more consistent with ability to pay than other sources of revenue. The principal advantage of earmarked tax revenue over general revenue is that the flow of funds is not dependent on periodic budget votes; the principal disadvantage is that a weak tax base (e.g., cigarette tax) will provide an erratic source of income.

Capital Expenditures and Investments

Whatever the system of financing, the distinction between capital and operating expenditures is important. Rapid obsolescence of equipment and facilities in today's technological society has complicated the problems of both operating and capital finance, but the capital problem is particularly critical because amounts well in excess of current income must often be committed in a given year. Paradoxically, the least capital-intensive branch of health care—the private office practice of medicine—is the one that most consistently makes a surplus from current earnings available for investment. Yet this surplus is seldom invested in health care facilities outside the physician's own practice; investment advisers in any capitalist country can show the practitioners of medicine that investment in real estate, mining, manufacturing, and other fields of business activity brings a far higher return than investment in hospitals and out-patient treatment centers.

Investment in the expensive major health facilities, therefore, often requires some form of subsidy in order to compete for capital. This can be in the form of charitable donations, particularly when favored by national tax legislation, by government loans at concessionary rates, and by direct government construction or cost-sharing grants that in turn are financed from government bonds. In periods when capital in general is in short supply and interest rates are high, the tendency is away from investment in low-yield activities. Even when capital is plentiful and interest rates are low, higher yield activities will attract the bulk of free market funds. As a result, health service facilities tend to rely on government more than on other sources of capital, and when government itself is unable to shoulder the full burden, the result is an undercapitalized and technologically underdeveloped health care system.

REFERENCES

1. Hamilton, James A. *Patterns of Hospital Ownership and Control.* Minneapolis: University of Minnesota Press, 1961.
2. Senate Committee on Government Operations. Subcommittee on Executive Reorganization and Government Research. *Federal Role in Health.* Report No. 91-809. Washington, D.C.: Government Printing Office, 1970.

ADDITIONAL READINGS

Primary

Anderson, O. W. "Medical Care: Its Social and Organizational Aspects. Health-Services Systems in the United States and Other Countries—Critical Comparisons." *New England Journal of Medicine* 269:839-843 and 896-900, 1963.
    A very interesting analysis of the several types of health services systems, ranging from the loose pluralistic one in the United States to the tight one in the Soviet Union and variations in between. The author favors the looser systems.
Evang, K. *Health Service, Society, and Medicine.* London: Oxford University Press, 1960.
    This little book presents in few but well-chosen words the main issues and main solutions to them in health services organization.
Hamilton, James A. *Patterns of Hospital Ownership and Control.* Minneapolis: University of Minnesota Press, 1961.
    A report of a study of the different types of hospital control in the United States. Government hospitals are compared with private nonprofit hospitals. Differing modes of administration are described.
Klarman, H. E. *The Economics of Health.* New York: Columbia University Press, 1965.
    A classic in the field of medical care and health economics. It reviews the literature on the work of economists in the health field and identifies the many economic problems in the health field awaiting examination.
Roemer, M. I. "General Physician Services under Eight National Patterns." *American Journal of Public Health* 60:1893-1899, 1970.
    This study identifies and compares two contrasting patterns for providing the services of general physicians. The "direct" pattern utilizing salaried physicians appears to serve social needs more effectively.
Senate Committee on Government Operations. Subcommittee on Executive Reorganization and Government Research. *Federal Role in Health.* Report No. 91-809. Washington, D.C.: Government Printing Office, 1970.

A detailed report of the many health programs and activities financed by the United States Government, including discussions of the provision of health services and the purchase of health services by the Department of Defense. Health activities in poverty areas are also covered.

Weinerman, E. R. "Research on Comparative Health Service Systems." *Medical Care* 9:272-290, 1971.

A scholarly review of what has been learned about different health systems by comparative studies. A selective bibliography is included.

Secondary

Berki, S. "Economic Effects of National Health Insurance." *Inquiry* 8:37-55, March, 1971.

Division of Medical Care Administration. *Medical Care Financing and Utilization.* Selected Revisions. U.S.P.H.S. Publication No. 947-1A. Arlington: Government Printing Office, 1967.

Falk, L. A. "Medical Care Organizations." *Journal of the National Medical Association* 45:34-37, 1953.

Fendall, N. R. E. "Organization of Health Services in Emerging Countries." *The Lancet* 2:53-56, July 11, 1964.

Glaser, W. A. *Paying the Doctor: Systems of Remuneration and Their Effects.* Baltimore: Johns Hopkins Press, 1970.

Murnaghan, J. H. and White, K. L., editors. "Hospital Discharge Data." *Medical Care* 8:Supplement, July-August, 1970.

Pan American Health Organization. *Financing of the Health Sector.* Scientific Publication No. 208. Washington, D.C.: Pan American Health Organization, 1970.

Piore, N. K. "Dimensions and Determinants of Health Policy: Rationalizing the Mix of Public and Private Expenditures in Health." *Milbank Memorial Fund Quarterly* 46:161-170, No. 1, Part 2, January, 1968.

Roemer, M. I. "Medical Care in Integrated Health Programmes of Latin America." *Medical Care* 1:182-190, 1963.

Roemer, M. I., editor. *Health Insurance Plans: Studies in Organizational Diversity.* Los Angeles: University of California, School of Public Health, 1970.

Roemer, M. I. and Friedman, J. W. *Doctors in Hospitals.* Baltimore: Johns Hopkins Press, 1971.

Schonfeld, H. K. "Standards for the Audit and Planning of Medical Care: A Method for Preparing Audit Standards for Mixtures of Patients." *Medical Care* 8:287-298, 1970.

Somers, A. R. "The Rationalization of Health Services: A Universal Priority." *Inquiry* 8:48-60, June, 1971.

Somers, A. R. *Health Care in Transition: Directions for the Future.* Chicago: Hospital Research and Educational Trust, 1971.

Vidaver, R. M. "Underfinanced Services in the Public Sector: The Interrelationship of Funding, Service Patterns, Manpower, and Allied Health Professions Education." *Medical Care* 9:169-181, 1971.

White, K. L. "Dimensions and Determinants of Health Policy: Organization and Delivery of Personal Health Services—Public Policy Issues." *Milbank Memorial Fund Quarterly* 46:225-258, No. 1, Part 2, January, 1968.

White, K. L. and Murnaghan, J. H. "Health Services Planning: Models and Means." *Health Services Research* 5:304-307, 1970.

III

Specific Methods in Plan Development

13

Organizations and Information Systems

WILLIAM A. REINKE

Individual words by themselves are quite useless until they have been molded into a language through which ideas are communicated. Likewise, it is not enough to catalog the existence of individual health resources. We must in addition consider the organization of these resources into useful health services. To illustrate the importance of organization, consider the effect of switching so simple a function as rabies control services from the sheriff to the agricultural commissioner, the health department, or the humane society (1). Organizational goals and individual attitudes within agencies vary widely; therefore, the results achieved can be expected to depend upon who is made responsible for the control services.

Organizations are essentially channels for the flow of information, ideas, and influence for the purpose of making decisions and taking action. To begin with, then, organization theory deals with *structural* matters of responsibility, authority, and the coordination of decisions and actions. Since the decision-making process hopefully utilizes quantitative, objective information, consideration must also be given to the nature of the *information systems* employed by an organization. Because individual ideas and influence likewise form an important input to the decision process, organization theory has come to have a strongly *behavioral* flavor.

These factors form a dynamic process whereby individual and organizational goals are examined and modified, and methods are devised for rewarding their achievement. Likert has observed that this process is ideally of such a nature that:

A. The relevant goals of persons in the organization, or related to it, develop so that these goals achieve a satisfactory level of compatibility between them;
B. The objectives of the entire organization and of its component parts are in satisfactory harmony with the relevant goals and needs of the great majority, if not all, of the members of the organization and of the persons served by it;
C. Each member of the organization has objectives and goals which have been established in such a way that he is highly motivated to achieve them and

221

which, when carried out, will result in his doing his part in enabling the organization to achieve its over-all objectives;

D. The methods and procedures used by the organization and its subunits to achieve the agreed upon objectives are developed and adopted in such a way that the members of the organization are highly motivated to use these methods to their maximum potentiality; and

E. The reward system of the organization is such that the members of the organization and the persons related to it feel that the organization yields them equitable rewards for their efforts in assisting the organization to achieve its objectives (2, p. 207).

ORGANIZATIONAL CHARACTERISTICS

From the foregoing introduction we discern four organizational features that bear closer scrutiny. In the first place, organizations are *formal structures;* yet, second, they exhibit nearly *lifelike* emotional qualities, as well as patterns of growth, development, and decay. Since they are made up of individuals, consideration must be given in the third place to *interpersonal* relationships and motivations. Finally, individual activities and organizational interests must be brought together in terms of *performance* measurement and control.

Formal Structure

The formal structure is first of all characterized by specialization because of the limited capacity of single individuals to perform the wide range of activities required in an organization. Although compartmentalized to some extent, the individuals must interact, and frictions inevitably arise as a result. Some stem from the functional interdependence among officials, whereas others are allocational conflicts. Problems of a functional nature arise whenever the actions of one individual or segment of the organization have repercussions upon the effectiveness of others, regardless of the type or amount of resources used. For example, decisions regarding the nature of a family planning program may have a substantial impact upon child-care programs under the direction of entirely different members of the organization. In contrast, allocational conflicts arise when two or more activities must be supported out of a single pool of scarce resources, so that an increase in the money allotted to one reduces the funds available to support the other.

Administrators have generally felt that arbitration of these conflicts is best resolved by a hierarchical type of organization structure. Embedded in the hierarchy is a system of formal rules designed to reduce to a minimum the cumbersome communication required in the appeals process. The formal rules are likely to cover a fairly wide range of behavior in recurrent situations for which precedents have been established. Beyond this range are, on the one hand, decisions deemed too important to make without prior review by higher authorities and, on the other hand, matters that are sufficiently inconsequential to permit lower level discretionary action.

Granted the general use of hierarchical structures, organizations differ markedly according to whether they employ a relatively "steep" structure or a "flat" one. In the former case we have a long chain of command with many layers, so that the administrator at the top receives only a limited amount of thoroughly screened information. Presumably, he is then able to give adequate attention to a small number of critical decisions that are made in the light of a broad overview of organizational activities, undistracted by petty details. The difficulty with a steep structure is that movement of information up and down the line may be accompanied by distortion or improper selection. Important information may reach a dead end, while some relatively inconsequential data may be unnecessarily passed on.

The obvious way to reduce this difficulty is to flatten the structure so that higher level administrators have direct contact with more subordinates. This can lead, however, to a deluge of information that cannot be assimilated and to an unwieldy "span of control." Flat hierarchies, therefore, tend to be useful only where decision-making and control can be largely decentralized.

Our discussion of organizational hierarchies has led us to consider chains of command. Earlier we spoke of the need for specialization within an organization. We must bring these two notions together and remark that not all the individual specialists have authority and responsibility in the chain of command, at least not in the strict sense. Thinking more broadly, one's status within an organization can come from the confidence he commands through his special knowledge or education as well as through his official position in the chain of command. Thus, there are "staff" personnel and "line" personnel who differ formally in three ways. ". . . staff members perform purely advisory functions, whereas line personnel have operational responsibility; each staff reports directly to its top-level boss, whereas most line officials report to their ultimate boss through hierarchical superiors; staff members are technical specialists, whereas line members are generalists" (3, p. 143).

It follows that "staff work influencing future action of organizations is based upon an ability to persuade" (4, p. 718), whereas line officials can rely upon formal authority. We must not overemphasize this distinction, however, for the effectiveness of any official is determined informally in large part through his ability to influence, rather than to command.

Lifelike Characteristics of Organizations

Organizational entities are far more than inanimate structures. Their observed rise and decline and their need for viability in the face of destructive forces cause them to have a dynamic, if not entirely animate, character. In the long run, they face extinction unless they can change and innovate. In the short run, however, they demand stability, which causes them to seek a comfortable routine. As a result organizations are continually in a state of tension. In some the forces of energy and movement are dominant, while others have a clearly sluggish nature. In short, organizations have metabolic levels much as individuals do. While the biochemistry of the former is not as well understood as it is for individuals, two "laws" are worth noting. The first is the *Law of Countervailing Goal Pressures,* which states: "The need for variety and innovation creates a strain toward greater goal diversity in every organization, but the need for control and coordination creates a strain toward greater goal consensus" (3, p. 150).

Much lip service is given to rewarding innovation, but unfortunately control and compliance are the more dominant characteristics of many organizations. To illustrate, Argyris has performed an extensive analysis of 265 corporation decision-making meetings at the board or presidential levels. Among the nearly 12,500 units of behavior identified from tape recordings, ". . . there were almost no instances in which executives took risks, experimented with new ideas, or helped others to experiment with new ideas" (5).

Second, we have the so-called *Law of Increasing Conservatism:*

> All organizations tend to become more conservative as they get older, unless they experience periods of very rapid growth or internal turnover . . . . They formulate more extensive rules, learn to perform their tasks more efficiently, broaden the scope of their activities, develop more rigid procedures, shift their attention from task-performance to organizational survival, and devote a higher proportion of their activities to internal administration (3, p. 31).

No doubt other "laws" could be formulated and instances could be found which would tend to invalidate the ones presented here. The point is, however, that organizations as entities possess rather predictable characteristics that extend beyond but are not entirely independent of those of the individuals in them.

Informal Nature of Organizations

The individuals themselves deserve attention, of course. In studying ways in which relationships among various health services and structures were modified in six different communities, Morris found that the major impetus to change could usually be traced back to one or two key leaders (6). Moreover, within a total agency there was often one guiding subgroup with religious or ethnic similarities.

Downs has postulated and discussed in some detail five different types of officials who fall into two broad classes (3, pp. 8-9). Each type is motivated differently by such factors as power, income, prestige, security, creativity, loyalty to an ideal or institution, and desire to serve the public interest.

A. *Purely self-interested officials* are motivated almost entirely by goals that benefit themselves rather than their bureaus or society as a whole. There are two types of such officials:
  1. *Climbers* consider power, income, and prestige as nearly all-important in their value structures.
  2. *Conservers* consider convenience and security as nearly all-important. In contrast to climbers, conservers seek merely to retain power, income, and prestige they already have, rather than to maximize them.
B. *Mixed-motive officials* have goals that combine self-interest and altruistic loyalty to larger values. The main difference among the three types of mixed-motive officials is the breadth of the larger values to which they are loyal. Thus:
  3. *Zealots* are loyal to relatively narrow policies or concepts, such as the development of nuclear submarines. They seek power for its own sake and to effect the policies to which they are loyal. We shall call these their *sacred policies.*
  4. *Advocates* are loyal to a broader set of functions or to a broader organization than zealots. They also seek power because they want to have a significant influence upon policies and actions concerning those functions or organizations.
  5. *Statesmen* are motivated by loyalty to society as a whole and a desire to obtain the power necessary to have a significant influence upon national policies and actions. They are altruistic to an important degree because their loyalty is to the "general welfare" as they see it. Therefore, statesmen closely resemble the theoretical bureaucrats of public administration textbooks.

Relating these categories of individuals to the Law of Increasing Conservatism, Downs observes that almost every organization goes through a period of rapid growth before reaching what he calls "its initial survival threshold." During the growth period the organization contains a high proportion of zealots who helped to establish it and climbers who have been attracted by its fast growth. Ultimately a high proportion of the organization's membership tends to be converted into conservers because of increasing age and the frustration of ambitions for promotion. The squeeze on promotions also tends to drive many climbers out of the organization into faster growing agencies if alternatives are available. From this point of view, then, the nature of individuals, with their private goals, combined with the more or less natural course of events, results in the organizational patterns of growth and decline, energy and stagnation that we have come to recognize.

Measurement and Control of Performance

The discussion thus far has repeatedly stressed the importance of goals. Our consideration of the nature of organizations, therefore, would be incomplete if we disregarded the extent of achievement of goals. For the present, we shall confine attention to a few basic principles of performance and control, postponing more detailed discussion to the sections on communications networks and information systems.

The measurement of performance is sometimes thought to be a matter of providing enough data so that alarms will sound when a need for control action arises. It is true that lack of control often results from lack of useful information. In addition, however, we must consider the quality of the data and the nature of the individuals who may be sounding the alarms. The point is that it is possible to take inappropriate action just as we sometimes fail to take needed action.

> There are no easy solutions to this problem. With so many "Chicken Littles" running around claiming the sky is about to fall, the men at the top cannot do much until "Henny Penny" and "Foxy Loxy" have also started screaming for help, or there is a convergence of alarm signals from a number of unrelated sources within the organization. Even the use of high-speed, automatic data networks cannot eliminate it. The basic difficulty is not in procuring information but in assessing its significance in terms of future events—from which no human being can eliminate all uncertainty (3, p. 93).

Experience with organizations quickly reveals that the magnitude of the control problem is closely related to the size of the organization. This experience can be formalized into three basic principles of organizational control, which go along with the two laws of organization cited previously (3, p. 130). First is the *Law of Imperfect Control:*

> No one can fully control the behavior of a large organization.

Second, we have the *Law of Diminishing Control:*

> The larger any organization becomes the weaker is the control over its actions exercised by those at the top.

Third, the *Law of Decreasing Coordination* states that:

> The larger any organization becomes, the poorer is the coordination among its actions.

COMMUNICATIONS NETWORK

In his comparison of health planning groups in six different communities, Morris noted a greater tendency for such bodies to be successful when they had already established a reputation for impartiality, objectivity, and wide community interest. Obviously this requires a broadly based communications network that systematically transmits accurate and sufficiently complete information. This is a big order and causes us to seek, first, to understand better the networks through which bits of information move and, second, to identify effective systems into which the bits can be assembled.

Information coming to a given individual can be forgotten or destroyed, retained for personal use, or passed on. If it is passed on, it can be forwarded in total, in part, or in some distorted manner. The individual deciding what to do with the information is affected by his own self-interest, his understanding of the organization's interests and goals, his perception of the real world, and his interpretation of those specific data on hand. Even a piece of concrete information may have a great deal of uncertainty attached to it. For example, one may learn that 112 cases of Asian flu have been reported during a certain period in an adjacent state and still be unsure when, where, how, or whether there will be a local impact. The greater the inherent uncertainty the more latitude officials have in interpretation. They tend to emphasize one ramification of the data as being most probable, not because it really is, but because the occurrence of that result would benefit them more than other possible outcomes.

We shall discuss these communications problems in three respects: the effect of information *screening*, the impact of *distortion,* and the nature of *redundancy.* As an integral part of the exposition we shall employ a model which, while admittedly artificial and oversimplified, will contribute to the understanding of the phenomena of interest.

In the model, we postulate a hierarchy of authority containing seven levels. We will assume that the officials on the lowest (G) level are actually out in the field. The information that they collect is sent to their F level superiors who screen it and relay the most salient parts to their superiors on the E level. The screening continues in this way until eventually the information reaches the top man in the hierarchy after having been screened six times in the process.

Carrying the model a step further, we assume that each official on the G level collects one unit of data in a single time period. We further suppose that the average span of control in the organization is four, i.e., that each individual above the G level has four subordinates on the average. This means that there are 4^6, or 4,096, units of data gathered at the G level during each time period.

Screening of Information

In order to appreciate the effect of screening, let us see what would happen if the average official forwarded only one-half of the information received by him. Then, 2,048 units of data per time period would be received at the F level, 1,024 at the E level, etc., until A would receive only 64 bits of information. The winnowing process would have removed 98.4 percent of the data originally generated. By comparison, if the average official screened out only one-fourth of the data received, official A would end up with 729 units per time period, more than 11 times the amount previously calculated.

The screening process is obviously essential if higher level officials are not to be inundated with communications. The process will be successful, however, only to the extent that unimportant information is screened out and useful data are forwarded for use in higher level decision-making. Let us suppose, initially, that only one-half of the information received at any level of the hierarchy is worthy of being forwarded and that one decision results from each item of information that passes through the organization. We assume further that officials tend to usurp authority, in that at each organizational level 20 percent of the information that should be passed on for action at a higher level is held for action at the lower level.

The flow of information and decision-making is then as shown in Fig. 13.1. At the bottom of the hierarchy (Level G), only 1,638 of the 2,048 items of information deserving the attention of superiors is forwarded. If Level G personnel are ineffective in acting upon this information, 410 inadequate decisions would be made at that level. In following the information screening upward to Level A, we find that the top executive receives only 17 of 64 units, or 27 percent of the vital information he needs. Furthermore, the accumulation of ineffective decisions, indicated by the circled numbers, reveals that 680 of the 4,096 organization decisions (17 percent) are ineffective.

On the contrary, some organizations are plagued by officials who are reluctant to take certain actions of which they are fully capable. Let us suppose that at each hierarchical level, 20 percent of the information that should be acted upon is instead forwarded to superiors. Thus in our illustration, 410 of the 2,048 decisions that should be made at Level G are passed upward, along with all of the 2,048 decisions that truly merit higher action. In this case, an information flow diagram analogous to Figure 13.1 would reveal that Level A receives the 64 units of information essential to effective action at that level and 22 additional items of data as well. The top-level executive is forced, therefore, to make 86 decisions (64 + 22), of which 22 could be made equally as well at a lower level in the organization. The ratio 22/86, or 26 percent, might be considered an index of inefficiency for Level A. In all, 807 of the 4,096 decisions are taken at an unncessarily high level under these circumstances, so that over-all organizational inefficiency is at a 20 percent level.

In practice, the screening of information may be imperfect in a manner which produces both ineffectiveness and inefficiency. Suppose we combine the two foregoing sets of circumstances to postulate a situation in which 20 percent of the information deserving upward transmittal is instead retained, while 20 percent of the information that could be retained for action is instead forwarded. The information flow diagram in this case reveals that 17 percent of the 4,096 decisions are handled inefficiently and a similar percentage are

Organizational Level	Status of Information*	Items of Information Meriting: Upward Transmittal	Items of Information Meriting: Action
A	Received		17
B	Forwarded	17	
	Held	(4)	21
	Received	21	21
C	Forwarded	42	
	Held	(10)	52
	Received	52	52
D	Forwarded	104	
	Held	(26)	131
	Received	130	131
E	Forwarded	261	
	Held	(66)	328
	Received	327	328
F	Forwarded	655	
	Held	(164)	819
	Received	819	819
G	Forwarded	1638	
	Held	(410)	2048
	Received	2048	2048

*20 Percent of Information Meriting Upward Transmittal is Retained.

Fig. 13.1. Hypothetical flow of information.

ineffective. Level A receives only 17 of the 64 vital items of information but receives 8 units of unnecessary information.

With calculations such as these, we begin to gain some appreciation for the practical implications of such things as steep and flat hierarchical structures, the principles of management by exception, and the advantage of clear-cut, formal decision rules.

Quality of Informational Flow

This screening process is likely to affect not only the quantity and type of information received at each decision point but its quality, i.e., its substantive content as well. The selection principles and interpretations applied by officials at the various levels may well be different. Hence, the information that finally reaches A will have passed through six filters of different quality, and the "facts" reported to A will be quite different in content and implication from the "facts" gathered at the lowest level.

To illustrate the potential magnitude of the resulting distortion, let us simply assume that each screening destroys a certain fraction of the true meaning of the information from A's point of view. If this fraction is 10 percent, then by the time the information passes through all six filters, only about 53 percent of it will express the true state of the environment as A would have observed it himself. In particular, if individuals at Level G were to initiate budget requests which were then reduced by 10 percent at each level, the final amount determined at A would be 53 percent of the original request.

Redundancy

As A comes to recognize that the information he is receiving is incomplete or distorted, he may try to establish more than one channel of communication reporting to him about the same events and topics. From one point of view this redundancy approach is wasteful, yet under the circumstances it may be quite productive.

Using an earlier illustration as a point of departure, let us suppose that an administrator receives from one source only one-fourth of the information he needs to have. A second, independent source of the same kind would likewise report one-fourth of the total, although he could expect a certain amount of duplication. The two sources combined could be expected to report to him seven-sixteenths of the total information needed, from the Additivity Law of Probability:

$$(1/4) + (1/4) - (1/4)^2 = 7/16$$

The second channel of communication, therefore, would increase the administrator's knowledge by 75 percent.

While our assumption of independence between the two channels of communication has been convenient, in practice the lack of independence may be by design, in order that competition may stimulate each of the two sources to become more productive of useful information.

INFORMATION SYSTEMS

Recent studies in the Rochester, New York, area have suggested that approximately 24 percent of total hospital operating costs may be assignable to information processing (7). Registered nurses and practical nurses spend as much as 40 percent of their time in processing or handling information, and student nurses spend as much as 30 percent of their time in similar tasks. From this and other evidence, we know that communications networks are active. We have no guarantee, however, that the many bits of information are integrated into an efficient over-all information system that actually improves the quality of the decisions made in the health planning process. On the other hand, we can be reasonably sure that the collection and processing of data will be costly and time-consuming, and that the amount of data which decision makers can absorb regarding any one problem is limited. For these reasons, we shall take a brief look at information systems in general and describe two systems which have gained considerable attention in recent years. A third system which has recently been developed is also outlined.

Perhaps the general exposition will be clearer if we begin at the level of the individual patient record. An ideal information system would contain a complete medical history, along with certain demographic and other relevant data for each individual in the system. Then each encounter between the health services and the patient could be made entirely effective in that all relevant historical information could be utilized and duplication of effort could be avoided.

At the same time, the individual records could be combined in order to produce useful economic, epidemiologic, and other analyses. For example, an up to date computerized evaluation of the relative effectiveness of various treatment procedures could be generated on the basis of far more information than a single physician could possibly assimilate (8). In the diagnosis and treatment of a patient, the physician would avail himself of both the basic record of the given patient and the analytical results from the entire information system.

In broader terms, the health planner is in a sense a "physician" who is attempting to diagnose health problems and to recommend appropriate kinds of treatment in the form of services and programs. He, too, must deal with an information system with three constituents: basic data collection and storage, processing and analysis, and recall and utilization. The required information consists of such things as population data from census records and manpower supply information coming from training institutions, tax records, and licensing authorities. These and other data are not only stored for direct access by the planning body but are summarized and analyzed in terms of population growth and migration patterns, hospital admission trends, physician utilization rates among various segments of the population, and other factors. The information users, then, are able to extract the information either from basic records or in interpreted form, and they in turn provide a feedback to the system for purposes of updating, revision, and control.

The need for such an information system was made clear by the National Commission on Community Health Services in its statement that:

.... the paucity of comprehensive health data on a national basis shows the nationwide need to develop an automated system of data collection, storage, and retrieval, not only on statistics of births, deaths, marriages, and reportable diseases, but in a far wider area pertaining to all facets of health and disease. Such information will provide the raw materials for the research projects so necessary in improving personal and environmental health services. Additionally, automatic data processing makes statistical data more valuable in measuring the effectiveness of programs, and in testing alternative models of action (9, p. 135).

Comprehensive computerized health information systems offer the potential of increased accessibility of data. There is a danger, however, that they may be so cumbersome and poorly integrated that the information they finally generate is no longer timely. The Commission recommends the establishment of regional centers and information clearinghouses that would be accessible not only to large medical centers but also to small hospitals, direct service health plans, and individual physicians in rural areas.

The value of information systems can perhaps best be judged following a description of specific forms that have been developed. First, we shall consider the broadly based planning-programming-budgeting system (PPBS). Then we shall discuss a somewhat narrower technique for program evaluation and review, one form of which is the familiar PERT.

Planning-Programming-Budgeting System

In its broadest sense, an information system should link together and entirely encompass the planning, implementation, evaluation, and control aspects of activity. In the past we have had well-developed financial accounting and budgeting systems oriented toward control, while at the other end of the spectrum, planning has often gone on at rather sophisticated levels. Frequently, however, disparity between the budgets and the plans has evidenced the lack of serious intention to implement the plans. As a result, budgets have usually been spelled out in terms of "object accounts," such as wages and salaries, travel allowances, and purchase of specified materials and equipment. They have thus stressed things to be acquired rather than services to be performed. They have shown in *what* ways agencies are spending money, but not *why*.

In recent years the planning and budgeting activities have been brought together into a system, PPBS, which includes a multi-year portrayal of anticipated program developments, along with a detailed budget covering the first year of this span (10). Annual reviews provide revisions of the multi-year plans and new budgets for the upcoming year.

In particular, PPBS is a five-step process of comparison and coordination involving:

1. Appraisals and comparisons of various government activities in terms of their contributions to national objectives;
2. Determination of how given objectives can be attained with minimum expenditure of resources;
3. Projection of government activities over an adequate time horizon;
4. Comparison of the relative contribution of private and public activities to national objectives;
5. Revisions of objectives, programs, and budgets in the light of experience and changing circumstances (11, pp. 26-27).

As the process is put into action, certain unique features emerge. In the first place, emphasis is given to *ends as well as means.* Consequently, the system contributes to the sharpening of objectives. Second, a comprehensive set of information is developed concerning the functioning of existing programs in terms of the amounts of resources being allocated to particular purposes, their costs, and the accomplishments of the programs. The system, therefore, emphasizes *quantitative,* but not necessarily monetary, *comparisons.* Third, the expected *costs and benefits* of alternative means to the desired ends are examined. Finally, a forward-looking, although tentative, plan emerges as the backdrop for annual *budgetary decisions.* The tentative plans are subject to modification for political or other nonquantitative reasons. The system is such, however, that the cost of such political intervention is made apparent.

The scope of PPBS is broad enough to permit programming to take place along several dimensions. The orientation may be in terms of major objectives such as voter appeal or increased productivity. On the other hand, classification might be made on the basis of the prospective beneficiary groups such as urban dwellers versus rural residents, or the aged versus children. Finally, distinctions might be made according to the timing of the benefits, recognizing that some programs soon produce results whereas others are investments in future benefits.

For a concrete illustration of the difference between program budgets and standard administrative budgets, we refer to two different compilations of United States government health expenditures compiled by Frankel for the 1965 fiscal year (12, pp. 229-230, 238-239). In Table 13.1 we find a listing of expenditures by agency, while in Table 13.2 we find the same funds listed according to the program category classifications which Frankel proposes. The most striking thing about the first table is the substantial involvement in health revealed to exist outside the Department of Health, Education and Welfare.

Table 13.2 has several interesting features from a programming standpoint. For one thing, it assists in delineating the choices available to the programmer. For example, research that extends our ability to immunize against communicable diseases will alter the balance between outlays for control and prevention versus treatment and restoration. In addition, the table raises questions about priorities. To illustrate, we note that research expenditures on chronic diseases and on diseases of age are more than three times as great as those on mental illness and comprise more than one-fourth of total health research expenditures. Yet, over one-half of the expenditures on long-term care are allocated to mental illness, and less than one-third goes for chronic diseases and diseases of age.

Admitting the advantage of linking the planning and budgeting activities, it might seem logical to revamp organizational structures to conform to program designs. Then program budgets would not be so radically different from the old-fashioned agency budgets. As a matter of fact, this suggestion should be taken seriously to whatever extent is possible. There are reasons, however, why we are never likely to witness a perfect one-to-one correspondence between programs and administrative agencies.

For one thing, existing organization patterns usually have deep historical roots that are not easily changed. A second, more rational argument against change is that current programming structures are not permanent, and stability in the organization may be worth the price of some inconsistency with the structure that contemporary logic may suggest. Third, occasions arise in which overlapping program structures are sensible, and in such cases a given organization is not likely to be able to do full justice to both of them. For example, the

Table 13.1
Estimated Federal Health Expenditures Classified by Agency, 1965

Administrative Budget by Agency	Estimated Amount (Millions of Dollars)
Department of Health, Education and Welfare	2867.9
Veterans Administration	1326.6
Atomic Energy Commission	93.1
Department of Agriculture	252.6
National Aeronautics and Space Administration	54.0
National Science Foundation	35.0
Housing and Home Finance Agency	29.2
Civil Service Commission	26.7
Department of State	1.0
Department of Labor	17.0
Department of Justice	11.8
Department of the Interior	15.8
Small Business Administration	2.8
General Services Administration	2.0
United States Information Agency	0.1
Public Works Acceleration (Presidential Fund)	87.0
	4822.6
Other	585.7
Total Net Budget Expenditure for Health	5408.3

Table 13.2
Estimated Federal Expenditures for Health and
Related Purposes, 1965

Category	Amount (Millions of Dollars)
Control and Prevention	
Infectious and allergic diseases	94.8
Neurologic and degenerative diseases	3.4
Chronic diseases and those of age	19.8
Accidents and occupational hazards	20.8
Food and drug hazards	153.9
Child health and nutrition	211.3
Other (including environmental health)	231.7
Total	735.7
Treatment and Restoration	
Rehabilitation and development	230.3
Chronic diseases	44.3
General illnesses	1,049.7
Other (including unallocable facilities costs)	328.2
Total	1,652.5
Long-Term Care and Domiciliary Maintenance	
Chronic diseases	4.7
Care of aged	249.4
Mental illness	412.0
Unallocable and other	105.7
Total	771.8
Training	
Infectious and allergic diseases	11.2
Neurologic and degenerative diseases	16.8
Mental illness	83.2
Chronic disease and those of age	32.2
Unallocable and other	184.6
(Allocable)	(49.5)
	328.0
Research	
Infectious and allergic diseases	58.9
Neurologic and degenerative diseases	69.6
Mental illness	92.3
Chronic diseases and those of age	325.4
Occupational and other hazards	3.7
Unallocable and other	563.1
(Allocable)	(89.9)
	1,113.0
Other	
Training and research combined	28.6
Unallocable–Overlap, two or more categories	193.0
Total	221.6
Grand Total	4,822.6

SOURCE: Adapted from: *The Budget of the United States Government for the Fiscal Year Ending June 30, 1965.* Appendix. Washington, D.C.: Government Printing Office, 1964.

communicable diseases control objective has both functional and regional connotations. In the comparison of alternatives and program *planning,* the functional view is important; on the other hand, *implementation* at the regional level may be more effective if a noncategorical organizational base is employed. Fourth and finally, we recall the specialization feature of organizations. With this in mind, it may be quite reasonable to organize a homogeneous set of activities into, say, a testing laboratory, which serves a variety of programs and objectives.

At this point, we may echo the thoughts of Frankel:

> This very extensive overlapping of agency responsibilities, together with the multiple responsibilities of some agencies, leads to concern over the possible adverse effects of competing interests and jurisdictional claims on the planning and implementation of programs. It also causes one to doubt whether there can exist in the administrative echelons the kind of over-all perspective that would seem indispensable if . . . health resources are to be rationally allocated (12, pp. 236-237).

Apart from these administrative difficulties, the PPBS approach raises at least three technical problems. First, it ultimately forces us to deal with *measurements* of unlike things (a case of measles prevented and a pneumonia cured, for example) that apply to different points in time. Second, the application of such measurement procedures requires *analytical skills* that are in short supply. Third, complex as the programming may be, it may touch upon only a *fraction* of the total problem. The far-flung federal health programs in the United States, for example, reflect only about one-eighth of total health expenditures.

Clearly, then, PPBS is not the final word in information systems. At the same time, however, we must admit that its systematic integrated view of planning and implementation problems certainly has great merit, even in the absence of precise, quantitative measurements.

Network Analysis

We now turn to the matter of monitoring a program in action. Generally, the program can be divided into a series of discrete *activities,* each with a well-defined end point. For example, the development of a multiphasic screening program might include such activities as the installation of an x-ray unit and the provision of a supply of Pap kits. The end point of such activities, or *events,* as they are called, might be identified by such statements as "x-ray unit in place" and "Pap kits on hand." Another general feature of programs is that the individual activities are *ordered* to some extent. The installation of the x-ray unit could not begin, for instance, until blueprints had been drawn up specifying locations for the various pieces of equipment. Under these conditions, a technique known as network analysis can be very useful.

We shall describe the technique with the aid of a hypothetical, oversimplified illustration. We suppose that a crisis has arisen which requires the construction, staffing, and supplying of a crude health center. Hopefully, this is to be accomplished within a 15 day period. The planning begins with a listing as in Table 13.3 of the individual jobs that must be performed. The listing consists of a brief description of associated events and arbitrarily assigned reference numbers. It is also necessary to record the expected time required to perform each of the tasks. Table 13.3 lists these times in days, although other time units can be used according to individual circumstances. Finally, considering the problem of sequencing, we must identify for each task the last job that must be completed before the one in question can start. For example, job No. 5, which involves the laying of brick to form the exterior wall of the building, cannot begin until the basic framework, identified with job No. 1, is in place.

Once the information of Table 13.3 is compiled, the network of Figure 13.2 can be diagrammed. Observe that this network records the individual events in their required sequence, and lists the estimated times involved. The network analysis can then proceed either from the diagram itself or, in more complicated cases, from a computerized analog of the network.

The first thing to note is that there are many paths leading from the start to the finish of the project. Presumably, one of these will require more time to traverse than any of the others, and will thus be of special concern. In the present illustration, this so-called *critical path* is the sequence 0-1-6-14 and is denoted by a double line. Only by finding ways to shorten jobs along the critical

Table 13.3
Hypothetical Health Center Activation Problem

Event Number	Event Description	Estimated Time (Days)	Predecessor Event
0	Start	—	
1	Building framework in place	4	0
2	Electrical wiring installed	2	1
3	Plumbing installed	3	0
4	Cement floor ready for use	2	3
5	Brick outer wall completed	6	1
6	Inside walls plastered and dry	10	1
7	Roof installed	2	1
8	Drug list authorized	4	0
9	Drugs ordered	1	8
10	Drugs received	7	9
11	Personnel authorized	2	0
12	Personnel recruited	3	11
13	Personnel trained	5	12
14	Health center operating–finish	2	2, 4, 5, 6, 7, 10, 13

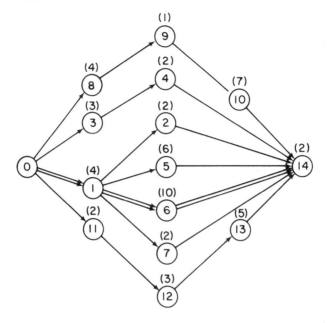

PATH	TIME	SLACK
0-8-9-10-14	14	2
0-3-4-14	7	9
0-1-2-14	8	8
0-1-5-14	12	4
0-1-6-14	16	0
0-1-7-14	8	8
0-11-12-13-14	12	4

KEY

(6) TIME (DAYS)

(5) EVENT NUMBER

Fig. 13.2. Activity network based upon Table 13.3.

path can the over-all project time be reduced. In our case, the estimated time required to traverse this path is 16 days, one more than the number initially allotted to the project.

Each path other than the critical one has *slack time,* which is the difference between the critical path time and that associated with the given path of interest. As an example, the estimated time required for path 0-11-12-13-14 is 12 days, which means that this path has four days slack time.

Such calculations are useful for two reasons. In the first place, the noncritical path with the least slack time gives evidence of the maximum reduction in total project time that can accrue from modifications of the critical path. Suppose, for example, that the project director in our illustration, recognizing job No. 6 to be critical, decides to consider the use of a more costly, prefabricated substitute for plaster. If this substitution reduces job No. 6 time from ten days to six, the time of the formerly critical path will be reduced by four days, but the total project time will be reduced by only two days. This is because path 0-8-9-10-14 will become critical, so that the only saving in project time will be the two days of slack formerly associated with this path.

The second use of slack time is to provide flexibility in the conduct of the project. Consider, for instance, the fact that path 0-11-12-13-14 has two days more slack than path 0-8-9-10-14. Both paths entail administrative red tape in the form of personnel authorization in the one case and drug authorization in the other. Recognizing the difference in urgency between these two administrative tasks, the project officer might choose to take early, perhaps costly, action to expedite the drug authorization, even at the expense of a slight increase in personnel authorization time. In order to visualize opportunities in this direction better, the project officer will probably compile a list of *late start* and *late finish* times for each job. These will indicate the maximum delay that can be tolerated in the initiation or completion of any activity without affecting the total project time.

The approach to network analysis that we have just described is called the Critical Path Method (CPM), which is one of the earliest and simplest forms. Perhaps the most important factor which it fails to recognize is the possibility of error in the time estimates. The Program Evaluation and Review Technique (PERT) is the best known approach that includes the error feature (13). In PERT applications, the estimator provides not only an expected time requirement for each activity but "most pesssimistic" and "most optimistic" estimates as well. The calculated required time is then a weighted average in which the best estimate is given four times as much weight as either of the other two. The range of possible error incorporated into the estimates is further used to calculate such probabilistic aspects as the likelihood of completion by the target date, most probable completion date, etc.

A number of other refinements will be mentioned only in passing, in order to indicate the many aspects of planning that can be incorporated into network analysis. PERT/COST adds the consideration of resource costs to the schedule produced by the PERT procedure. As we have seen in our simple illustration of plastering, time can often be purchased at a price. Apart from this, the allocation of expenditures is important in itself. Similarly, PERT/MANPOWER recognizes the importance of personnel allocation and utilization.

In view of the fact that a plan usually includes several projects, a technique known as Resource Allocation and Multi-Project Scheduling (RAMPS) has been developed (14). Finally, for cases in which results can be achieved in a variety of ways, the alternative sets of activities can be analyzed by means of Decision CPM (15).

Greater sophistication in approach may produce more meaningful results, but it also requires more and better information and greater analytical effort. Even in its simplest form, however, network analysis, like program budgeting, is useful in providing a framework for the orderly consideration of complex problems.

Functional Analysis: The Functional Information Generating System

The third information system, which is designed more specifically for health services, is the Functional Information Generating System (FIGS) developed in a multinational study of health center functions (16). The conceptual framework underlying the Functional Information Generating System uses health functions as a bridge between a community's health needs and available health resources. The number, scope, and definitions of the functions are somewhat arbitrary. The main consideration is that they represent semi-independent areas of health concern without regard for traditional administrative divisions. At present, two applications of this methodology for health planning seem practical, as well as a further application for health services research. First, as a descriptive exercise, functional analysis reveals gross inefficiencies and anachronisms which can be adjusted in accordance with needs and priorities. Second, by obtaining repeated measurements over time within this functional framework, it may be possible to establish an evaluative process that will facilitate continuing adjustment of health services to changing health status by concentrating on the bridge between these two areas. From the research point of view, such periodic functional analyses carry the potential of permitting assessment of the effectiveness of alternative service program packages in field trials. Table 13.4 presents the streamlined FIGS format developed through field research in India, Turkey, and Taiwan. It represents one minimum array of health needs and services information necessary for meaningful comprehensive appraisal.

Functions

This system accommodates 11 functions (as seen in the middle section of Table 13.4). The first four—medical relief, personal preventive services, maternity services, and family planning—are personal services stimulated by the felt needs of the consumers of the services. A second set of five functions—communicable disease control, environmental sanitation, mass population control, mental health, and general health education—are basically services stimulated through provider initiative. A third set consists of two functions—internal administration and liaison—which are nonspecific with respect to particular services but which facilitate the conduct of all operational responsibilities.

Needs

Table 13.4 is organized so that health needs are classified and quantified on the left side, channeled through the functional grid which runs down the center of the figure, and then related to the services as indicated on the right side. It should be clear that in order to specify magnitudes of need, one must collect information regarding related factors. For example, the need for maternity care is dependent upon the birth rate, but other factors (maternal and neonatal death rates, pregnancy complications) are also relevant. Needs have been defined according to a data flow through three stages: first, the form in which data were most readily collected; second, grouping into categories providing a logical transition to service programs; and third, the numbers in each category requiring service with different units, e.g., people, deaths, households, or special facilities such as pumps.

Services

The analysis of services (right side of Table 13.4) requires at least three types of measurement: (1) number of client contacts or other service units; (2) time spent in rendering the service; and (3) cost. Individual service categories to be analyzed in this manner depend upon technical considerations relating to the providers and upon relevant characteristics of the clients. Technically, for example, it is useful to analyze medical relief services in terms of patient consultations (diagnosis and advice), injections, dispensing of drugs, and other forms of treatment. Service contacts are enumerated separately for members of the particular services system being studied, for other health profession providers, and for lay sources of service such as family and friends. Time and cost allocations usually are of interest only for the system being studied or evaluated. Time can be allocated among auxiliary workers, middle level workers, and upper level workers. In allocating costs, a distinction should be made between personnel cost, other recurring costs of operation, and capital cost.

Uses of Functional Information Generating Systems

The system provides a means of assessing all aspects of needs, resources, and functions. As part of the analysis of needs, data on population characteristics and mortality and morbidity levels (for adequate population base) constitute the basic information input and will provide, for example, a distribution of estimated annual episodes of illness per person and per 100,000 population for the area under study. Information generated on utilization of services (through community surveys, health center records, or other sources) leads to various estimates which can be used in assessing the health care system. Such data, for example, will include figures for both the total number of persons with health problems and the total number seeking care. Subtracting the latter figure from the former will give the total number lacking service and thus presumably with unmet needs. Measures of the extent and nature of activities and services of the health center can be derived from data in the segments of the format under service units and time expended per level of worker. Analyses might be made,

Table 13.4

Needs			FUNCTIONS	Services
Data collected	Categories	Numbers		Type of service units
Diagnostic complaint Duration	Grade 1 Grade 2 Grade 3 Grade 4 Grade 5	Patients	MEDICAL RELIEF	Diagnosis— advice Injection Dispensing Other treatment
Birth rate Morbidity Infant mortality rate Ages 1-4 mortality rate Immunization status Nutritional status	Growth and development Maintenance and promotion Protection	Persons	PERSONAL PREVENTIVE	Routine examination Immunization Nonspecific Nutrition
Birth rate Complication rate	Antenatal Natal Postnatal	Deliveries	MATERNITY	Antenatal Delivery Postpartum
Marital status Living children and sons Knowledge, attitudes, practices	Spacing Limitation	Eligible couples	FAMILY PLANNING	Motivation Acceptance by contraceptive method Follow-up
Clinical morbidity Disease prevalence Vectors Environmental conditions	Surveillance Primary prevention Immunization Vector control Mass or local treatment	Population of house- holds	COMMUNI- CABLE DISEASE CONTROL	Surveillance visits Surveys Immunization Treatments Environmental control
Morbidity Water sources and uses Sanitation practices and facilities Crowding and housing	Availability and purity of water Waste disposal Food preparation Clean air Adequate housing	Specific facilities	ENVIRON- MENTAL SANITATION	Provision of facilities Motivation and education in use Maintenance
Rate of population growth Relation to economic development Relation to social services	Community development Population Education Economic factors	Population units	MASS POPULATION CONTROL	Economic incentives Educational measures Social change Legal support Administrative facilities

Functional Information Generating System (FIGS)

	Services								
Client Characteristics	Numbers of contacts			Time			Cost		
	System under study	Other practitioners	Layman	Auxiliary	Middle	Upper	Personnel	Other recurring	Capital
Age Sex Socioeconomic status									
Age Socioeconomic status									
Risk level Complications									

Living children
  and sons
Educational and
  socioeconomic
  status									

Persons Households Community									
Household composition Community character- istics Socioeconomic status									
Cultural character- istics Social organization Economic status Educational status									

Table 13.4 —*Continued*

Needs			FUNCTIONS	Services
Data collected	Categories	Numbers		Type of service units
Morbidity for mental illness Institutional admissions Cultural patterns Specific situational pressures	Stress charac-teristics Mental development Protection from drug dependency Protection from alcohol dependency	Persons	MENTAL HEALTH	Diagnosis (community and personal) Prevention and treatment
All of above Community structure Existing belief and knowledge Cultural pattern	Knowledge of health hazards Favorable disposi-tion to action Understanding appropriate action	Persons Households Schools Communi-ties	GENERAL HEALTH EDUCATION	School, mass media, group meetings Organization of individual contacts Community organizations
Data system Information requirements Staff (size, config-uration) Physical resources (size, configuration)	Supervision Organization and coordination of services Manpower maint. and development Financial accountability Evaluation	Manpower facilities Budget Reports	INTERNAL ADMINIS-TRATION	Planning, supervision, training Information control —Personnel —Inventory —Financial —Operations Evaluation
Channels of authority and administrative relationships Program responsibilities Consumer knowledge, satisfaction Referral patterns	Coordination with other admin-istrative units Program coordina-tion and role identification with other providers Facilitation: consumer rapport	Adminis-trative units	LIAISON	Referral meetings Administrative contacts Reports

Table 13.4–*Continued*

	Services								
Client Characteristics	Numbers of contacts			Time			Cost		
	System under study	Other practitioners	Layman	Auxiliary	Middle	Upper	Personnel	Other recurring	Capital
Age Sex Cultural characteristics									
Age Sex Cultural characteristics									
Personnel characteristics Political patterns									
Other health services Nonhealth agencies Consumers									

for example, on (1) the percentage time distribution among activities (direct service, support or administrative service, or travel) by type of worker, (2) the percentage contribution of each worker to a given function, regardless of the service content, or (3) differences in time allocation of individual categories of workers to a single service or function. Data recorded in accordance with the model can be combined and recombined to enable researchers to carry out increasingly detailed and sophisticated analyses.

In brief, then, the possible uses of this functional analysis method as applied to health planning can be summarized as follows:

1. In a cross-sectional survey, functional analysis provides a quantitative description of health needs and resources in a population group, thereby permitting better priority setting and allocation.

2. In a continuing planning process, repeated functional analysis can measure change in health status and provide evaluation of health services, especially as new measures are introduced.

3. In a comprehensive analytic system which includes cost accounting, functional analysis provides a basis for cost-effectiveness comparisons.

REFERENCES

1. Blum, H. L. "Research into the Organization of Community Health Service Agencies—An Administrator's Review." *Milbank Memorial Fund Quarterly* 44:52-93, No. 3, Part 2, July, 1966.
2. Likert, R. "A Motivational Approach to a Modified Theory of Organization and Management." In: Haire, Mason, editor. *Modern Organization Theory.* New York: John Wiley & Sons, Inc., 1959.
3. Downs, A. *Bureaucratic Structure and Decision Making.* Memorandum RM-4646-1-PR. Santa Monica, California: Rand Corporation, 1966.
4. Fleck, A. C., Jr. "Evaluation of Research Programs in Public Health Practice." *Annals of the New York Academy of Science* 107:717-724, 1963.
5. Argyris, C. "How Tomorrow's Executives Will Make Decisions." *Think:* 18-23, November-December, 1967.
6. Morris, R. "Basic Factors in Planning for the Coordination of Health Services." *American Journal of Public Health* 53:248-259 and 462-472, 1963.
7. Fanwick, Charles. "Systems Development as a Part of Planning for Health Enterprises." pp. 66-81. In: *Planning for Health: Report of the 1967 National Health Forum.* New York: National Health Council, 1967.
8. Ledley, R. S. "Computer Aids to Clinical Treatment Evaluation." *Operations Research* 15:694-705, 1967.
9. National Commission on Community Health Services. *Health Is a Community Affair.* Report of the National Commission. Cambridge: Harvard University Press, 1966.
10. Novick, David, editor. *Program Budgeting.* Cambridge: Harvard University Press, 1965.
11. Smithies, A. "Conceptual Framework for the Program Budget." In: Novick, D., editor. *Program Budgeting.* Cambridge: Harvard University Press, 1965.

12. Frankel, M. "Federal Health Expenditures in a Program Budget." In: Novick, D., editor. *Program Budgeting.* Cambridge: Harvard University Press, 1965.
13. Arnold, M. F., editor. *Health Program Implementation through PERT.* San Francisco: Western Regional Office, American Public Health Association, 1966.
14. Lambourn, S. "Resource Allocation and Multiproject Scheduling (RAMPS)—A New Tool in Planning and Control." *The Computer Journal* 5:300-304, 1963.
15. Crowston, W. and Thompson, G. L. "Decision CPM: A Method for Simultaneous Planning, Scheduling and Control of Projects." *Operations Research* 15:407-426, 1967.
16. Reinke, W. A., Taylor, C. E., and Parker, R. L. "Functional Analysis of Health Needs and Services." In: *Proceedings of the Sixth International Scientific Meeting of the International Epidemiological Association,* Primosten, Yugoslavia, September, 1971. (In press)

ADDITIONAL READINGS

Primary

Dalkey, N. C. *The Delphi Method: An Experimental Study of Group Opinion.* RM-5888-PR. Santa Monica, California: Rand Corporation, June, 1969.
Discussion of an increasingly important method for establishing group consensus.
Downs, A. *Bureaucratic Structure and Decision Making.* RM-4646-1-PR. Santa Monica, California: Rand Corporation, October, 1966.
A systematic analysis of the principal features of bureaucracy.
Frazier, T. M. "The Questionable Role of Statistics in Comprehensive Health Planning." *American Journal of Public Health* 60:1701-1705, 1970.
Critical appraisal of the questions: Do we really need hard data in health planning; Are we properly using what we have?
Levy, F. K., Thompson, G. L., and Wiest, J. D. "The ABC's of the Critical Path Method." *Harvard Business Review* 41:98-108, 1963.
A simplified exposition of an important scheduling technique.
March, J. G. and Simon, H. *Organizations.* New York: John Wiley & Sons, 1958.
A classic on the principles of organization.
Planning-Programming-Budgeting Guide. Revised edition. Ottawa: Queen's Printer for Canada, 1969.
Lucid account of PPBS in English and French.
Shull, F. A., Jr., Delbecq, A. L., and Cummings, L. L. *Organizational Decision-Making.* New York: McGraw-Hill Book Co., 1970.
Another approach to group process.

Secondary

Arnold, M. F. *Health Program Implementation through PERT.* San Francisco: Western Regional Office, American Public Health Association, 1966.
Bauer, Katherine G. *Problems and Perspectives in the Design of a Community Health Information System.* Final Report of the Project for the Preliminary

Design of a Health Information System for Boston. Cambridge, Massachusetts: Joint Center for Urban Studies of M.I.T. and Harvard University, February, 1969.

Derry, J. R., Lubin, J. W., Laird, O. M., Carrell, C., Chelew, P. G., and Ribak, N. "An Information System for Health Facilities Planning." *American Journal of Public Health* 58:1414-1421, 1968.

Gaines, C. W. "The Role of the Management Person in a Health Agency." *American Journal of Public Health* 59:663-665, 1969.

Haire, M., editor. *Modern Organization Theory*. New York: John Wiley & Sons, Inc., 1959.

Kissick, W. L. "Planning, Programming and Budgeting in Health." *Medical Care* 5:201-220, 1967.

McKean, R. N. *Public Spending*. New York: McGraw-Hill Book Co., 1968.

Merton, W. "PERT and Planning for Health Programs." *Public Health Reports* 81:449-454, 1966.

Michael, J. M., Spatafore, G., and Williams, E. R. "A Basic Information System for Health Planning." *Public Health Reports* 83:21-28, 1968.

Miller, R. W. "How to Plan and Control with PERT." *Harvard Business Review* 40:93-104, 1962.

Mott, B. J. F. *Anatomy of a Coordinating Council: Implications for Planning*. Pittsburgh: University of Pittsburgh Press, 1968.

Noble, J. H. "Designing Information Systems for Comprehensive Health Planning." *Inquiry* 7:34-40, 1970.

Peters, R. J. and Kinniard, J. *Health Services Administration*. London: E. and S. Livingstone Ltd., 1965.

Planning-Programming-Budgeting: Guidance for Program and Financial Plan. Revised edition. Washington, D. C.: Government Printing Office, March, 1969.

Quade, E. S. *Systems Analysis Techniques for Planning-Programming-Budgeting*. Publication No. P-3322. Santa Monica, California: Rand Corporation, 1966.

Rosner, M. M. "Administrative Controls and Innovation." *Behavioral Science* 13:36-43, 1968.

14

Decision Theory, Systems Analysis, and Operations Research

WILLIAM A. REINKE

Even in the most developed countries, health needs outstrip health resources. Even our technical capacity to satisfy these needs exceeds our economic capability to do so. As a result, we find increasing support for the position that technical research must be accompanied by analysis at the operating level so that limited resources—human, physical, organizational, and informational—are used most effectively.

As we formulate the analysis, we are inevitably struck by the number and variety of interrelated relevant factors that must be included. Many must be regarded as intangibles, and even the quantitative factors are often difficult to measure, highly variable, and steeped in uncertainty. To illustrate, the extent to which a new 300-bed hospital would affect the health status of the surrounding community cannot be assessed directly. Even if we resort to indirect measures such as bed utilization rates, we may be discouraged by fluctuations in usage and the difficulty of forecasting. Rather than being a source of discouragement, however, these facts of life should motivate us to identify patterns, so that we can to some degree control the statistical variation. To state this in the popular jargon of the day, we are espousing systems analysis that will provide "well organized information, analysis of alternatives, and methods of evaluating consequences of decision-making practices" (1, p. 66).

ELEMENTS OF THE DECISION PROCESS

For purposes of roughly sketching the essential elements of the decision process, let us suppose that we face the problem of staffing a rural maternal health center. Alternative staffing patterns can be shown schematically by a "decision tree" such as Figure 14.1.

At point D_1 a decision must be made from among three contemplated alternatives:

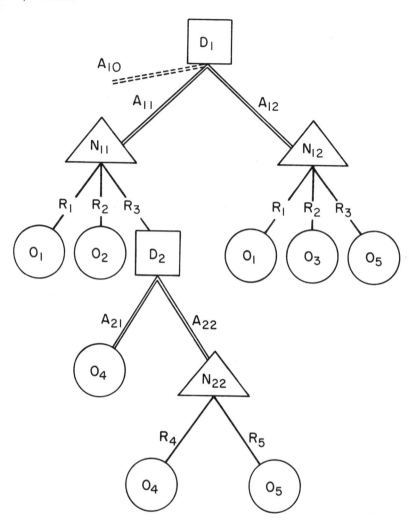

□ D = DECISION
  A = ACTION VARIABLE
△ N = NATURE
  R = RANDOM VARIABLE
○ O = OUTCOME

Fig. 14.1. Hypothetical decision tree.

A_{10}—Operate the health center as a "self-serve" delivery facility without staff;

A_{11}—Employ a midwife only;

A_{12}—Retain a physician as well as a midwife.

Alternative A_{10} is clearly unacceptable and would normally be excluded from the decision tree. There are usually so many possible choices that the decision maker must restrict himself to valued alternatives. In the interests of simplicity, we have included only two such alternatives at D_1.

Choices A_{11} and A_{12} are called *action variables*. In general, action variables are the alternatives that are subject to the discretion of the decision maker. In addition, there are *random variables* beyond the decision maker's control. They might be thought of as the acts which are subject to the discrimination of nature, i.e., chance. In fact, decision theory is sometimes conceived as a game which pits the decision maker against nature. The decision maker attempts to prepare himself against the uncertain acts of nature in such a way that those acts are most rewarding or least damaging to him.

In our illustration, pregnancy outcome is an important random variable. We shall distinguish among three possibilities:

R_1—Routine pregnancies;

R_2—Complications present which require special medical attention;

R_3—Complications present which require special medical and surgical attention.

The decision maker cannot know in advance whether all cases in the next (specified) time interval will be routine or whether complications will be encountered. In effect, after he selects action A_{11} or A_{12}, nature gets a "turn" at N_{11} or N_{12} to select (at random) condition R_1, R_2, or R_3.

The combined responses of the decision maker and nature produce a number of possible *outcomes*. In compiling the present list, we assume that a midwife cannot handle surgical complications at all, and that she treats medical complications with less skill than a physician would. Thus, we arrive at five possible outcomes:

O_1—Routine deliveries only;

O_2—Medical complications inadequately treated;

O_3—Medical complications skillfully treated;

O_4—Surgical complications unattended;

O_5—Surgical complications attended.

In the event that a complicated case is encountered with only the midwife present at the health center, we suppose that the opportunity exists to seek treatment at a neighboring hospital. Thus, we have a second decision point D_2, with alternatives:

A_{21}—Do not seek hospital care;

A_{22}—Seek hospital care.

Even if hospital services are sought, delays or other problems in reaching the hospital may cause service there to be essentially unavailable. We have two new chance conditions, therefore:

R_4—Hospital service unavailable;

R_5—Hospital service available.

One of the more complicated paths of Figure 14.1 is $D_1 N_{11} D_2 N_{22} O_5$. This describes a situation in which the decision maker decides to employ a midwife only (A_{11}), but surgical complications (R_3) arise, so that he makes a second decision to seek hospital treatment of the complications (A_{22}); this story ends happily, as hospital treatment is successfully accomplished (R_5).

While we do not propose that the decision process need always be displayed as graphically as in Figure 14.1, the decision tree does point out elements of the process clearly and systematically. The attempt to reach a specified goal is characterized by decision points (D) at which the decision maker may take discretionary action and points (N) at which nature, or chance, intervenes to produce results that are beyond the control of the decision maker. The discretionary actions (A) are known as action variables, while responses (R) beyond the decision maker's control are called chance, or random, variables. A sequence of action and chance variables eventually leads to an end point or outcome (O). The path that leads to an outcome point is called a *consequence.* Since different paths may lead to the same outcomes, there are likely to be more consequences (means) than outcomes (ends). Figure 14.1 contains eight consequences and five outcomes.

The decision maker's *strategy* is defined by the combination of action variables he selects. In our illustration, the selection of A_{11} could lead to decision point D_2 and a choice between alternatives A_{21} and A_{22}. Combination $A_{11} A_{21}$ depicts one strategy, while $A_{11} A_{22}$ defines a second. The third and final strategy embodied in the figure is alternative A_{12} alone.

The decision maker's choice of strategy will depend upon the alternatives perceived and his assessment of the outcomes that might result. This assessment will involve the *valuation* he places upon the various outcomes and the *likelihood* that given strategies will produce particular outcomes.

SYSTEMS ANALYSIS

In order that a comprehensive list of reasonable alternatives may be assembled, the decision maker must take an imaginative open-minded view of the entire system involved. The individual patient usually approaches the physician with a particular problem that has arisen from certain symptoms. In his diagnosis and treatment, however, the competent physician deals with the entire physical, emotional, and social system at hand. Similarly, the administrator often calls attention to a particular trouble spot, and the systems analyst responds with a broad analysis of the many interrelated factors that have a bearing upon the original problem.

Steps

In proceeding with the systems analysis we must first identify the *elements* of the system. These include the characteristics and health needs of the inhabitants served by the system, the existing manpower, facilities, and organizational base, and the underlying laws, regulations, practices, and procedures which must be reckoned with.

Once the system elements have been identified, their *interrelationships* must be established to determine how the elements perform or, quite as important, how they fail to perform. This means that the roles of specific types of health workers cannot be assumed in advance, but must be analyzed in relation to health needs in the particular situation under investigation and with respect to the monetary, organizational, and facilities constraints that exist. The systems approach also stresses the interrelationships between health officials and politicians, between health agencies and others, and among health agencies, as for example between clinics and hospitals.

Next, a careful operational statement of *goals* is required to guide the system into the proper channels for accomplishment. The goals must be defined in terms of the operations that will have been realized when the goals are attained.

At this point, the systems analyst should be prepared to develop an analytical *model*, along with a graphic description of the system and its subsystems.

The model serves as a base for the consideration of possible *modifications* of the system. Expert professional opinion in a variety of disciplines can be utilized to select promising alternatives, but underlying the assessment must be a set of clearly defined criteria for evaluation in order that the systems analysis does not become a series of off-the-cuff private statements of opinion.

The assessment of alternatives should lead to the *selection* of an improved set of relationships designed to provide a more efficient and logical operation of the system in terms of its functional characteristics and capabilities. The selection process may be hampered by a lack of available information in certain areas. Thus, for example, a determination of the prospects for increasing use of chronic care facilities may require studies of existing facilities along with present and future needs. Observe, however, that the information gathering will be limited to those investigations which make an effective contribution to the understanding of the system potential and thereby affect decision-making. In the end, of course, these decisions may be further affected by political, social, or cultural constraints. The analysis should include an evaluation of the impact of the constraints and prospects for their removal.

In summary, systems analysis requires:

1. Recognition of the system elements;
2. Identification of the interrelationships among elements;
3. A statement of goals;
4. Development of an analytical model;
5. Consideration of alternative system modifications;
6. Selection of one of these alternatives.

Application to Health Services

While the components of systems analysis may fit together logically enough, the approach may appear rather abstract for something no more clear-cut than the health services system. We should not be deterred, however, for we do have available some rather specific guidelines that can be useful in the analysis. There are, for example, the attributes of good medical care proposed by Dr. George James: competence, comprehensiveness, continuity, patient-family focus, community orientation, and timeliness. Further, our system must certainly embody the medical activity sequence of prevention, detection, diagnosis, treatment or cure, rehabilitation, and long-term care. Traditional institutional forms—public health agencies and hospitals—have been clearly inadequate in these terms. The "system" modifications that have evolved to try to fill the gaps have included "community clinics of great variety, out-patient departments in various roles, emergency rooms which serve few emergencies, 'experimental' extended care capabilities, and the institutionally isolated nursing homes of poor standards, limited staffing, and minimum effectiveness" (1, p. 83).

A more rational systems analysis might produce a model which would indicate that:

> ... departments of health and similar agencies should focus attention upon disease detection and prevention; out-patient departments and related clinics should evolve to recognizable institutions devoted to specialization in early diagnosis and early treatment; hospitals as such may thus perfect a traditional treatment and teaching role; extended care should not be met by a quasi-independent institutional form in close relationship to the hospital but specializing in post-clinical treatment; ambulatory care needs should be met by comprehensive community clinics where the four functions above cited are counterparted or represented, or coordinated as the case may be, for the benefit of the patient and the community; finally, chronic care requirements should be met by an institutional form quite as formalized as the hospital (1, p. 87).

Multidisciplinary Approach

The comprehensive approach that we have described requires a multiplicity of talents that no one individual possesses. This leads to the need for a multidisciplinary team which Andersen has suggested should at least consist of a public health administrator, an epidemiologist, a mathematician, a statistician, and a social scientist (2). On larger teams the general social scientist would be replaced by an economist and a sociologist, and a sanitary engineer and an educational specialist would be added.

OPERATIONS RESEARCH

We may appreciate the systems concept, but its identification in practice is made difficult by the fact that most entities that we contemplate are really parts of something bigger. Thus, we may visualize a regional system of hospitals, but this is not unrelated to other health agencies in the area, and even the totality of health services is not entirely independent of the prevailing educational, social, political, and economic systems. As we broaden our scope of attention, however, analytical problems mount to the point where our thinking tends to become very fuzzy; therefore, we must not carry systems analysis too far. On the other side, however, we must point out that the development of analytical procedures, along with computers, has provided a vastly increased base for systems analysis.

Nature

At the heart of these procedures is the need for experimentation, which suggests the use of the scientific method that has proved so useful in the laboratory. A distinctive feature of operational problems, however, is that the experimenter outside the laboratory usually is unable actually to manipulate and control his environment. As a result, operations research is essentially the application of the scientific method to artificial representations of real life situations. These representations are either in the form of mathematical models to be studied analytically or simulations of actual experience under hypothetical conditions.

In either case, relevant input variables are related to operational achievements. In the health field, the inputs might include the total health budget; its geographic and functional breakdown; inflow and outflow of personnel; quantity and quality of training; inflow, storage, and consumption of drugs and supplies; and distribution of all types of health services and institutions. Operational achievements might include such things as clinic attendance, vaccinations performed, number of childbirths assisted, wells constructed, drugs distributed, and other such activities. In the mathematical models, the input-output relationships are made explicit and an appropriate analytical technique such as differential calculus or linear programming is applied in order to determine the optimum relationship in some sense.

To illustrate the difference between the analytical and simulation approaches, let us suppose that a clinic wishes to study the average length of time per patient visit. This is an operational achievement that is related to patient arrival patterns and service times required. Both input factors might be considered random variables that can be expressed mathematically as specific probability distributions. The analyst could then determine mathematically, for example, the amount by which average service time must be reduced in order that not more than 10 percent of the patients seen would be required to spend a total (service + waiting) of more than one-half hour at the clinic.

In case patient arrivals are affected by bus schedules, weather conditions, and other factors that are difficult to combine into a single mathematical formulation, the analyst may resort to simulation. The simulation would first employ a random device to determine for each hypothetical moment of time under consideration whether or not a patient "arrived" at the clinic. This operation would produce an accumulation of patients in the hypothetical waiting room that would be "served" sequentially, with a random device again being employed to determine the service time consumed and hence the waiting times required of other patients. A given experiment involving a predetermined segment of time would provide evidence of the operating achievements to be expected in practice under the conditions simulated. These results would perhaps be compared with those from other experiments in which the hypothetical conditions had been altered in some way.

Methodology and Areas of Application

A good bit of the flavor of the operations research approach can be gained from concrete illustrations. We shall consider three widely different problem areas: appropriate drug inventory levels, hospital size and location, and ideal combinations of health manpower. Just as these represent major health problem areas, the techniques to be applied are fundamental to the operations research kit of tools. Nevertheless, we must emphasize that the description of both problems and techniques is highly simplified and artificial.

Supplies Inventories

In deciding how much of a particular drug to order at one time, one must recognize two conflicting factors. On the one hand, a certain fixed cost of ordering is associated with the necessary paperwork and transportation of the material. This suggests that costs might be reduced by ordering large quantities infrequently, rather than small quantities more frequently. On the other hand, large order quantities mean large inventories which require costly storage and the use of working capital that might be employed profitably elsewhere. The way in which these two individual costs vary according to order quantity is shown in Figure 14.2. The curve depicting their sum, also shown in Figure 14.2, reveals

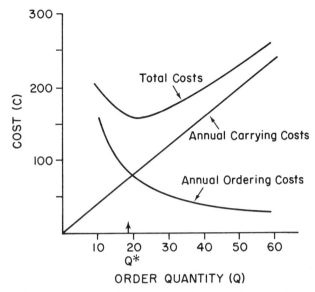

Fig. 14.2. Economic order quantity: supplies inventory.

that there is an ideal compromise resolution of the two conflicting forces at the order quantity level designated Q*. In practice this quantity need not be determined graphically, for application of the differential calculus has produced the equation:

$$Q^* = \sqrt{2SU/I},$$

where

Q* = minimum cost order quantity;
S = fixed costs of supplying an order;
U = annual usage of the item in question (in units); and
I = cost of carrying one unit of the item in inventory for one year.

In general, the higher the ordering cost, the higher the order quantity, and the higher the carrying cost, the lower the order quantity.

Suppose that two similar drugs, A and B, are each priced at $40 per case, with 100 cases of A being used per year compared to 25 cases of B. Experience has shown that the placement of an order costs $16 and the annual carrying cost after delivery is 20 percent of the purchase price. Hence,

$$2S/I = (2)(16)/8 = 4, \quad \text{and} \quad Q^* = \sqrt{4U}.$$

From this, the minimum cost order quantity of A (Q^*_a) is $\sqrt{(4)(100)}$ or 20. For B, the Q^*_b is $\sqrt{(4)(25)}$ or 10.

Given these minimum cost order quantities, an order for 20 cases of A should be placed on 5 occasions during the year and for 10 cases of B on 2.5 occasions during the year. If, on 5 occasions during the year, an order is placed for 20 cases of A, stocks will vary between 0 and 20 cases, averaging 10. The ordering plus carrying costs for A will thus be

$$(5)(16) + (10)(8) = \$160.$$

Corresponding costs for B will be $(2.5)(16) + (5)(8)$, or $80 per year.

Since A and B have been defined as similar drugs, we might consider standardization on a single product C, where C is a replacement for both A and B. Then

$$Q^*_c = \sqrt{(4)(100 + 25)} = 22.$$

Annual costs of ordering and storing this single item would amount to $179, compared with the total of $240 calculated above for A and B.

As we extend this simple illustration to more complex and real dimensions, we can see numerous opportunities and difficulties in assembling the combination of drugs that most effectively satisfies varied needs of different severity in a reasonably standardized manner.

Facility Size and Location and Utilization

The problem of standardization of drugs and supplies has its counterpart in the question of merger of separate facilities. A number of relevant factors beyond our present range of interest must enter this kind of consideration, but an important one to which we can address ourselves is the need to provide for variations in utilization. A rule of thumb suggests that accommodation to this variability will be satisfactory if the number of hospital beds provided exceeds the average usage level by three times the square root of the average. Hence, if there were an average demand for 200 beds, capacity should be

$$200 + 3\sqrt{200} = 242 \text{ beds.}$$

Then, if two hospitals are operated to serve an average demand of 200 beds each, they should each contain 242 beds, or 484 in all. In contrast, a single unit would require only

$$400 + 3\sqrt{400} = 460 \text{ beds.}$$

Moreover, if, say, one-fourth of the admissions could be scheduled and therefore removed from the influence of chance variation, total capacity could be reduced to

$$100 + [300 + 3\sqrt{300}] = 452 \text{ beds.}$$

Another important aspect of facilities planning is that of the referral relationship between scattered clinics and district hospitals. Suppose that five clinics are to relate to three such hospitals, with clinic referral loads and hospital capacities for acceptance of referrals as shown in Table 14.1. Certain referral patterns are likely to be more costly than others due to factors of transportation and inconvenience. To the extent that the cost differentials can be quantified and are constant, a form of linear programming, the *transportation technique*, can be very useful. In the illustration summarized by Table 14.1, the optimal arrangement can be shown by this technique to be as displayed in Table 14.2. The actual mechanics of the technique are discussed elsewhere (3), but the important element is that it provides an economical basis for allocation of resources in the face of various limiting constraints. For example, the constraint in this instance is hospital capacity.

Table 14.1
Data for Assessing Clinic-Hospital Relationships

Hospital	A	B	C	D	E	Hospital Capacity
	Unit Costs—Clinic to Hospital					
X	10	20	5	9	10	90
Y	2	10	8	30	6	40
Z	1	20	7	10	4	80
Clinic referrals	30	50	40	60	30	210

(Header spanning A–E: Clinic)

Table 14.2
Optimal Solution for Clinic Referrals: Based Upon Data of Table 14.1

To Hospital	A	B	C	D	E	Hospital Utilization
X			40	50		90
Y		40				40
Z	30	10		10	30	80

(Header spanning A–E: From Clinic)

Manpower Mix

In considering the application of operations research to the health manpower question, we shall call upon the widely publicized *linear programming technique*

(4). The simplex and other procedures have been developed for providing solutions to linear programming problems. Our interest, however, is not in describing a given procedure, which in practice would be applied via computer anyhow. Instead our intention is to provide a basic understanding of the nature of the approach. A graphic portrayal is most useful for these purposes, but this limits us to two dimensions, i.e., two variables. Let us consider, therefore, the problem of determining the ideal mix of doctors and nurses that should be trained and practicing in 1980 (Figure 14.3).

In order for a problem to exist, we must face certain constraints that limit our freedom of action. For example, a number of professionals who are now active or in training will still be available in 1980; therefore, it seems reasonable to insist that our solution provide for at least this minimum number of each category of workers. If this amounts to 80 physicians and 150 nurses, we block off the portions of Figure 14.3 that depict less than these amounts.

Upper limits on available funds and facilities may be of even greater concern. Suppose not more than $800,000 is expected to be available monthly to support physicians at $1,500 each and nurses at $400 each. Expressed mathematically, this means that

$$1,500D + 400N \leqslant 800,000.$$

The limiting case, where $1,500D + 400N = 800,000$, is drawn in Figure 14.3.

With respect to training facilities, we anticipate the capability to train 225

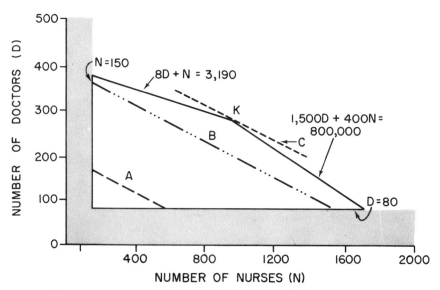

Fig. 14.3. Illustration of linear programming: manpower mix.

new doctors and 600 nurses. The ratio can be altered, but every doctor added to or deleted from the pipeline will reduce or increase the corresponding capability of training additional nurses by a factor of 8. With some algebraic manipulation, we can translate this condition into the limiting relationship

$$8D + N = 3,190$$

as noted in Figure 14.3.

Finally, let us suppose that we are able to determine that the service rendered by health workers is such that each doctor produces five service units for every one contributed by each nurse. This, in effect, states that

$$5D + N = S,$$

where S is the number of service units and is to be maximized. A series of parallel lines can be constructed to indicate various manpower mixes that will yield given service levels. Line A of Figure 14.3, for example, depicts service levels of 1,000, whereas line B portrays levels of 2,000.

We see that increasing service levels are associated with higher lines on the graph; therefore, we wish to find the highest line that contains some point that has not been blocked out as being unacceptable. This is line C, which barely touches corner K and indicates that the optimum mix consists of 280 physicians and 950 nurses. Plans should be made, therefore, to train 200 new physicians and 800 new nurses.

In addition to selecting optimum solutions to problems involving linear relationships, the linear programming technique is useful in analyzing the impact of the constraints imposed. We might wish to know, for example, how much the solution would be affected if the maximum budget were raised from $800,000 to $1,000,000. This would permit the relevant restraining line to be raised, thereby unblocking a portion of Figure 14.3 and admitting service level lines higher than C. In particular, the further analysis (not shown in the figure) reveals that the corner then associated with the new optimum would suggest that most of the additional funds be put into the training of nurses in view of the relatively low demands which they place upon the limited training facilities.

In part, our illustration is unrealistic because some of the relationships of interest are not, in fact, linear. Thus, a more complex form of mathematical programming might be more appropriate. Moreover, we have failed to recognize the dynamics of the situation with respect to the timing of training increments and the uncertainties of future needs. These elements can be incorporated into the analytical model by means of a technique known as *dynamic programming* (5). The more complex our statement of the problem, of course, the more sophisticated must be the solution. As a result, an admittedly oversimplified approach can often serve as a useful first approximation to the appropriate course of action, provided there is recognition of the weaknesses in the assumptions being made.

Other Problems

Problems dealing with medical stores, facility construction, and manpower training are quite typical of those that attract the attention of health planners. There are numerous other important concerns, however, which likewise lend themselves to the application of operations research. Several deserve brief mention, apart from any attempt to detail the particular techniques involved.

In the stores area, one may wish to go beyond optimum ways of supplying current demands to a review of the demand structure itself. For example, an analysis of physician drug prescription patterns has been reported from the United Kingdom (6).

The structure of this problem is in turn similar to those involving the routing and scheduling of patients and personnel. In personnel scheduling, one is often forced to review workload levels and the allocation of tasks, which are typical operations research problems. Job descriptions and performance are intertwined with training programs and turnover ratios, which have also been studied (7). Personnel problems likewise become entangled with facilities and organizational matters, as for example in the question of geographic area to be served by a midwife, public health nurse, or sanitarian.

More predominantly, types of problems involving facilities include such things as the allocation of beds among services, facility layout, and the effect of early hospital discharge upon out-patient and extended care facilities.

In an earlier discussion of resources, we included organization and information systems. These areas, too, offer opportunities for the fruitful use of operations research. The prime example in the information area is the effective use of records, both for administrative evaluation, control, and decision-making and for patient diagnosis and management.

As we critically appraise the organization and scope of health services, we must deal with matters of selection from among competing or complementary programs, the integration of specialized services (perhaps developed earlier on an emergency basis) into the general health services structure, and the desirability of organizing care on an "intensity of need" basis.

Perhaps we can best summarize the content of systems analysis and operations research by citing the need for a comprehensive functional analysis of the activities and impact of an entire health services system. This leads to a number of operations research applications to many interrelated substudies of the types we have listed, all of which are designed to answer the one basic, ageless question: "Who does what and how well to whom, and who gets paid for it?"

REFERENCES

1. Parks, R. B. and Adelman, H. M. *System Analysis and Planning for Public Health Care in the City of New York.* Paramus, New Jersey: System Development Corporation, 1966.
2. Andersen, S. "Operations Research in Public Health." *Public Health Reports* 79:297-305, 1964.
3. Churchman, C. West, Ackoff, Russell L., and Arnoff, E. Leonard. *Introduction to Operations Research.* New York: John Wiley & Sons, Inc., 1957.
4. Ackoff, R. L. and Sasieni, M. W. *Fundamentals of Operations Research.* New York: John Wiley & Sons, Inc., 1968.
5. Bellman, Richard. *Dynamic Programming.* Princeton: Princeton University Press, 1957.
6. Horvath, W. J. "British Experience with Operations Research in the Health Services." *Journal of Chronic Diseases* 17:779-788, 1964.
7. Flagle, C. D. "Operational Research in the Health Services." *Annals of the New York Academy of Sciences* 107:748-759, 1963.

ADDITIONAL READINGS

Primary

Andersen, S. "Operations Research in Public Health." *Public Health Reports* 79:297-305, 1964.
Some examples of the role of operations research in public health.
Halpert, H. P., Horvath, W. J., and Young, J. P. *An Administrator's Handbook on the Application of Operations Research to the Management of Mental Health Systems.* National Clearinghouse for Mental Health Information Publication No. 1003. Washington, D.C.: Government Printing Office, 1970.
Simplified presentation of operations research methods with concrete examples related to health.
McKean, R. N. *Efficiency in Government through Systems Analysis.* New York: John Wiley and Sons, Inc., 1958.
Basic reference on systems analysis in public service areas.
Raiffa, Howard. *Decision Analysis. Introductory Lectures on Choices under Uncertainty.* Reading, Massachusetts: Addison-Wesley Publishing Co., Inc., 1968.
Reasonably nontechnical presentation of the principles of decision theory.
Reinke, W. A. "The Role of Operations Research in Population Planning." *Operations Research* 18:1099-1111, 1970.
Suggested applications of operations research and decision analysis approaches to the population area.

Secondary

Ackoff, R. L. "Toward a System of Systems Concepts." *Management Science* 17:661-671, 1971.

Ackoff, R. L. and Rivett, P. *A Manager's Guide to Operations Research.* New York: John Wiley and Sons, Inc., 1963.

Arnold, M. F. "Uses of Management Tools in Health Planning." *Public Health Reports* 83:820-826, 1968.

Baumol, W. J. *Economic Theory and Operations Analysis.* Englewood Cliffs, New Jersey: Prentice Hall, 1961.

Black, Guy. *The Application of Systems Analysis to Government Operations.* New York: Frederick A. Praeger Publishers, 1968.

Churchman, C. W., Ackoff, R. L., and Arnoff, E. L. *Introduction to Operations Research.* New York: John Wiley and Sons, Inc., 1957.

Dahl, T. "Operations Research on Health Care in Chile: An Experiment." *International Journal of Health Services* 1:271-284, 1971.

Feldstein, M. S. *Economic Analysis for Health Services Efficiency: Econometric Studies of the British National Health Service.* Amsterdam: North-Holland Publishing Co., 1967.

Flagle, C. D. and Lechat, M. F. "Statistical Decision Theory and Selection of Diagnostic and Therapeutic Strategies in Public Health." *Proceedings of the Third International Conference on Operations Research, Oslo.* London: English Universities Press, 1963.

Horvath, W. J. "British Experience with OR in the Health Services." *Journal of Chronic Diseases* 17:779-788, 1964.

Revelle, C., Feldmann, F., and Lynn, W. "An Optimization Model of Tuberculosis Epidemiology." *Management Science* 16: B190-B211, December, 1969.

Stimson, D. H. "Utility Measurement in Public Health Decision Making." *Management Science* 16:B17-B30, October, 1969.

15

Methods of Planning the Distribution of Personal Health Services

VICENTE NAVARRO

Planning for personal health services involves four steps, closely related but conceptually different: the elaboration of the plan, its acceptance by those affected, its implementation, and its evaluation. This chapter reviews the methods used in the first step, the elaboration of the plan. It deals with planning for adequate and appropriate distribution of health resources. The methods described have been developed in a variety of situations that differ in time, location, and scope of concern.

METHODS BASED ON MORBIDITY

Clearly the level and structure of morbidity are important determinants of health resources utilization and thus form a possible basis for planning. Such planning has three requirements: (1) to survey the extent and character of morbidity in the subject population; this morbidity can be either "perceived" by the individual or "defined" by the health professional; (2) to translate the morbidity information into a need for certain health services; and (3) to prescribe the types and amounts of health resources required to provide the services needed.

Several investigators in different countries have conducted such morbidity studies, either in general populations or in specific ones, e.g., hospital populations (1-5). Whereas the morbidity data have been quantitative, their conversion into measurement of health resources needed usually has relied on subjective judgment, i.e., "expert professional opinion."

Among the more detailed studies is that reported by Popov from the Soviet Union (6). This study involved several cities and rural districts in which experts on delivery of medical care considered that demand for personal health services had been met, i.e., there were no waiting lists for hospitalization. For the survey, every member of the community was provided with a card on which all utilization of medical and hospital facilities was recorded for an undetermined period of time. Following this utilization survey, a health examination survey was carried out by medical specialists on the whole population. The return rate for this survey was high but precise figures were not given. Elderly people, in particular, were reluctant to cooperate in such studies.

The objective of this massive health investigation was to determine the extent of the "iceberg of need," the submerged as well as the visible parts, on the basis of a professional definition of "need." From a comparison of the findings of these two surveys of utilization and need, estimates were made of the extent of "overuse," "underuse," and "misuse" of health resources. To make these judgments, utilization standards were defined by experts on the delivery of medical care. They calculated, for instance, the average number of hospital beds required per year per 1,000 population from the formula:

$$K = [A \times R \times P \, (N-3\sqrt{N})/365 \times N \times 100]$$

Where

K is the average number of hospital beds required per 1,000 persons per year,
A is the morbidity (conditions or persons) per 1,000 persons estimated from the "utilization" and "need" surveys,
R is the percentage of A (conditions or persons) judged by the experts to require hospitalizaton,
P is the average length of hospital stay in days,
N is the average number of currently available beds in all hospitals in the region under survey per year.

In this mathematical formula two assumptions are made: first, that the number of beds available equals the number of beds demanded and, second, that the demand for beds, reflecting the number of hospitalizations, follows a Poisson distribution.

Among the limitations commonly attributed to this method of estimating potential demand for health services, based on measures of need determined by morbidity surveys and defined by expert standards, are the following.

First, it uses as the basis for planning, the highly subjective concept of "need," instead of the more objective one of "demand." The fact that need exists does not imply that it will be expressed as demand for services.

Second, adequate morbidity data are scarce. In a recent review of morbidity statistics said to be available in 98 countries, Abel-Smith comments that "administration and planning of services in most countries lack this kind of basis (morbidity and utilization statistics) to an extremely serious extent" (7, p. 28). The present reality is that ". . . health administrators faced at first with the virtual necessity of doing without an adequate numerical basis for their decisions have now come to feel that they can dispense with statistical information. The results of this may be seen in many countries today where the available services bear very little relation to the health needs of the communities they are supposed to serve" (7, p. 26).

The main reason for this scarcity of data is the high cost of obtaining reliable morbidity information. This cost, however, should be weighed against the benefits obtained from the data, including appraisal of the effects of medical and social intervention.

Third, this method requires a consensus of medical opinion on how best to care for each condition. This consensus is difficult, if not impossible, to reach in many cases.

METHODS BASED ON MORTALITY

In their calculation of required health resources, some authors have preferred to plan on the basis of mortality data rather than morbidity data. The reasons given for this preference are (1) mortality statistics are more reliable than morbidity statistics; (2) mortality data are available annually for most localities, whereas morbidity data are not similarly obtainable; and (3) when morbidity data are available, translation into health resources required to meet "need" and/or "demand" involves the difficult process of establishing criteria for services.

The assumption made in all planning based upon mortality data is that the ratio of health resources utilization to mortality is constant. Technological, demographic, and socioeconomic changes (among others), however, condition changes in utilization as well as changes in mortality, and hence the validity of the hospital bed utilization/mortality ratio may be questioned.

STRAIGHTFORWARD EXTRAPOLATION

Among the methods designed to calculate the health resources required to meet future demands, the most frequently used has been application of the present health resources/population ratio to the future population size. This method takes into account only increased demand due to demographic growth. It assumes that the work-loads carried in the past are the best and most objective guide to the requirements of the future. Sometimes this demand is "corrected" to exclude overuse and include underuse, according to expert judgment. Since this correction depends upon the criteria selected, it may reflect valuations concerning the purposes to which the health resources should be put.

Bailey introduced the concept of the "critical number of beds," which has been widely used in England (8). This is the number of beds that will just keep pace with current demand. It is calculated by noting the change in the length of the waiting lists for hospital admissions over a given period of time, and adding this change to the satisfied demand, i.e., the patients actually admitted to the hospital during the same period. Provision is then made for additional beds to compensate for variability in admissions. Elective admissions are assumed to follow a normal distribution, whereas nonelective admissions are considered to follow a Poisson distribution.

Recently, Drosness and his associates published one of the first studies in the United States on variations in daily hospital bed census in Santa Clara County, California (9). They concluded that for all hospital bed units studied (medical, surgical, obstetrical, and pediatric) a normal distribution gives a more accurate description of variation in daily census than does a Poisson.

Planning based on extrapolation methods can be criticized because it tends to perpetuate, and even magnify, inefficiencies. Moreover, it fails to take account of shifts in demand related to socioeconomic changes in the population or to scientific and technologic developments in medicine. A further reservation about the use of these methods has been created by Roemer's and Newell's findings that supply appears to promote demand, although Rosenthal and Sigmond have questioned these findings (10-13). This divergence of opinion seems to indicate that there is as yet no clear understanding of the effect that supply has upon demand for hospital beds.

METHODS BASED ON ANALYSIS OF DEMAND

A more sophisticated approach than simple extrapolation either of present demand or of ratios of resources to population is that based on analysis of present demand. This method represents, in fact, market analysis of consumer use. Brooks and his colleagues predict future demand by multiple regression analysis of 117 variables, including demographic data, mean life expectancy, mean effective buying income, average length of stay in hospital, average occupancy rate, ratio of physicians to population, and others (14). Monthly figures are collected for each of these variables for five years, and then multiple regression techniques are applied to establish the relation between the number of patients in each hospital department and the 15 to 20 most important factors. The number of patients expected per month in each department can be predicted by estimating the value of the factors for that month. The number of beds needed by departments or by the whole hospital is estimated by multiplying the number of patients per month by the average length of stay and dividing by the average number of days in a month.

Feldstein and German use two methods: first, extrapolation from present trends of supply and demand; second, in relation to estimates of population growth, analysis of selected socioeconomic factors that affect utilization (15). By predicting the future level of these factors they derive estimates of future hospital utilization.

Reinke and Baker have developed a new analytical method, the multisort technique, that improves the analysis of the effects of multiple variables on utilization (16). Multiple regression techniques frequently overlook or inadequately identify nonlinear effects and interactions. Analysis of variance has proved useful in handling interaction, but uneven distribution of observations among cells tremendously complicates the computational procedure. The multisort technique, on the other hand, is an approximation procedure that simplifies computations while maintaining most of the benefits of the analysis of variance approach.

Swedish workers base their estimates of required medical and hospital resources upon a demographic analysis of hospital utilization. Because of the polarized age distribution of the country they are particularly interested in differences in utilization by different age groups. Swedish health planners, therefore, use an index—the "consumption unit"—defined as the number of visits per 100 persons for each age group divided by the mean number of visits (for the whole population). For estimating future demand, this gives differences in utilization by different age groups rather than by the number of persons.

An example of this approach is illustrated for Göteborg in Table 15.1. By multiplying the consumption unit for each age group by the number of people in Göteborg in each age group in 1963, 1970, 1975, and 1980, the total number of

Table 15.1
Annual Number of Consumption Units per Person in the City of Göteborg (1967)

Age Group	Number of Visits per 100 Persons (V)*	Number of Consumption Units (C.U.)** per Person
0-15	125.0	0.540
16-19	154.0	0.665
20-29	196.9	0.850
30-39	236.0	1.019
40-49	274.9	1.187
50-59	311.1	1.343
60-66	345.2	1.491
67 and over	308.9	1.334
Mean Number of Visits ($\overline{V}$)	231.6	

* Data taken from National Insurance Board Study, 1963.
** C.U. = $V/\overline{V}$; for example: C.U. for Age Group 0-15 = 125.0/231.6 = 0.540.

consumption units for the region may be estimated. By taking into account differences in the consumption of medical and hospital services by different age groups, the method gives more detailed estimates of future consumption than those estimates based on the growth of the entire population.

METHODS BASED ON DISTRIBUTION

The concepts of distribution and coordination refer to the geographical and functional relationships between resources and the population served. To study these characteristics two methods have been used: the "facilities-centered" and the "population-centered" approaches.

Facilities-Centered Approach

In the facilities-centered approach, a group of facilities, usually hospitals, is surveyed to define the population served by these hospitals. This method involves collecting information about hospital discharges according to patients' places of residence for each of the hospitals serving the community or region under study. From this information estimates can be made of the extent to which each small area (e.g., county, commune, municipality) is served by each facility. By estimating projected changes in the populations of each of the areas served, one can predict future hospital utilization and thus future requirements for the whole region. This method suffers from the defect that it does not take into account the influence of selective bias in choosing a hospital on the part of residents in given areas.

Schneider in the United States has described a conceptual model for evaluating the location efficiency of physicians' offices and hospitals, using a facilities-centered approach in his analysis (17). Locational efficiency measures hospital operating costs that are attributable to its location.

Population-Centered Approach

The population-centered method is based on the analysis of the current patterns of hospital utilization by a defined population. The initial step is to define the survey population as the residents of a particular geographical area. The pattern of bed utilization for this specified population is then determined. This involves analyses of bed utilization data from hospitals both inside and adjacent to the defined area. Current use of hospital beds is measured rather than demand for beds. This method has been used more often for planning hospital beds than for manpower planning. It has the advantage of fostering the idea of community care, with the hospitals as an essential but not the only component.

Combinations of Both Approaches

In a number of instances, the facilities-centered and population-centered approaches have been combined; recent work in Göteborg is especially noteworthy in this respect (18). There it was decided to centralize the superspecialities, e.g., neurosurgery, in one teaching hospital, which would be the principal medical center of a region. Using hospital utilization experiences of different surveyed populations, as well as experts' opinions, the authors defined the desired ratio of superspecialty beds to population. By defining the minimal desirable size for the superspecialty units in regional hospitals, they were able to define the optimal size of a region. For example, if the experts defined the minimal size of a neurosurgery unit as 60 beds and the suggested number of beds for neurosurgery patients per 100,000 persons as 5.5, then the minimal size of a region that could generate enough patients to support a neurosurgery unit would be $(60 \times 100,000)/5.5 = 1.1$ million persons.

With respect to geographic distribution and size of regional centers, these authors attached primary importance to the accessibility of the regional hospital center for the population living in the region (18). The constraints chosen as the basis for selection were travel times and costs. No person within a region should have to travel more than four hours round trip by car or public transport. The travel times for alternative locations of regional centers were represented graphically on isochrone maps. If travel cost instead of time is used, isochrone maps also perform the role of travel cost maps (isodapan maps), since travel cost is proportional to travel time. The isochrone maps for each alternative location were placed over the population projection maps for each future year. The population living within each travel time zone was then estimated. The location chosen was that which minimized aggregate travel times and costs.

METHODS BASED ON SYSTEM PERFORMANCE

Conceptually, at least, the planning of personal health services could be based upon analysis of the performance of the system. In this method the required resources would be determined by the amount and type needed to achieve a defined output, measured in terms of performance such as reduction or control of death, disease, disability, discomfort, and so forth. Effectiveness is the relationship between input and output in the system performance method.

In practice, more analytical studies of health services have been concerned with productivity, expressed in terms of efficiency, than with effectiveness. In most cases the precise relationships between inputs and outputs of the system are not known; even less is known about methods of quantifying them. No evidence is available, for example, to show that by providing X units of prenatal care one will save Y children's lives.

In the absence of more objective measurements, use has been made of expert opinion in the system performance models. Such is the case in the method used by the Centro de Estudios de Desarrollo (CENDES) and the Pan American Health Organization (PAHO) in health planning (19). In this method the main goal is to decrease mortality by disease categories, subject to the constraint of cost. Although morbidity could be taken into account also, only mortality is considered, owing to the lack of data on the former. The first step is to establish a priority rating for each cause of death by disease category based on the incidence of death, i.e., the proportion of total deaths due to each disease category. Second, the relative importance of the disease category is measured by an arbitrary score based on age at death and the degree to which premature deaths caused by this disease could be prevented. This preventability is defined either by experts' opinions or epidemiological studies.

For nonreducible morbidity and related nonreducible mortality, two alternatives are considered: in the so-called "minimum alternative," the required future resources are calculated by extrapolation of current demand generated by these diseases; in the "maximum alternative," the future requirements are defined by experts' opinion of what resources should be provided to care for prospective demand, regardless of cost.

For reducible morbidity and mortality, the needed resources are divided into preventive and curative. The number of preventive resources required is defined by expert opinion of standards of prevention needed, according to the "minimum alternative," to keep morbidity and thus mortality at the current ratios, or according to the "maximum alternative," to reduce morbidity and mortality as much as possible, regardless of cost. The number of curative resources required is based in both alternatives on the ratio of utilization to mortality, i.e., "a correlation between the mortality rate for each reducible disease and the hospital and consultation rates for the same disease" (19, p. 63).

In the United States, the Division of Indian Health has developed a planning method that defines its objectives as quantifiable reduction of morbidity and mortality (20). Determination of health problem priorities is based on a Health Problem Index, which takes into account mortality and disability for each category of disease. The resources required are determined by the plan of action chosen, based upon a cost-benefit analysis of the different alternatives. The difficulties in applying similar approaches in open health services systems, in contrast to the closed system of Indian Health Services, have been discussed by Kissick (21).

METHODS BASED ON SYSTEM STRUCTURE

These methods are based upon knowledge of the internal relations among the system's components. Consideration must be given both to the productivity of individual components and to the dynamic aspects of referral and transferral. After defining the system dynamics in terms of transitional probabilities, one can calculate the likelihood that specific types of patients will follow a particular course from one part of the system to another, e.g., from ambulatory to hospital in-patient to nursing home status.

Navarro, Parker, and White have described such a planning model (22). Based upon the Markovian process, it is used to predict resource requirements under a variety of hypothetical situations and to estimate the best alternative medical care strategy for reaching a desired goal in the presence of a defined constraint.

The advantage of these mathematical models in planning is that they allow greater clarity and precision than purely intuitive methods. Further, the use of probability models is essential to describe chance patterns of occurrence. The models are valid and useful, of course, only to the extent that they are realistic.

REFERENCES

1. Lee, Roger I. and Jones, Lewis W. *The Fundamentals of Good Medical Care.* Chicago: University of Chicago Press, 1933.
2. Kalimo, E. and Sievers, K. "The Need for Medical Care: Estimation on the Basis of Interview Data." *Medical Care* 6:1-17, 1968.
3. Forsyth, G. and Logan, R. F. L. *The Demand for Medical Care.* Nuffield Provincial Hospitals Trust Publication. New York: Oxford University Press, 1960.
4. Barr, A. "The Extent of Hospital Sickness." *British Journal of Preventive and Social Medicine* 12:61-70, 1958.
5. Logan, R. F. L. "Assessment of Sickness and Health in the Community: Needs and Methods." *Medical Care* 2:173-190 and 218-225, 1964.
6. Popov, G. A. "Questions of Theory and Methodology of Health Services Planning." (In Russian). A brief summary appears in: Burkens, J. C. J. "The Estimation of Hospital Bed Requirements." *World Hospitals* 2:110-113, 1966.
7. Abel-Smith, B. *Morbidity Statistics. A Report on Current Practice in Member Countries of the World Health Organization.* Eleventh Meeting, Expert Committee on Health Statistics, 7-13 November 1967. Geneva: World Health Organization, 1968.
8. Bailey, N. T. J. "Statistics in Hospital Planning and Design." *Applied Statistics* 5:146-157, 1956.
9. Drosness, D. L., Dean, L. S., Lubin, J. W., and Ribak, N. "Uses of Daily Census Data in Determining Efficiency of Units." *Hospitals* 41:45-48, passim (December 1) and 65-68, passim (December 16), 1967.
10. Roemer, M. I. "Bed Supply and Hospital Utilization: A National Experiment." *Hospitals* 35:36-42, 1961.
11. Newell, D. J. "Problems of Estimating the Demand for Hospital Beds." *Journal of Chronic Diseases* 17:749-759, 1964.
12. Rosenthal, G. D. *The Demand for General Hospital Facilities.* Monograph No. 14. Chicago: American Hospital Association, 1964.
13. Sigmond, R. M. "Does Supply of Beds Control Costs?" Letter to the Editors. *Modern Hospital* 93:6, 1959.

14. Brooks, G. H., Beenhakker, H. L., and McLin, W. C. "A New Development in Predicting Hospital Bed Needs." *International Nursing Review* 11:33-39, 1964.
15. Feldstein, P. J. and German, J. J. "Predicting Hospital Utilization: An Evaluation of Three Approaches." *Inquiry* 2:13-36, 1965.
16. Reinke, W. A. and Baker, T. D. "Measuring the Effects of Demographic Variables on Health Services Utilization." *Health Services Research* 2:61-75, 1967.
17. Schneider, J. B. *Measuring the Locational Efficiency of the Urban Hospital.* Philadelphia: Regional Science Research Institute, 1967.
18. *The Regional Plan of Health Services for Göteborg. Health and Hospital Planning.* (In Swedish). Göteborg: Council of Göteborg, 1966.
19. Ahumada, J., *et al. Health Planning: Problems of Concept and Method.* Scientific Publication No. 111. Washington, D.C.: Pan American Health Organization, 1965.
20. *The Principles of Program Packaging in the Division of Indian Health.* Silver Spring, Maryland: U.S. Public Health Service, Bureau of Medical Services, 1966.
21. Kissick, W. L. "Planning, Programming, and Budgeting in Health." *Medical Care* 5:201-220, 1967.
22. Navarro, V., Parker, R., and White, K. L. "A Stochastic and Deterministic Model of Medical Care Utilization." *Health Services Research* 5:342-357, 1970.

ADDITIONAL READINGS

Primary

Anderson, Odin W. and Kravits, Joanna. *Health Services in the Chicago Area—A Framework for Use of Data.* Research Series No. 26. Chicago: University of Chicago, Center for Health Administration Studies, 1968.
    A monograph describing a model for planning a comprehensive health services system for a large metropolitan area using both existing data and estimates from national or regional studies. Basically a sociological case study, focusing on the characteristics of the population, morbidity and mortality patterns, numbers and distribution of facilities and personnel, utilization patterns, and financing and payment patterns. Extensive Appendix lists sources of data for the area under study.
Engel, Arthur. *Perspectives in Health Planning.* New York: Russell Sage Foundation, 1968.
    A series of lectures delivered at the London School of Hygiene and Tropical Medicine by the former Director-General of the National Board of Health of Sweden, covering "Health Planning in a Changing Society;" "Statistics and Health Planning" (with emphasis on collecting good statistical information not only on services and their function but also on output of training programs and current availability of medical manpower, as well as changing patterns of disease and disability); "Mass Screening for Asymptomatic Disease as a Public Health Measure;" and "The Swedish

Regionalized Hospital and Health System" (its function, growth and transition are presented briefly as an introduction to Swedish methodology and experience).

Feldstein, M. S. "An Aggregate Planning Model of the Health Care Sector." *Medical Care* 5:369-381, 1967.

Description of an early econometric model for planning in the health sector. Its application is illustrated by an example drawn from a study of demand and supply of hospital beds. This model allows planners to take the effects of supply into account more readily than do other methods of planning hospital facilities.

Navarro, V. "Methodology on Regional Planning of Personal Health Services—A Case Study: Sweden." *Medical Care* 8:386-394, 1970.

Methods used by Swedish health planners to regionalize personal health services are described, including estimating future demand (with the help of a "consumption unit index") and determining the size of a region and its geographic distribution of resources. Accessibility to a regional center is the determinant variable in deciding on center location, and in terms of a cost-efficiency approach, the best location will be the one that minimizes aggregate travel times and costs.

Vacek, M. and Skrobkova, E. "Methods of Planning Health Services in Czechoslovakia." *Milbank Memorial Fund Quarterly* 44:307-317, No. 3, Part 1, July, 1966.

Brief description of the health planning procedures used in Czechoslovakia for 1966-1980, which is basically a combination of the analytical method (analysis of morbidity in a population according to diagnosis) with the experimental method (assessing demand for health services at experimental bases around the country under conditions similar to those anticipated for the time interval that is the target of planning). Advantages and disadvantages of each approach are noted.

Secondary

Barr, A. and Davies, J. O. F. "The Population Served by a Hospital Group." *Lancet* 2:1105-1108, November 30, 1957.

Community Health Service, Department of Health, Education, and Welfare. *Conceptual Model of Organized Primary Care and Comprehensive Community Health Services.* U.S.P.H.S. Publication No. 2024. Washington, D.C.: Government Printing Office, 1970.

Donabedian, A. *Aspects of Medical Care Administration.* Ann Arbor: University of Michigan, School of Public Health (in press).

Godlund, S. *Population, Regional Hospitals, Transport Facilities and Regions.* Stockholm: The Royal University of Lund, Department of Geography, 1961.

Michigan Department of Public Health. "Planning Kit: Health Department Programs Plan for 1969-70." March, 1969.

Miller, J. E. "An Indicator to Aid Management in Assigning Program Priorities." *Public Health Reports* 85:725-731, 1970.

Milly, George H. *Computer Simulation Model for Evaluation of a Health Care Delivery System.* National Center for Health Services Research and

Development Report Series. Washington, D.C.: Government Printing Office, 1970.

Navarro, V. "The City and the Region." *American Behavioral Science* 14:865-892, 1971.

Nuffield Provincial Hospitals Trust. *A Balanced Teaching Hospital.* London: Oxford University Press, 1965.

Wenkert, W., Hill, J. G., and Berg, R. L. "Concepts and Methodology in Planning Patient Care Services." *Medical Care* 7:327-331, 1969.

Williams, W. J., Covert, R. P., and Steele, J. D. "Simulation Modeling of a Teaching Hospital Outpatient Clinic." *Hospitals* 41:71-75, November 1, 1967.

IV

Selected Categories of Health Planning
Requiring Special Considerations

16

History and Special Features of Mental Health Planning

PAUL V. LEMKAU and WALLACE MANDELL

HISTORICAL PERSPECTIVE

Mental health services have responsibility for dealing with individuals whose behavior has been outside the limits of tolerance of the culture in which they live or who are so uncomfortable because of symptoms best understood as due to psychiatric illness that they present themselves for care. Concern for the prevention of various mental illnesses has a long history, although the development of psychodynamics in the last 75 years has led to accentuated interest in prevention (1). In the last few decades, sociodynamics, a concern with the ecology of man as a factor in etiology of deviance, has also increased interest in prophylaxis (2).

The mental illnesses are usually considered divisible into two classes: those in which the symptoms are directly related to structural or physiological pathology and those in which such pathology is not demonstrable or known. Psychodynamics and sociodynamics are more closely related to the latter group, often called functional, although they also often supplement the understanding of illness of the first category.

Early Planning

Planning for services to persons whose behavior is disordered may be found in very ancient times. An Egyptian physician was called to Mesopotamia to consult about a mental illness, and King Saul's psychosis called for clear planning on how to deal with the situation, the prescription being music therapy. Plato's *Republic* includes references to the care of those of unsound mind, noting that they are the responsibility of their families. Ancient Greek law provided ways to deal with cases of senile psychoses.

Treatment of mental illnesses in hospitals began very early, at first probably without clear separation of these illnesses from other types of disease. As early as the seventh century A.D., however, the separation of behavior disorders from other types of diseases began. This separation has continued through the centuries, so that two systems of hospitals now exist in most parts of the world, one primarily for diseases other than psychiatric, the other for the treatment of mental illnesses.

With the increase in medical knowledge in the last century, both in psychiatry and in medicine in general, this separation has begun to be deplored. The reunification of hospitals and their adaptation for the management of acute and chronic psychiatric illnesses has become a legitimate aim of planning medical services for populations, although in many areas there is much ambivalence about it (3, 4).

During the Middle Ages, practically all hospitals in the western world became charitable agencies operated by religious organizations. As such, their support by the political authorities was largely indirect, through gifts to the Church. When this pattern began to fail after the Renaissance, hospitals, particularly psychiatric hospitals, came directly under government support and control. This has been especially true in the United States, where the great majority of psychiatric beds have been operated by political authorities since the start of the nation. The reasons for this are extremely complex but must include the fact that, historically, mental illnesses and chronicity have been associated. The cost of treatment was so high that only government could support it through general taxation (5, 6).

Pre-World War II Efforts

Until the end of World War II in the United States and in much of Europe as well, planning for mental health services was almost entirely a matter of the accumulation of problems until they reached a point of explosive severity, coupled with the emergence of a leader to instigate reforms. The names of the leaders are a part of psychiatric history: Weyer, Chiarugi, Pinel, the Tukes, Dorothea Dix, Clifford Beers, and many others. For the most part, little long-term planning took place; what happened was a series of emergencies with some resultant improvements but no steady advance.

In the USSR, the national health services apparently were the subject of nationwide and more continuous planning than elsewhere (7).

Post-War Changes

World War II had allowed the care of psychiatric patients to reach a low ebb. In the United States, the financial and manpower stringencies of the war years fell very strongly on these never-popular institutions. The result was a series of blatant newspaper exposés of conditions. Needed reforms were made in many areas of the country on the basis of hastily prepared programs. The publicity and the exposure of the miserable conditions in many hospitals resulted in the direct involvement of many legislators and other governmental officials in the problems of the care of psychiatric patients and in planning to meet the obvious needs. This, in turn, led to continued concern and more continuous surveillance of services and to long-term planning.

In Europe, the war's destruction led to the development of new methods of delivering services. The Netherlands had suffered great damage to its ports. Psychiatric hospital beds were also in very short supply because of destruction and lack of construction. The government wished to give priority to construction of income-producing facilities rather than hospitals beds and asked its psychiatrists to devise services which would make the need for beds less pressing. Querido, in Amsterdam, proposed and built a system of emergency and supervised home care to meet the needs* (8). In practice it proved so successful and so advantageous to patients that it spread throughout the Netherlands and to many other parts of the world.

In England, psychiatric beds had not been destroyed, but economic stringencies forced more efficient use of beds. T. P. Rees,† Duncan Macmillan (9, pp. 29-39), and others, in response to this need and also influenced by the psychodynamic and sociodynamic concepts mentioned earlier, developed new systems of care. In Amsterdam, the administrative center of the new system was the health department; in England, the psychiatric hospital was the administrative and planning center, built, of course, into the general administration of the National Health Service.

Hospital reforms (including the unlocking of psychiatric hospital doors, ready accessibility to the community, and the development of industrial therapy schemes) spread widely over the world, particularly affecting the United States and Canada. In France, Sivadon and others developed plans for extramural services and partial hospitalization for defined parts of metropolitan populations (10).

These reforms and the subsequent introduction of new drugs which allowed better pharmacological control of psychiatric symptoms led to marked reduction in the length of psychiatric hospitalizations and to a reduction in the number of hospitalized patients. In the United States, the rate of psychiatric hospitalization in state mental hospitals reached its peak in 1945 at 409 per 100,000 population; it has since fallen continuously, and in 1966 was 287 per 100,000. The trend in actual numbers of patients is not so striking because of population increases. It is worth noting, however, that 522,000 patients were in psychiatric

---

* Querido, A. Discussion before the New York City Community Mental Health Board, December 6, 1955 (unpublished).

† Rees, T. P. Discussion before the New York City Community Mental Health Board, November 7, 1956 (unpublished).

hospitals in 1945. The peak in numbers was reached in 1955 when psychiatric hospitals had 634,000 patients. By 1966 the number had fallen to 556,000 (11).

Postwar reforms in the United States were not confined to hospitals. Out-patient treatment had come to be well known through the development of child guidance clinics after 1920 (12, 13).

Freudianism was widely accepted in the United States and its psychodynamic and developmental concepts furnished a base for prophylactic developments. Clifford Beers had been successful in capturing public attention for the mental health field (14). The military experience, accentuating early and definitive treatment, was influential in setting the stage for the foundation of planning mental health services in the United States.

RECENT MENTAL HEALTH LEGISLATION IN THE UNITED STATES

Mental Health Act of 1946

The United States National Mental Health Act was passed by Congress in 1946 and funded in 1947. It aimed (1) to relieve the manpower shortage through training programs for all members of the psychiatric treatment team, (2) to extend psychiatric knowledge through research, and (3) to aid the states in establishing out-patient services. The law also established the National Institute of Mental Health as a permanent part of the health system of the country and, within it, advisory groups whose function, among others, was to fulfill the need for continuous surveillance and long-term planning. The act called for state agencies to be designated for similar purposes. Initially, the National Mental Health Act specifically avoided the financial and administrative problems of psychiatric hospitals, leaving these to the states. In recent years, psychiatric hospitals have received both training grants and funds to finance demonstrations for hospital improvements, but the federal government still avoids the core problem of state-supported psychiatric hospitalization.

President's Joint Commission on Mental Health and Disease

Action for Mental Health, published in 1961, was the result of several years of study of the problems of mental health programming in the United States and made recommendations for future development (15). This report leaned strongly in the direction of continued separation of patients with general medical and psychiatric problems, while its Canadian counterpart took the opposite view, recommending the general hospital and its services as the base upon which the system of psychiatric services should be built (3).

As a result of the publication of *Action for Mental Health* and of President Kennedy's interest in the field of the mental illnesses and mental retardation, Congress responded with three basic pieces of legislation which pertain directly to mental health planning. The first provided funds to the states for a two-year study to result in a mental health plan. The guidelines for this operation were such that professionals and laymen were required to collaborate in a long-term plan for mental health services. The expectation was that, once established, the planning groups would become an integral part of state machinery, and in most instances this happened.

Shortly after mental health planning was written into law, the second step was taken through passage of a similar law applying to the field of mental retardation. This was also a result of the recommendations of a presidential commission and was carried out in much the same way (16). The fact that mental health and mental retardation legislation were separate packages, together with certain scientific discoveries in the retardation field which stimulated more widespread interest in that field (17), has tended to separate mental retardation planning from mental health planning in many areas. Indeed, in some places the two fields became quite separate in administrative structure.

Community Mental Health Center Act of 1963

The third action of Congress was to provide financing for the development of a system of mental health centers. The Community Mental Health Center Act of 1963 offered matching funds for the construction of such centers and was amended in 1965 to provide a subsidy, decreasing proportionally over time, for staffing the centers. The national goal was 2,000 community mental health centers, each serving a specified population so that everyone would have available an array of psychiatric services. As of 1970, about 350 centers were said to be in operation. The goal of the centers is to make psychiatric treatment available to all persons needing it early in the development of behavior disorders and, whenever possible, to provide for treatment with minimal interruption of family and work patterns and with minimal loss of social skills (18).

The community mental health center approach called for a program capable of providing continuous care through multiple treatment programs in each community; these programs would be organized under the same administration, although not necessarily under the same roof. Each center was required to have five basic component services: in-patient service, partial hospitalization (day hospital service), emergency service, out-patient service, and consultation and education service. Other services, including specialized diagnostic services, rehabilitation, research, evaluation, and training, were considered desirable but not required by the guidelines (19).

Partnership for Health Act of 1966

The trends toward the separation of mental health from general health services and toward fragmentation of the field itself into mental illness and mental retardation (with alcoholism, drug addiction, and so forth as special categorical problems) have been considered unwise by many who see the health field as integral. This influence was apparent in the passage by Congress in 1966 of Public Law 89-749 (the Partnership for Health Act), which provided for a nationwide effort in comprehensive health planning at the state and regional levels. This Act, however, had a special provision specifying that a certain percentage of the funds available should be spent in mental health planning, indicating that the integration could not be made complete.

SPECIAL FEATURES OF MENTAL HEALTH ACTIVITY IN THE UNITED STATES

Review of the history and philosophy of mental health legislation provides some understanding of the special problems encountered in this health area. Fuller understanding, however, requires a more direct description of the important conditions relevant to a given place of interest. We shall confine our attention here to the United States and discuss two important issues: (1) the priority assigned to mental health as a result of its great cost and (2) the broad involvement of nonhealth as well as health agencies in mental health activities.

Cost of Mental Health Services

Nervous and mental conditions rank third among the causes of limitation of activity among all chronic diseases. Mental illness accounts for 7.8 percent of all individuals who suffer any activity limitation (20). According to statistics on sales of medications, one out of seven people in the country is taking tranquilizers. Since these are among the more expensive drugs, the dollar cost for drugs alone is substantial.

The cost per episode of illness cared for in a state mental hospital in 1968 was approximately $4,500. Thus, the 350,000 reported episodes generated expenditures of $1.6 billion. For every 86 patients hospitalized in public mental institutions in 1960, 14 others were hospitalized in private facilities. If we can extrapolate this relationship to 1970, we can assume that 90,000 patients per day were cared for in private facilities during the latter year. Using an estimated cost of $40 per patient day we add $1.3 billion to the $1.6 billion public cost to arrive at a figure of $2.9 billion as the total cost for care of the mentally ill during the year 1970. Economists estimating the cost of illness also calculate the loss in taxable income as part of the cost of illness load (21).

Since these figures relate only to hospitals, they do not measure total expenditures on what is usually recognized as mental ill health. Furthermore, they fail to account for the role of general practitioners and other health and nonhealth workers in promoting mental well-being.

Granted that mental health problems are highly visible and costly in the United States, the next point of interest is the acknowledged primary responsibility which state governments have for the provision of mental health services. These two factors go far toward explaining both the interest in mental health planning that has developed in this country and the many political connotations attached to such planning.

Multiplicity of Functions and Agencies in Mental Health

For our purposes, four broad categories of societal institutions can be identified which impinge on the mental health delivery system. First are standard-setting agencies such as legislatures, courts, and religious organizations. Second are the educational institutions designed to provide skills and attitudes necessary for competent economic performance and adherence to societal standards. Third are agencies devoted to the control and rehabilitation of criminals. Fourth are the health agencies designed to cure and prevent illnesses.

These agencies all encounter individuals who are beyond the ability of the agency to influence or contain without substantial disruption of their own pattern of functioning. They have usually developed subunits which specialize in diagnosing and treating patients, or in referring the special categories of individuals who are unusual or who cannot be managed by that agency. These special units are usually staffed by mental health personnel. These agencies thus have vested interests in determining how funds for mental health services are apportioned and what the lines of administrative authority will be.

Two illustrations of this are the educational system and the correctional system. Educational systems use methods which are reasonably effective for the majority of children. For those who are irregular in attendance, difficult to manage in class, or learn slowly, "control and correction" agencies have been developed within the educational system. This puts education squarely in the mental health arena. The remedial education, compensatory education, and vocational training programs have not been effective in preparing the lowest socioeconomic urban groups, who are concentrated in the central areas of cities, to fit into the American occupational structure.

The correctional system for those who do not obey the laws in the United States operates through prisons, labor camps, and probation and parole agencies at each governmental level. On any day in this country, roughly three million people are in the hands of the correctional system—a system which obviously operates on principles designed to be effective with large numbers of individuals.

Clearly the correctional system confronts a substantial number of individuals who cannot be managed, much less corrected, by the mass techniques used. Many of these individuals are defined as "residual deviants" of concern to the mental health planner.

On occasion, many other societal agencies, finding that they are entirely unable to handle a given individual, refer him to an available mental health agency for definition of his particular problem, as well as for control and rehabilitation. As a result, these agencies have a vested interest in the distribution and availability to them of mental health facilities as resources.

Mental health planning thus involves the interests of many societal agencies and institutions which vie for resources. It also must address issues which are broader than the specific needs of particular agencies. In fact, the norms established by legislatures, courts, and religious, educational, and health institutions may in themselves create significant stresses which lead to psychological disorders. Examples of such norms are enforced early retirement restrictive to older citizens or those which lead to elimination from the educational system of children from poverty backgrounds.

Mental health planning, therefore, must also involve review of the societally controllable policies which impinge on vulnerable populations to increase disability.

REFERENCES

1. Brosin, Cameron. "Psychodynamics." In: Whitehorn, J. C., editor. *The Psychiatrist. His Training and Development.* Report of the 1952 Conference on Psychiatric Education, Ithaca. Washington, D.C.: American Psychiatric Association, 1953.
2. Lemkau, Paul V. *Mental Hygiene in Public Health.* Second edition. New York: Blakiston Division, McGraw-Hill Book Co., 1955.
3. Tyhurst, J. S., Chalke, F. C. R., Lawson, F. S., McNeel, B. H., Roberts, C. A., Taylor, G. C., Weil, R. J., and Griffin, J. D. *More for the Mind—A Study of Psychiatric Services in Canada.* Toronto: The Canadian Mental Health Association, 1963.
4. Maryland State Planning Commission, Committee on Medical Care. *Report of the Subcommittee on Organization for Health.* Publication No. 109. Baltimore: State Planning Department, 1960.
5. Deutsch, Albert. *The Mentally Ill in America—A History of Their Care and Treatment from Colonial Times.* Garden City: Doubleday, Doran & Co., 1937.
6. Gorman, Mike. *Every Other Bed.* Cleveland: World Publishing Co., 1956.
7. Wortis, Joseph. *Soviet Psychiatry.* Baltimore: Williams & Wilkins Co., 1950.
8. Querido, A. *Early Diagnosis and Treatment Services in the Elements of a Community Mental Health Program.* New York: Milbank Memorial Fund, 1956.
9. Macmillan, Duncan. "Hospital Community Relationships." In: *An Approach to the Prevention of Disability from Chronic Psychoses.* New York: Milbank Memorial Fund, 1958.

10. Sivadon, P. "Transformation d'un Service d'alienes de Type Classique en un Centre de Traitement Actif et de Readaptation Sociale—L'experience de Ville-Evrard, France." *Bulletin of the World Health Organization* 21:593–600, 1969.

11. Bureau of the Census. *Statistical Abstract of the United States.* 88th edition. Washington, D.C.: Government Printing Office, 1967.

12. Witmer, H. *Psychiatric Clinics for Children.* New York: The Commonwealth Fund, 1940.

13. Bahn, A. K. *Methodological Study of Population of Out-Patient Psychiatric Clinics, Maryland, 1958-59.* Public Health Monograph No. 65. U.S.P.H.S. Publication No. 821. Washington, D.C.: Government Printing Office, 1961.

14. Beers, Clifford W. *A Mind That Found Itself.* Garden City: Doubleday, Doran & Co., 1953.

15. Joint Commission on Mental Illness and Health. *Action for Mental Health.* Final Report. New York: Basic Books, 1961.

16. U.S. President's Committee on Mental Retardation. *A First Report to the President on the Nation's Progress and Remaining Great Needs in the Campaign to Combat Mental Retardation.* M.R. 67. Washington, D.C.: Government Printing Office, 1967.

17. Lemkau, Paul V. "Prevention in Psychiatry." *American Journal.of Public Health* 55:554–560, 1965.

18. American Public Health Association. *Mental Disorders: A Guide to Control Methods.* New York: American Public Health Association, 1962.

19. National Institute of Mental Health. *CMHC: The Comprehensive Community Mental Health Center.* Publication No. 5009. Washington, D.C.: National Clearinghouse for Mental Health Information, 1969.

20. National Center for Health Statistics. *Chronic Conditions Causing Activity Limitation.* U.S.P.H.S. Publication No. 1000, Series 10, No. 51, Table A, p. 3. Washington, D.C.: Government Printing Office, 1969.

21. Fein, R. *The Economics of Mental Illness.* New York: Basic Books, 1958.

ADDITIONAL READINGS

Primary

Cohn, Sidney. *The Treatment of Alcoholics: An Evaluative Study.* New York: Oxford University Press, 1970.
> A balanced description of the organization of treatment programs for alcoholism at the state and political subdivision levels as well as at the treatment level.

Connery, Robert H. *The Politics of Mental Health.* New York: Columbia University Press, 1968.
> Description and analysis of the process of getting mental health programs established in several metropolitan centers in the United States. Detailed interrelationships of power and service groups are described.

Panzetta, A. F. *Community Mental Health: Myth and Reality.* Philadelphia: Lea and Febiger, 1971.
> Built upon the experience of a mental health center in Philadelphia, the author uses this example to extract basic principles and ideas useful in planning.

Susser, M. *Community Psychiatry, Epidemiologic and Social Themes.* New York: Random House, 1968.
> Combines the findings of the epidemiology of the mental illnesses with factors involved in evolving mental health programs in communities, with major illustrations drawn from experience in Great Britain.

Secondary

Halpert, H. P., Horvath, W. J., and Young, J. P. *An Administrator's Handbook on the Application of Operations Research to the Management of Mental Health Systems.* Bethesda: National Institute of Mental Health, 1970.

Kramer, Morton. *Applications of Mental Health Statistics: Uses in Mental Health Programmes of Statistics Derived from Psychiatric Services and Selected Vital and Morbidity Records.* Geneva: World Health Organization, 1969.

May, P. R. A. "Cost-Efficiency of Mental Health Delivery Systems. I. A Review of the Literature on Hospital Care." *American Journal of Public Health* 60:2060-2067, 1970.

May, P. R. A. "Cost-Effectiveness of Mental Health Care. II. Sex as a Parameter of Cost in the Treatment of Schizophrenia." *American Journal of Public Health* 60:2269-2272, 1970.

May, P. R. A. "Cost-Efficiency of Mental Health Care. III. Treatment Method as a Parameter of Cost in the Treatment of Schizophrenia." *American Journal of Public Health* 61:127-129, 1971.

Mental Disorders: Guide to Control Methods. New York: American Public Health Association, 1962.

17

Selected Environmental Health Problems in the United States

CORNELIUS W. KRUSÉ

This brief essay on environmental health problems is particularly related to recent events in the United States, where 100 years of effort has resulted in the virtual disappearance of water-borne and milk-borne diseases, yellow fever, malaria, and other diseases associated with work environments. In most developing countries, on the other hand, if a single program were chosen which would have the maximum health benefit, which would rapidly stimulate social and economic development, and which would materially improve the standard of living of people, that program would be an adequate and safe water supply with provision for running water into or adjacent to each house.

Environmental health management policies are solely for the purpose of preventing disease and injury. The basic science is ecology, the object is population, the method is epidemiology, and the control is primarily administration and engineering. The whole enterprise rests upon a foundation of law and is implemented through codes, rules, regulations, and standards imposed upon a person or bodies responsible for the creation of potential hazards to health. In the United States, the police power of the state has long been used to enforce regulations concerning health, safety, morals, and public order.

Today we are witnessing tremendous popular interest in conserving our national resources and the quality of our environment. As developed countries have discovered, highly productive industry and agriculture accumulate unwanted or spent waste products throughout heavily urbanized areas. Exotic contaminants of all sorts are carried by air and water, and these products may be potentially detrimental to human health. "Pollutants" complicate the regulation of products for human consumption. They limit desirable living space and interfere with cleanliness and full enjoyment of the natural environment. These environmental management problems are geographical, with little regard for the boundaries of political subdivisions, and it is logical that the federal government intervene and assist the states in obtaining a uniform program of environmental improvement. Although current federal laws recognize the states' primary responsibility in abating "pollution," there has been much effort to impose tighter standards than states want and to expand the enforcement powers of the federal government.

Basic to comprehensive health planning is the notion that local entities historically have served the urban population efficiently and economically. They have provided safe public water supplies and the collection and disposal of liquid and solid wastes. Public and private agencies such as water districts, sanitary districts, cities, towns, villages, commissions, and authorities are responsible for planning, financing, constructing, and operating such facilities which are under state regulation and standards. The urban crisis which smoldered during the World War II years and finally erupted in the 1950's was of such dimensions that the historical system of management was unable to react rapidly and effectively. The problem was complicated in that the most vocal and popular pressures concentrated on pollution control, which relates more to wildlife conservation than to the environmental health problems of exploding urban complexes. The unexpected and unplanned phenomenal urban development on raw land at the fringes of central cities found local governmental units unable to engineer, finance, and administer the water, waste water, and other public services that are essential to public health.

Environmental health planners may have difficulty in concentrating exclusively on identifiable health problems because of the current demand for recognizing the impact on man of the "total environment" or the interrelationships among physicochemical, biological, and social environmental factors. Ultimately, planners of all sorts will have to face up to the need for improved scientific organization of space on earth. To do so, there must be widespread understanding and application of the principles of common planning. The first principle of common planning is that some of the sources of the world's resources—air, water, land, energy, and human—are *exhaustible*, while other sources are either *inexhaustible* or *renewable.* By choosing the least exhaustible sources of supply—namely, the most efficient processes which use the air and water—economic civilization may be sustained, but not without scientific management and redistribution of population, industry, and agriculture. Although attempts have been made on a regional basis, man has yet to apply successfully the principles of common planning anywhere; perhaps the real challenge is the development within man of a sense of responsibility and moral obligation to cooperate more fully with nature through the intellectual abilities not available to any other being.

Experts in health already have an awareness of the influence of the total environment; for example, overdeveloped versus undeveloped regions in a given area lead to wide disparities in usable wealth with which public health may be purchased. Environmental health planners cannot afford to be diverted by elegant debates regarding the exhaustion of natural resources; they must guide the planning process around management schemes which honestly promise better health. Although not a popular view, eliminating septic tanks and cesspools in built-up urban areas commands a higher health priority than reducing the discharge of phosphates and other nutrients into lakes and streams. Construction of sanitary land fills on swamp land for the disposal of urban refuse could benefit human beings more than could an undisturbed swamp ecosystem. Health experts are not sanguine regarding the delicate balance of factors sustaining life in the biosphere. They generally welcome the increased awareness of the role of exotic microchemical pollutants. These are some of the problems in natural resource conservation; hopefully, intelligent and objective planning and abatement programs will evolve to reduce the overfertilization of our waters and to preserve wet lands and endangered wildlife species. The point is that none of these programs contributes significantly to human problems such as infant mortality rates in the inner cities or provision of safe water supply and excreta disposal for millions of residents of "septic tank suburbia."

The first order of priority of planning the environment for health benefit would be the protection of water for community water supply, fish and shellfish propagation, swimming and recreation, and other appropriate uses. Water carriage collection and disposal of domestic and industrial sewage follow closely in order of priority. The next priority area is that of air pollution control. During unfavorable meteorological conditions in highly industrialized areas, air pollutants may reach concentrations that are hazardous to human health. Ample reasons exist, in addition to health, for clearing the atmosphere. Refuse collection and disposal are of less health impact but of high esthetic, sanitary, and convenience value. Due to the enormous volumes involved, waste disposal presents the greatest threat to air, water, and soil. The problem of rodents and insects of public health importance is not as critical as the nuisance odors and unsightliness associated with solid wastes of domestic, commercial, and industrial origin. Comprehensive environmental health planning in such areas as occupational health and safety, food and milk control, radiation protection, and low cost housing will not be discussed here because, aside from the housing problem, the need for long-range planning in anticipation of meeting future needs is not as critical as the priority areas listed above.

THE WATER PROBLEM: WATER SUPPLY

Adequacy of Water

Water, unlike natural resources such as fossil fuels, is an inexhaustible resource on earth. The supply available for use is a function of rainfall potential. Rainfall is not uniformly distributed but varies geographically, ranging from too much to no rainfall at all. The original source of rain water is the ocean. The water evaporates into the atmosphere and the water vapor is carried by the winds over land and sea where it falls as rain, snow, or hail. In the United States (excluding Alaska and Hawaii) the average precipitation is 4300 billion gallons each day. Of this amount, an estimated 1200 to 1250 billion gallons per day represents infiltration and runoff which replenish the ground water storage level and replenish streams and lakes. The larger fraction of the precipitation is returned to the atmosphere as water vapor through evaporation from soil and water surface and through transpiration from vegetation.

An estimated 324 billion gallons of fresh water is discharged into the oceans each day, leaving a flow of 876 to 926 billion gallons per day in ground and surface storage. It is not economically feasible for much of this fresh water to be pumped or withdrawn since the levels of lakes and streams must be maintained for navigation, hydroelectric power, fish and wildlife, water sports, and natural beauty. The estimate most frequently given by water resource experts is that a sustained dependable supply from the ground and surface water for irrigation, industrial, and domestic purposes varies from 300 to 325 billion gallons per day.

The "prophets of doom" are quick to note that the withdrawal of fresh water in the United States is almost 300 billion gallons per day now and that surely we face exhaustion of our fresh supply. The fallacy sometimes employed by groups who wish to promote schemes for desalting the sea or seeding clouds is the idea that all water "withdrawn" is "consumed" and is thus unavailable for reuse. A look at the 1968 National Water Assessment given in Table 17.1 should clear this misconception. The critical values to be compared with available supply are the numbers in the "consumed" column. Furthermore, were it not for the practice of "making the deserts bloom" which is now evaporating 86 percent of all the fresh water consumed in the United States, there would be little reason for future concern. Uses other than irrigation return 90 percent of the water withdrawn to the rivers and lakes for downstream reuse. The future problem is to be sure that the water to be returned for reuse is of satisfactory quality.

Each year during the hot summer months, many American communities are forced to restrict water just when it is most needed. Actually, they are not short of water but, as discussed below, they are short of facilities to collect, treat, and deliver water to those who need it. The United States will never run out of water for domestic uses. With the Hudson River flowing by its doorstep, New York City, for example, need never experience a water shortage. Nor, with proper water resource management, should any of man's needs for fresh water be in jeopardy.

Growth of Water and Sewerage Systems

One good indication of the standard of living and general level of health is the percent of total population served with public water supply and sewerage

Table 17.1
Fresh Water Use in Billion Gallons per Day

Category Use	Withdrawal	Consumed	Returned for Reuse
Irrigation	112.6	91.5	21.1
Steam-electric cooling	84.5	0.8	83.7
Industrial	46.4	7.5	38.9
Municipal (domestic-commercial)	23.7	5.4	18.3
Rural domestic and farm	2.4	1.6	0.8
United States Total	269.6	106.8	162.8
Percent	100%	40%	60%
Available dependable supply		300	
Percent of supply unused		64%	

SOURCE: Water Resources Council. *First National Assessment 1968.* Washington, D.C.

utilities. The figures given in Table 17.2 show the remarkable growth of piped water supplies in the United States during the past four decades. This statistic comes from the census question regarding "water and toilet in the house." Having piped water or a flush toilet does not mean that public facilities are used; it may mean that any of the possible combinations of public and private on-lot systems are employed. The fact that, by 1970, 94 percent of the population of the entire United States, rural and urban, has plumbing in the home reflects the extent of rural electrification and the growth of urbanization in this country. The extension of public water and sewers into built-up suburban areas is progressing slowly. Nevertheless, about the same number of wells and septic tank systems were added during the last decade as were replaced by public facilities. The most disturbing fact is that 13 to 15 million citizens in the United States are still without modern sanitary conveniences. Most of these are poor people living in rural tenant farms, fringes of the less developed small urban centers, and Indian reservations.

The most important activity of the environmental health planning process is to instigate at the state level a mechanism for integrating the plans for water and sewerage utilities. The past long-range planning effort, with a few exceptions, has not looked at the advantages of developing economical service areas which disregard local political boundaries. The United States is operating too many small systems whose services are less than satisfactory. By putting the small utilities into large regional organizations, such nations as England and Holland were able to have proper administrative, technical, and financial supervision. This goal will not be easy to attain in the United States without mechanisms for communication among the strange mixture of concerned ghetto and conservative suburban residents and the provider groups such as public works agencies and political leaders.

Table 17.2

Growth of Water and Sewerage Systems in the United States

(Estimated Population in Millions)

	1940		1950		1960		1970	
	Pop.	%	Pop.	%	Pop.	%	Pop.	%
Piped Water Supplies	98.3	74.5	125.0	82.8	165.4	92.9	192.0	93.8
Public and private utility	85.0	64.4	92.0	61.0	134.0	75.3	160.0	78.2
Home and farm systems	13.3	10.1	33.0	21.8	31.4	17.6	32.0	15.6
Non-Piped Water Supplies	33.7	25.5	26.0	17.2	12.6	7.1	12.7	6.2
Total	132.0	100.0	151.0	100.0	178.0	100.0	204.7	100.0
Water Carriage Sewerage	84.8	64.2	113.0	74.5	160.0	89.8	190.0	92.5
Public sewers	72.0	54.5	80.0	53.0	111.0	62.3	140.0	68.5
Septic tank and cesspool	12.8	9.7	33.0	21.5	49.0	27.5	50.0	24.4
Non-Water Carriage, Privy	47.2	35.8	38.0	25.5	18.0	10.2	15.7	7.3
Total	132.0	100.0	151.0	100.0	178.0	100.0	204.7	100.0

Based on: U.S. Bureau of the Census. 16th Census Reports: 1940. Housing, Vol. II; U.S. Census of Housing: 1950, Vol. I; 1960, Vol. I; and 1970, preliminary census data. Washington, D.C.: Government Printing Office.

One successful device for bringing the communities together is a sanitary facilities fund, with legislation for appropriating state money for improving and extending sanitary services in the state through matching grants. At one time, it was felt that federal funds would supply the financial assistance needed for upgrading water and sewerage services. It became clear, however, that federal funds disbursed to local public work projects through the Departments of Interior and Housing and Urban Development represented only "seed money" which has had the effect of encouraging communities to wait for federal money, rather than to assume the financial responsibility for their own problems. State regulatory agencies feel that without some offer of financial assistance, comprehensive planning will not proceed. In Maryland, for example, the facilities fund act requires that each county adopt and submit for approval by a certain date county-wide plans for public water and waste facilities. Financial assistance for planning and matching construction funds (state and federal) are contingent upon an approved long-range plan.

Present Status of Public Water Supply

Despite the remarkable post-World War II progress, the private and municipal water works industry is in trouble in meeting both recurring water shortages and in maintaining the quality of water delivered to consumers. The greatest challenge of the future is for the communities to finance the enormous construction expenditures required to overcome current deficiencies, obsolescence, and demand by future population growth.

In its periodic check of adequacy of public water supply capacity, the U.S. Department of Commerce came to the conclusion that in 1963 one-third of the American population was served by systems which were deficient or near-deficient in meeting current demand. In each instance, the problem was due not to natural shortages but to deficiencies in facilities for transmission, storage, and treatment. The estimated annual construction requirements for the water utilities in the United States is given in Table 17.3.

Table 17.3
Average Annual Construction Requirements for Water Utilities, 1967-1980
(Millions of 1966 Dollars)

Region	Deficiencies	Obsolescence, Depreciation	Population Growth	Total
Northeast	$103	$156	$269	$528
North Central	112	171	293	576
South	109	166	286	561
West	77	118	203	398
Total	$401	$611	$1051	$2063

Assistance from the federal and state governments has been slow in coming to the water works industry. If the industry is to continue to support and finance itself with a minimum of public assistance as it has done in the past, it must stop being proud of slogans like "water cheaper than dirt" and begin to be ashamed of the poor service caused by low water rates. New standards of quality and service will result in higher cost to the consumer. Of concern is the knowledge that while municipal and privately owned water utilities must expend $2.1 billion annually to meet standards, the federal contribution to solving water supply problems is only $2.3 million per year.

Economic Considerations of Water Supply Systems

Many factors determine the cost of community water, including the source of supply, degree of treatment required, total usage, and variations in usage. The water usage or demand is a function of domestic, commercial, industrial, and public needs. The national public water consumption expressed in average gallons per capita per day or percent of average daily usage is given in Table 17.4.

Variation in usage depends upon size of lots and reaches a peak during lawn sprinkling in the summer months. The maximum water consumption in a day and hour is usually 180 percent and 265 percent, respectively, of the average daily use. A reliable water system's distribution and storage capabilities must be designed for peak usage of water.

Annual Costs

Annual cost methods of analysis involve finding the uniform annual cost for recovering capital and providing for maintenance and operation expenses. Capital recovery is variously termed interest plus depreciation or amortization charges. The usual method for computing these charges is to calculate the annual interest (at rate i) on the initial capital cost (K) and the end of year deposit (R)

Table 17.4
National Public Water Consumption

Use	Average Gallons per Capita per Day	Percent of Average Daily Usage
Domestic	60	40
Industrial*	32	21
Commercial	21	14
Public	15	10
Waste or loss	22	15
Total	150	100

*Does not include "process" water.

to a hypothetical sinking fund that accumulates at compound interest for the period of analysis (n years) to equal the initial cost. Adding these charges and the operation and maintenance costs (OM), annual cost becomes

$$AC = Ki + R + OM, \ or$$
$$AC = Ki + [Ki/(1 + i)^n - 1] + OM.$$

In developing generalized cost data for fresh water supplies, unit costs have been computed from the annual cost incorporating a constant load building factor. A factor of 0.75 has been applied for storage, transmission, and conventional treatment cost by dividing the annual cost (AC) by the design capacity Q (in millions of gallons per day, or mgd) times d (365 days per year). Thus, the unit cost, or cost per million gallons, is

$$AC/0.75Qd.$$

Capital costs per capita are most difficult to interpret because the figure often does not reflect the actual quantity of water used by the individual and is merely computed on the basis of total population and cost. Capital cost per mgd capacity for the United States is given in Table 17.5.

Table 17.5
Cost in 1000 Dollars per Capacity in Millions of
Gallons per Day

Capacity (mgd)	Collection and Distribution	Treatment	Total
0.1	$1,715	$865	$2,580
1.0	1,654	400	2,050
10.0	1,354	186	1,540
100.0	974	86	1,060

BASED ON: United States construction from 1956 to 1965, adjusted to 1970 cost, by *Engineering News Record Index*.

The annual unit cost of water which includes debt service (amortization of capital cost), operation, and maintenance averages 33¢ per 1000 gallons in 875 municipally owned water utilities. If the systems were built at today's construction cost and interest rates, the unit cost of water would be as follows (Table 17.6).

Anyone can see the economic advantage of the large capacity system in both capital cost and operation and maintenance cost to the consumer. These economic considerations should offer incentives for the smaller systems to join in regional water supply programs.

Table 17.6
Total Annual Cost in Cents per 1000 Gallons

Capacity (mgd)	Debt Service	Operation and Maintenance	Total
0.1	46¢	33¢	79¢
1.0	37	13	50
10.0	28	5	33
100.0	19	2	21

Interest i = 5%; period n = 30 years.

THE WATER PROBLEM: WASTE WATER COLLECTION AND TREATMENT

Public sewerage (collection and disposal) has always fallen behind public water supply because of the difficulties of establishing an equitable source of revenue to meet bond obligations. In addition, the stigma associated with such operations makes it, along with solid waste management, unable to function with the dignity and effectiveness of most public utilities such as power, water, and telephone. There is nothing to sell except service. The revenue for the construction, operation, and maintenance has been found best in a sewer service charge system. The philosophy of the service charge based on water consumption, which is added to the water bill, provides an equitable self-supporting system of sewerage.

Responsibility for pollution control and abatement rests with those individuals, industries, and municipalities who withdraw water, use it, and return it to our streams, lakes, oceans, and underground sources of water. Only a part of the water pollution problem comes from municipal and industrial sewage treatment effluents; much of the undesirable pollutants reaching natural waters come from all kinds of land use practices. To mention a few: the chemical runoffs from agriculture lands, spills in railroad and highway accidents, contaminants from the air, construction erosion, leaking of mine tailings, and many other exotic materials difficult to intercept and treat.

Many state regulatory agencies welcomed the participation of the federal government in the water pollution field. They anticipated financial support for construction, upgrading of control agencies, and the development of comprehensive river basin schemes. However, the Water Pollution Control Act of 1948 concentrated efforts only on the abatement of stream pollution and in so doing encouraged states to forbid extensions of or connections to existing public sewers until certain pollution abatement requirements had been met. Since small subdivision systems were looked upon with disfavor, the act contributed to the most massive septic tank building program the world has ever seen.

Conservation interests, unhappy with the progress in stream pollution abatement, began in 1956 to appropriate annual sums for stimulating the construction of waste water treatment work. Nevertheless, the gaps between the amount of federal money authorized, appropriated, and actually expended were great—despite the proclamation of the need for more action.

The total capital outlay for waste collection and treatment in the United States is an enormous sum and averaged about $1.5 billion per year during the 1960's. Even so, the backlog to overcome deficiencies at the end of 1969 was $4.4 billion. The capital investment in the water pollution control area for 1968 is given in Table 17.7.

It should be emphasized that, in the period from 1956 to 1969, the total federal grant funds for construction were $1.1 billion while during the same time the total investment in sewerage by municipalities and industry was about $20 billion.

Table 17.7
Comparative Investment Outlays for Waste-Handling Purposes
1968

Investment Category	Millions of Current Dollars
New waste treatment plants	$180
Expansion, upgrading, replacement	189
Interceptors and outfalls	284
Collecting sewers	550
Industrial waste treatment	529
Total Capital Outlay	$1,732

SOURCE: Federal Water Pollution Control Administration. *The Economics of Clean Water.* Washington, D.C.: Government Printing Office, 1970.

Cost of Community Sanitary Sewerage

The cost of community sanitary sewers increases considerably with increasing lot size. The per dwelling unit cost in many instances varies inversely as the square root of the areal density of population. Thus, a sewer for dwellings on one acre (43,560 square feet) lots will cost three times more than for dwellings on a minimum size lot of 5,000 square feet. In addition to lot size, the variation in sewer cost depends upon topography, amount and character of excavation, need for pumping, and availability of a receiving stream for the treated effluent. Good conditions indicate a topography favorable for gravity flow with a minimum of excavation and blasting and a nearby receiving stream. At the other extreme, poor conditions represent steep topography requiring much pumping, extensive excavation with rock blasting, and long conveyance to a suitable disposal waterway.

The following estimated costs of community sewers are based on a model community having 10,000 square foot lots, with 3.5 persons per dwelling unit and capital cost amortized for a 30-year period with interest at 5 percent (Table 17.8).

Table 17.8
Sewage Collection Cost per Dwelling Unit (1970)

		Cost per Dwelling Unit per Year		
Condition	Capital Cost	Debt	Operations and Maintenance	Total
Good	$728	$48	$2	$50
Average	1,020	66	3	69
Poor	1,330	86	4	90

SOURCE: Engineering News Record Construction Cost Index.

Treatment Costs

Today, the stream standards adopted in most states require complete treatment including chlorination of effluent. The cost includes the unit operations for both liquid and sludge, but the cost of land is not included (Table 17.9). The sewage flow has been assumed to be 350 gallons per day per dwelling unit.

It can be seen that the cost shared by the large population densities (small lots) has economic advantages in both collection and treatment cost. The cost for extending sewer service into the suburban areas is quite high because of the

Table 17.9
Cost of Treatment (1970)

Plant Capacity mgd	Capital Cost		Cost per Dwelling Unit per Year		
	mgd	Dwelling Unit	Debt	Operation and Maintenance	Total
0.1	$1,670,000	$580	$38	$3	$41
1.0	800,000	280	18	1	19
10.0	535,000	187	12	1	13
100.0	290,000	102	6	1	7

SOURCE: Engineering News Record Construction Cost Index.

trend to large lot size and sparse population density. Experience indicates that reliance upon water rates alone for producing the necessary capital is insufficient and that front foot assessments must be charged to all benefiting property whether developed or not.

The principal limitation to the extension of the conventional water-carriage sewer system to fringe areas has been its high cost. Although requiring a greater amount of initial investment, community sewers as opposed to the installation of individual on-lot systems would in most instances have resulted in substantial long-term saving. In comparing the relative cost of community sewers to individual on-lot systems, it is necessary to take into account the cost of renewal, revamping, or replacement as well as installation costs. The state and local subdivision regulations exercise control over the design, construction, and maintenance of on-lot systems. The codes are written with minimum lot size restrictions for septic tank schemes based on soil percolation time. These tests attempt to evaluate the suitability of the soil to adsorb the settled sewage effluent. Poor soil conditions may be offset by costly adsorption systems but the space requirements may be so large as to discourage housing developments where public water and sewerage is unavailable.

Table 17.10
Average Cost of Septic Tank and Adsorption Systems (1970)

Soil Condition	Percolation (Minutes)	Total Cost		Renewal Period (Years)	Cost per Dwelling Unit per Year
		Tank	Adsorption		
Good	5	$551	$ 212	27.5	$ 60
Average	20	551	1059	17.5	176
Poor	50	551	1430	12.5	195

SOURCE: Engineering News Record Construction Cost Index.

The average cost of septic tank and adsorption systems according to soil condition and percolation time is presented in Table 17.10. The annual cost per dwelling unit, unlike public sewers, is independent of lot size but requires sufficient lot space for the adsorption system and replacement. The total cost includes cost of tank installation and present worth of sludge removal costs, the cost of adsorption system installation and its present worth of replacement at designated time intervals, with interest at 5 percent.

THE AIR POLLUTION PROBLEM

The threat of air pollution to man's health was recognized over 120 years ago by Lemuel Shattuck in his *Report of the Massachusetts Sanitary Commission.* This report served as both a basis and a goal for organized public health work in this country for many years. The effects of atmospheric pollution on health were not clearly demonstrated, however, and through the years only sporadic attacks at the local level were made under general nuisance abatement laws and ordinances based on the density of smoke emitted from chimneys. The 1948 disaster in Donora, Pennsylvania, in which 20 aged residents in a population of 14,000 died from the effects of industrial fumigation, resulted in the passage in 1955 of the first federal air pollution control legislation (PL 84-159). At that time, no state had an ongoing program and it is no wonder that pollution of the air is regarded as a recently discovered environmental problem.

Actually, reduction of smoke (by fuel conversion from coal to oil or gas) was markedly lowering the soot and fly ash problem throughout the major urban centers, but the Los Angeles "smog" (now known to be photochemical in origin) was the cause for the current nationwide emphasis on air management. Population and industrial growth and a high degree of dependence on the automobile have greatly complicated the traditional stationary sources of pollution associated with power plants and industrial processes. Initially, this air pollution law of 1955 (PL 84-159) stated that the control of the air pollution sources was a state and local responsibility and largely provided assistance to the states in the form of technical advice, research, and training. A second act passed by Congress in 1960 (PL 86-493) authorized the Public Health Service to study the problem of automobile exhausts. By then it became evident that to get air pollution control going, much more comprehensive federal programs would be needed, including financial assistance to state and local governments. The Clean Air Act in 1963 (PL 88-206) greatly expanded the federal programs to assist the states in appraising their problems, initiating state legislative authority, and assisting state regulatory agencies in organizing and carrying out programs "tailor made" for the region. The Clean Air Act was amended in 1965 (PL 89-272), expanded in 1966 (PL 89-675), and again amended in 1967 as the Air Quality Act (PL 90-148); for the first time, it authorized federal money to state and local agencies to start and maintain effective air pollution control programs and to set standards for emission of pollutants for certain motor vehicles. States could get financial aid only if the governor agreed to follow the federal procedure for establishing ambient air and emission standards and abatement implementation plans.

The first step in controlling air pollution is to determine the areas of the country where atmospheric ventilation is poor and the capacity to dilute the pollutant is frequently impaired. The United States has been divided into eight atmospheric areas based on long-term studies of meteorological factors that affect transportation and diffusion of airborne pollutants. The southern California coastal region is the only area where ventilation is persistently reduced, although ventilation is frequently reduced in the mountain states, both east and west, during the fall and winter months. In addition, the states east of the Mississippi River have occasional periods of poor ventilation. The plains states west of the Mississippi River from Texas to the Canadian border have conditions leading to good pollution dispersion. Unfortunately, very little or no consideration was given to air pollution dispersion when some of the population and industrial growth developed in areas such as Los Angeles, Pittsburgh, and Birmingham. Today, considerable thought must be given to the location of any heavy, potentially dirty industries. Electric generating stations, both fossil fuel and nuclear, will be outside high population density areas where ventilation and other ecological considerations will enter into site selection.

After the atmospheric areas were set, the next move by federal agencies was to designate air quality control regions within states or interstate. Air quality criteria are promulgated showing the effects of pollutants on health, vegetation, and materials. Armed with this information, the state must set regional standards acceptable to the federal Environmental Protection Agency, which has taken over the National Air Pollution Control Administration's work. Following the development of air quality standards, the state must implement abatement plans by setting specific emission levels for source pollutants. This entire procedure is to be accomplished step by step for all pollutants according to a specific timetable. As of July, 1970, air quality control regions had been designated to include 40 major metropolitan areas of an anticipated 90 regions. So far, criteria and control documents have been issued for five pollutants—namely, sulfur oxide, particulates, carbon monoxide, hydrocarbons, and photochemical oxidants. Seventeen states had submitted standards for approval and only ten had been approved. No implementation plans have yet been approved. Obviously, no enforcement can take place until plans are approved and underway.

Evidence is mounting that the current federal-state air pollution program is too cumbersome. Another amendment to the Clean Air Act may initiate:

1. Nationwide ambient air quality standards;
2. Greatly tightened emission standards for new automobiles by 1975;
3. Use of latest available techniques on all new sources of pollution;
4. Authority for land use and transportation planning;
5. New avenues for making sure the air pollution control law is enforced.

As mentioned under water and waste water management, the absence of adequate appropriations at the federal and state levels—despite laws—will mitigate against results anticipated by comprehensive planning. In fiscal 1969, the federal authorization was $185 million, but only $88.7 million was appropriated. For 1970, despite the authorization of $179.3 million, only $108.8 million was appropriated. The cost of air pollution control is borne by the ultimate consumer whether in the cost of power, automobiles, or other products of industry. The per capita federal cost for research, training, regulation, and enforcement is running about one dollar per year.

A preliminary phase of reconnaissance for a city, metropolitan area, or region is needed to size up the magnitude and nature of the problem, including the sources of pollution, which are generally divided into five categories: transportation, industry, power plants, space heating, and refuse disposal. The amount of emission of the five sources is usually given in tons per year of carbon monoxide, sulfur oxide, hydrocarbons, nitrogen oxide, and particulate matter. In general, such analysis will show that the major sources of carbon monoxide, oxides of nitrogen, and hydrocarbons are in vehicles powered by the internal combustion engine. Central-station generation of electricity is the principal source of oxides of sulfur, and the principal source of particulate matter is industrial processes. Statistics of this kind are impressive but give little information on the atmospheric concentration level and frequency. This information, which is determined by air monitoring, is necessary when standards for control are being set.

The air pollution control regions are being established on meteorological and topographical bases and may be visualized as large volumes of atmosphere in which air pollution is to be controlled. Various mathematical air quality models are being developed for forecasting the atmospheric concentration of a pollutant based on diffusion and transport of the pollutant emission under meteorological conditions of the region. Regional control will become increasingly important in air shed management just as in water basin management.

The interrelation between the environmental adjustments required for the control of water, air, and land make the comprehensive overview an absolute necessity in planning. The decisions made must be compatible with the objectives of better human health and the total resource base. The current fad of zero economic growth cannot realistically be a solution to the problem, knowing the enormous costs of providing health-related environmental controls. The long-range planning of the development of our urban complex to keep pace with the demands of an ever-increasing population is more than just an issue of health and survival but rather an issue of quality of life. The ultimate cure calls for heroic reorganization of urban designs, involving the total systems approach in restructuring housing, transportation, industry, and energy along more efficient and conservative lines. Health planners cannot wait for the research, mathematical models, and social and political changes that young people use as a philosophical base to attack the conventional system. In the United States, we have been diverted too long from things we know how to do; with planning, we should never have fallen so far behind.

THE SOLID WASTE PROBLEM: COLLECTION AND DISPOSAL

Unlike air pollution or waste water, which flow away from the sources of production, solid wastes pile up at the source unless mechanically hauled away.

The term solid waste is defined as unwanted residues of natural or manmade resources and of human activity which are handled in the solid state. Such expressions as "garbage" or "trash" are inaccurate since these comprise but a minute fraction of the solid waste problem.

Estimates developed by the Departments of Health, Education and Welfare and Interior, the Bureau of Solid Waste Management, and the Bureau of Mines suggest that 4.3 billion tons of waste were produced in the United States in 1969. This is a staggering production of some 118 pounds of solid waste per capita per *day*—an almost unbelievable figure until one realizes that most of it originates from agriculture and livestock (62.5 pounds per capita per day) and mining and mineral processing (30 pounds per capita per day). These wastes, along with other industrial residues such as fly ash, slag, metals, rags, and paper, comprise the private collection and disposal problem. The category of residential, commercial, and institutional solid wastes are part of the public services undertaken by either public or private refuse collection and disposal organizations.

Economic Considerations

The collection and disposal of urban refuse is the most expensive recurring public program next to the operation of schools. In the United States in 1969, $3.5 billion was spent handling 190 million tons, an average of $18 per ton. This does not include the private sections of industry and agriculture, which would be over one billion dollars per year. The residential, commercial, and institutional wastes are the clearest threat to health in that they provide food and harborage for disease vectors such as rats, flies, and mosquitoes and contribute to air pollution through burying dumps, poor incinerators, and nuisance odors. A source of considerable public outrage is the litter problem and unsightliness along streets, highways, beaches, and parks, which costs $88 per ton to collect and dispose of, or more than four times the cost of residential programs.

Collection

The cost of collection represents 80 percent of the total waste program. In general, people have been willing to pay the cost of removing refuse from their premises either through general tax revenues or special collection fees. The latter does not provide the much needed service for the urban poor who are unable to pay the collection fee. The amount of refuse collected will average about four pounds per capita per day. Actually, the total production figure is reported to be seven pounds, but this includes all collected wastes such as tree trimmings, demolition debris, and discarded appliances and automobiles which are sometimes a part of the public program.

Collection is a door-to-door manual labor program essentially unchanged from the horse-drawn wagon days. The major advance is in the "packer" vehicle which saves space by compacting waste on a three-to-one ratio and thus saves on the number of necessary trips to the disposal site. To save on production travel time, transfer stations are now employed. These provide large hauling vans which receive several packer loads and can more economically transport refuse to disposal sites. Housing projects with containers and institutions with shredders or compactors are cost-saving and eliminate the need for small incinerators which are notorious air polluters.

The cost of collection reflects the prevailing cost of labor and trucks and the haul distance. Below (Table 17.11) is tabulated the cost for mixed refuse per ton collected and per capita per year in the northeastern United States, assuming an urban area with 30 or more houses to the acre and two collections per week.

Table 17.11
Refuse Collection Cost

Haul Distance One Way (in Miles)	Cost per Ton*	Cost per Capita per Year**
4	$ 9.50	$6.65
8	10.50	7.35
12	11.20	7.85
16	11.50	8.05
20	12.50	8.75
24	13.50	9.45

* Labor, maintenance, and amortization of trucks (no disposal).
** Based on 1,400 pounds per capita per year.

Disposal

The average cost of disposal of refuse is about $4 per ton. Of the annual 190 million tons of residential, commercial, and institutional solid wastes collected, 146 million tons (77 percent) is deposited on unsanitary open dumps. About 25 million tons (13 percent) is made into proper sanitary land fills. Another 15 million (10 percent) is incinerated for volume reduction and the ash deposited on the land. The obvious pressure on disposal practices in the United States is that governments can no longer place the collected refuse in open dumps. Land for such dumps within economical hauling distance is already exhausted, and even distant sites operate under strong protest from citizen groups. People are not so willing to pay the cost for refuse disposal once it has been removed from sight. When properly done, sanitary land fill, which is nothing more than an engineered technique of burying compacted refuse, can reclaim marginal land, such as marshes, into attractive public parks. Improperly done, it can result in nuisance gas odors and vermin. The stigma associated with these operations contributes to the whole syndrome of poor administration and personnel, including poor pay, high rates of accidents, illness, absenteeism, and labor turnover. The cost of refuse disposal, exclusive of the cost of land, is given in Table 17.12.

Table 17.12
Refuse Disposal Cost

Operation	Cost per Ton	Cost per Capita per Year
Sanitary land fill		
Full day machine (s)	$0.45	$0.31
Less than full day	1.50	1.05
Incineration with pollution controls		
(>50 tons per day capacity)	$5-$10	$3.50-$7.00

Although small incinerators are used for commercial and industrial purposes, the resulting cost and air pollution problem has caused control agencies to ban such installations along with backyard trash burning. Generally, successful municipal incinerators have an average capacity of 300 tons per day, which limits the installation to larger cities unless the smaller jurisdictions join together in a regional disposal unit.

Recycling and Reuse

The task of solid waste management is that of either local governments or private enterprise. One common criticism is that those in charge are reluctant to utilize new ideas of salvage, recycling, and reuse. It is quite evident that organic composts may be made and returned to the soil, or that paper and glass can be salvaged, processed, and recycled. The disposal of automobiles is an excellent example of the complexities involved. Almost 97 percent of the revenue from the junked car is from the sale of spare parts that are removed. Scrap hulks, on the other hand, are not in as great demand by the mills and foundries as they were before the basic oxygen and electric induction processes of making steel were introduced. The cheapest means of preparing the stripped, junked car is to compress it in a great hydraulic press into bales contaminated with glass, chrome, plastic, upholstery, and other foreign material. This scrap yields a very low price. A better price for scrap may be made by shredding automobiles and separating the contaminants. There is money to be made in salvage, and private enterprises are already so engaged. The problem is to elevate these operations to an industry status with appropriate controls, so that they will be welcomed in the community rather than serve as a source of citizen protest. New and improved technology will emerge as wastes are recycled and reused.

The comprehensive environmental health planning process encourages the joining of communities in the solutions of common solid waste management problems. The federal government did not enter this field until the passage of the Solid Waste Disposal Act (Title II of PL 89-272) in 1965. Under this act, grants will be made for state and interstate solid waste planning. Planning operational systems, along with reclamation and reuse as a future goal, offers the solution to a problem which is characterized by inadequacies of attention, function, and application.

READINGS

Primary

Atkisson, A. and Gaines, Richard S. *Development of Air Quality Standards.* Columbus, Ohio: Charles & Merrill Publishing Co., 1970.
> This book, useful for both air pollution expert and nonexpert, deals with how air pollution standards are set, what must be known, and how to interpret various constraints (such as political, organizational, and legal). Abatement strategy is discussed, and mathematical models are presented for forecasting the results of varying strategies of air pollution abatement.

Bureau of Community Environmental Management. *Environmental Health Planning.* U.S.P.H.S. Publication No. 2120. Washington, D.C.: Government Printing Office, 1971.
> Comprehensive guidelines addressed to environmental health administrators and planners for stimulating review, evaluation, and planning of programs; linkage of programs to targets; and coordination of progress with other public and private efforts toward obtaining and maintaining a healthful environment.

Cleary, E. J. *The ORSANCO Story.* Baltimore: Johns Hopkins Press, 1967. This work deals with the history, organization, and achievements of the largest successful stream conservation agency, the Ohio River Valley Water Sanitation Commission, which involves eight states. Solving problems by the regional and basin approach is encouraged.

Consumer Protection and Environmental Health Service. *Environmental Health Planning Guide.* 1968 revised edition. U.S.P.H.S. Publication No. 823. Washington, D.C.: Government Printing Office, 1969.
> A guide designed to assist in evaluating health-related services and facilities from a planning standpoint. Its use should provide the community with a better view of the factors contributing to a healthful environment, now and in the future.

National Academy of Science. *Waste Management and Control.* Publication 1400. Washington, D.C.: National Research Council, 1966.
> A committee report giving its findings and recommendations on the national problem of pollution. The objective is to set forth the nature of the pollution problem and how it interacts with all living things and to suggest where science and technology can effectively assist in reducing and controlling pollutants.

National Academy of Science, Committee on Pollution. *Alternatives in Waste Management*. Publication 1408. Washington, D.C.: National Research Council, 1966.
> Sets out alternatives in waste management which might provide better long-range solutions to pollution problems than conventional means.

Strobbe, Maurice A. *Understanding Environmental Pollution*. St. Louis: The C. V. Mosby Co., 1971.
> A volume consisting of selected papers by various authors concerned with environmental pollution. Its purpose is to supply a text in support of biology, botany, and zoology courses in ecology and to provide a source of information on the current status of technological aspects of environmental quality for students of both the sciences and humanities.

U.S. President's Science Advisory Committee, Environmental Pollution Panel. *Restoring the Quality of Our Environment*. Washington, D.C.: The White House, 1965.
> Commonly known as the Tukey Report, after the chairman of the panel, Princeton Professor John W. Tukey. Although somewhat out of date, it still represents a balanced study of pollution problems distinguishing between what is known and what is not, along with recommendations necessary to assure lessening of the deterioration already here and to prevent unacceptable levels in the future.

Secondary

Banks, H. O. "Comprehensive Health Planning in Relation to Environmental Problems. I. Environment: Conflict and Compromise." *American Journal of Public Health* 61:1972-1979, 1971.

Cleaning Our Environment. The Chemical Basis for Action. A Report by the Subcommittee on Environment Improvement. Washington, D.C.: American Chemical Society, 1969.

Cost of Clean Air. First Report of the Secretary of Health, Education and Welfare. Washington, D.C.: Government Printing Office, 1969.

Council on Environmental Quality. *Environmental Quality*. First Annual Report. Washington, D.C.: Government Printing Office, 1970.

Degler, Stanley E. and Bloom, Sandra C. *Federal Pollution Control Programs: Water, Air, and Solid Wastes*. Washington, D.C.: Bureau of National Affairs, Inc., 1969.

Engdahl, Richard. *Solid Waste Processing. A State-of-the-Art Report on Unit Operations and Processes*. Environmental Control Administration, Bureau of Solid Waste Management, Report No. Sw-4c. U.S.P.H.S. Publication No. 1856. Washington, D.C.: Government Printing Office, 1969.

Federal Water Pollution Control Administration. *Economics of Clean Water*. Summary Report. Washington, D.C.: Government Printing Office, 1970.

Johnson, C. C. "Environmental Control Should Be Included in Comprehensive Health Planning." *Hospitals* 43:86-90, May 16, 1969.

Kurz, A. T. "Comprehensive Health Planning in Relation to Environmental Problems. III. Health Department Participation in Planning for Action." *American Journal of Public Health* 61:1982-1987, 1971.

Michael, J. M. "Systematic Planning for Environmental Development." *American Journal of Public Health* 60:1205-1212, 1970.

National Center for Air Pollution Control. *Storage and Retrieval of Air Quality Data (SAROAD)*. PHS-APTD-68-8. Washington, D.C.: Government Printing Office, 1968.

Peloquin, E. J. "Comprehensive Health Planning in Relation to Environmental Problems. II. Catalytic Comprehensive Health Planning." *American Journal of Public Health* 61:1979-1982, 1971.

18

Family Planning and Health Planning

CARL E. TAYLOR

No grouping of specialized health activities has surged more rapidly into prominence in recent years than family planning. Health services have for many centuries concentrated on mortality and morbidity control. In fact, population growth was considered one of the goals of organized health services. Now that death rates have fallen or are falling, health personnel must face the reality that it is as much of a challenge to work toward an ecological balance between numbers of births and quality of life as it has been to control disease and reduce the number of deaths.

Health workers should realize that we know little about why death rates have fallen. General economic development seems to have been a more potent force than the work of doctors (1, 2). The clearest evidence comes from retrospective analyses of the vital statistics of Europe, especially England, over the last few centuries (3, 4). The steady downward slope of death rates started when economic conditions began to improve and before the discovery of modern health measures.

When we turn from a perspective of centuries for the demographic transition in Europe to present patterns in developing countries, there is a frequently stated presumption that the current rapid mortality decline is because health measures have become more effective. Again, health workers should recognize with some humility that even our most dramatic health measures are merely synergistic with general development processes. A classic case study is Frederiksen's analysis of mortality data from Ceylon. When trend lines are followed over long periods rather than just during selected short-term intervals, it is clear that what first seemed to be a dramatic drop in mortality because of the introduction of DDT for malaria control in 1947 in actuality merely represented a return of Ceylon's death rate from a wartime high back to a long-term secular trend (5).

With mortality having declined at unprecedented rates, both because of the rapid spread of modernization and because of better health measures, we need new ways of bringing birth rates more rapidly into balance with death rates at the low levels characteristic of development (6). All health services in past

311

centuries depended on individualized responses of medical practitioners to the spontaneous demands of those who could pay. Similarly, family planning practice was highly individualized and available mainly to the educated and the affluent. Birth rates tended to follow the decline of mortality rates, but with a lag period of several generations (7). We are even more uncertain about the reasons for the decline of birth rates than we are for the decline of death rates (4, 8).

Population growth has become one of the strongest forces influencing social change in the modern world. Economic planners and development experts became aware of the impact of population growth when censuses and statistical returns showed that increases in GNP and other indices of development were being neutralized by a rapid increase in population. As this quantitative increase was recognized to be contributing to massive social and political complications there has been a somewhat reluctant and delayed recognition of the need for programs to keep population growth down to a reasonable balance with other growth indices.

Demographers and development planners have tended to use health services as a convenient scapegoat, claiming that health personnel have been too efficient. It is somewhat ironic that many of these same population experts subsequently have urged that family planning be removed from "domination" by health services because of the inefficiency and low status of health ministries. A collective guilt feeling has become evident in international agencies such as The Rockefeller Foundation and United States Agency for International Development. The first indication of an over-response to this dilemma was a sharp reduction in support for international health programs. After a few years large allocations of funds were made to population programs with predictable interpretations by officials of developing countries.

Gradually, a more balanced approach is now developing in international thinking about family planning programs. Health planning and population planning need to be closely integrated. Both have overlapping circles of interest. Population planning also must develop close program linkages with agriculture, labor, industry, urban affairs, education, mass media, and many other agencies and forces for social change. Although this presentation concentrates on the health aspects of family planning, it must be recognized that population planning has many other interfaces.

BROAD GOALS OF FAMILY PLANNING PROGRAMS

The dramatic increase around the world of efforts to expand family planning services has the fascinating feature that the various proponents give diverse reasons for their support. Acceptance of family planning by individuals or groups results from combinations of goals that shift with time. Stated rationales for population policy are determined mostly by traditional and historical commitments. While we understand little enough about individual motivations, we know even less about what makes certain population goals important to groups of people. The influence of national and ethnic strivings is clearest in the worldwide phenomenon that minority groups consider family planning programs to be genocidal in intent. Examples are found in the reactions of African countries toward international agencies, among the Black Panthers in the United States, and among some caste groups in Indian villages.

Three broad categories of goals for family planning programs have been defined (9).

Health Goals

Perhaps the earliest and almost universally accepted rationale for family planning is because it improves health. The point will be made in the next section that interactions between health and family planning are two-way in that health activities also promote the effective utilization of family planning services. Even in societies where group attitudes may be strongly pronatalist, there is a high probability that the need for family planning to protect the health of mothers, children, and the family as a unit will be readily accepted. Health workers concerned with the care of poor families were among the earliest advocates of family planning.

Human Rights Goals

Various societies have set up diverse controls on the basic right of couples to choose when and whether to produce a child. The social ramifications depend on the balance in responsibility for child care between the family and society. As patterns of reproduction have become increasingly controllable, social decisions about individual freedom are being made according to a wide range of national or group definitions of human rights. Included in this range are such considerations as (1) whether the availability of family planning services should be determined by socioeconomic status with the poor being less able to plan their families than those more affluent; (2) whether women should continue to carry the major responsibility for pregnancy and child rearing, especially at the cost of hazards to their own health and personal development; (3) in the larger social group, who is going to bear the cost of providing necessary social benefits for large numbers of children in populations where dependency ratios are already unfavorable; and (4) how do these human rights arguments affect the availability of specific family planning methods, especially abortion?

Individuals coming from democratic and egalitarian societies often assume that they pay most attention to human rights. It is of interest, however, that some Russian authorities claim that the USSR had the first national program for family planning and that it was based on human rights arguments (10). In spite of Marxist policy being clearly pronatalist and anti-Malthusian (11), contraception and abortion were made available under Soviet health services in the 1920's as part of the general move toward giving more rights to women and promoting health.

Population Control Goals

In the past several years an active altercation has developed between proponents of family planning and of population control. Kingsley Davis seems to have started the debate by stating that traditional family planning approaches were irrelevant to broad demographic concerns (12). Using the general definition that family planning makes it possible for individuals to have the number of children they want, he posed the broad social issue that people on the average want too many children. Population control then would be defined as measures for adjusting people's wants in family size to society's needs. Considerable enthusiasm for such views has led to multiple proposals for social engineering through economic, legislative, and social measures (13-17).

Population control rhetoric has two broad implications for health workers involved in family planning. First, doctors should realize that they are being criticized for being unresponsive to population goals. The medical profession tends to be intrinsically conservative and resistant to organized family planning movements, even though caring for the family planning needs of individual patients. Similarly, the World Health Organization was, in the mid-1950's, one of the first United Nations agencies in which efforts were made to promote national family planning programs. Because of vehement objections by European countries and the United States, WHO fell considerably behind some other United Nations groups in their support of active programs for family planning in the 1960's.

The second and presently more pertinent consideration for health workers is that no fundamental conflict exists among the three major goals of family planning. If properly synchronized they can be synergistic and compatible. The reproductive goals defined by health planners are fundamentally similar to those defined by social planners concerned with human rights and by demographic and economic planners advocating population control. Conversely, economic planners must be made to see that health planners do not really obstruct their goals—that we recognize that population growth neutralizes per capita benefits and that an increase in per capita GNP promotes better health. Health ministries have typically been handed the population problem by planning groups because no one else was better prepared to handle the problem. The fact that progress has not been immediately evident is due mainly to the difficulties of the problem. Better results in the future can be achieved by working together rather than competing.

SPECIFIC HEALTH OBJECTIVES OF FAMILY PLANNING PROGRAMS

Importance of Denominators in Health Planning

Family planning influences the denominators of vital statistics while health planning in general is concerned with numerators. In health statistics the denominators have generally been taken as given and attention has been focused on ratios of diseases to population, deaths to population, physicians to population, hospital beds to population, etc. Several centuries of research and effort have been devoted to changing numerators. We need to recognize that population denominators are also important in health planning. Demographic considerations must be taken into account in manpower planning so that projections can be related to increases in population size. Some lessons have, hopefully, been learned from the innumerable examples of hospitals which were built without allowing for population increase or shifts in distribution.

Now health planners must begin to think in terms not only of taking denominators into account but also of deliberate programs to modify population size and distribution. The health planner would then be directly involved in the broad goals of population control for health purposes. Health planners must begin to understand ways in which demographic variables interact and also start to develop new tools to analyze these interactions in field programs (18).

Hyperfertility as a Health Problem

Health workers have given insufficient attention to the numbers and spacing of pregnancies as public health problems. A WHO Scientific Group defined a wide range of health aspects of family planning (19). Most apparent are the many diseases which make pregnancy a direct and serious health hazard for mothers; examples range from such systemic conditions as heart disease and anemia to local pelvic and genito-urinary abnormalities. Even without overt disease, however, the health of mothers is affected by large family size, high parity, pregnancy under 18 or over 35 years of age, short intervals between pregnancies, and inadequate care and nutrition during pregnancy and lactation. Many studies show that high and frequent parity increase morbidity and mortality of both mothers and children (20-23). In fact, calculations have been done to show that about one-quarter of the childhood mortality would be prevented by limiting and spacing births (24).

Health planners should actively promote family planning as one of the more effective health measures now available, especially in developing countries where maternal and child mortality and morbidity are still high.

Promotion of Family Planning through Integration with Health Services

Acceptance and utilization of family planning can be markedly increased by improved health and better health services (25, 26). Family planning tends to be a delicate and somewhat unfamiliar subject to those population groups in most need. Parents will be more likely to accept advice from health workers who have demonstrated their competence and concern by caring for illnesses of children or helping mothers during pregnancies. Greater efficiencies can be achieved by combining personnel and facilities for health and family planning services, with both being done better when done together.

There is a complex group of poorly understood interactions between health and family planning that are essentially attitudinal. Better health promotes an orientation to the future characterized by the optimistic view that planning is worthwhile (1, 27). Parents who have a reasonable expectation of life will not only plan ahead but also have more drive and motivation in the intangible entrepreneurial characteristics necessary for development. These attitudes may be essential both for economic development and for family planning acceptance. Perhaps the most direct mechanism for such attitudinal change results from improved child survival. Some 15 years ago we began to point out that there is no reason to expect parents to stop having children until they have reasonable assurance that those they already have are going to survive. Evidence to support this common sense view is now gradually being accumulated (28; 29, pp. 196-200).

STAGES OF FAMILY PLANNING PROGRAMMING

Level of Development of Country and of Its Health Services

In family planning programming a prime consideration is recognition of the need for appropriate phasing. The population problem has taken a long time to develop. Similarly, it may take some time to get birth rates back into balance with death rates by deliberately planned efforts. The necessary phasing of population programs so as to introduce at appropriate times those elements which are most essential must be defined according to the stage of development of a country and of its health services.

Dramatic successes in rapid acceptance of family planning have occurred in situations such as Taiwan, Korea, Singapore, Hong Kong, and Malaysia, where general development and health services had already moved to a fairly advanced stage of coverage (30). A major gap in the broad front of development was apparent in the lack of attention given to family planning services. These countries were still in the demographic lag period since the spontaneous forces of progress which had brought birth rates down in Europe had not yet had time to establish a similar secular trend. When family planning was introduced under these circumstances, a rather prompt and general utilization occurred.

By contrast, some of the countries which are most overpopulated are those where family planning has no such framework of general development and health services into which it may fit. The peoples of some of the crowded countries have made remarkable personal adaptations to high population density at low levels of general development. Obviously, lessons learned in countries at the stage of development of Taiwan and Korea cannot be directly applied for many reasons, one of which is their lower death rate. The greatest need in countries at the earlier stages of development is to define combinations of health and family planning services that will be optimum for their conditions. Because of the severe limitation of resources and the high population density, the determination of priorities should be based on more than just which health program will have the greatest impact on death rates. This means that some dramatic epidemic disease programs may have to be developed in better balance with combinations of MCH and family planning services. A major objective in such priority determination will be to bring both death and birth rates down with the shortest lag period.

In countries which consider themselves to be seriously underpopulated, such as those in sub-Saharan Africa (31, 32), priority adjustments may be even more local. Crowded urban conglomerations may need focused concentration on family planning and maternal and child care. By contrast, sparsely populated rural areas may be made suitable for human habitation by programs specifically for controlling malaria, schistosomiasis, and onchocerciasis. It should also be recognized, of course, that the world needs to retain large areas where humans leave room for nature. As disease control opens new areas, other measures must be established to limit immigration so that there will not be an immediate rush to clear forests and start farms. As the benefits of better health are brought, even to groups such as the Masai or Karamajong, family planning should be included quietly; otherwise their own populations will grow so rapidly as to cause ecological deterioration.

Similar principles relating to the stage of development also apply to special groups within countries. In the United States much attention has been given to determining if there really are five million poor women who do not have access to family planning services as claimed (33). For comprehensive planning, such priority setting is important because the selective discrimination of not having family planning can seriously hold back the progress of poor families.

The Natural History of Family Planning Program Development

The First Response to Family Planning Services

In countries or social groups where family planning has not been readily available, family planning can start by merely providing services in response to existing demand. With great uniformity, some 10 to 15 percent of women will come eagerly whenever word spreads that births can be limited. The only health education needed at this stage is to tell women where to go.

This spontaneous and immediate response has repeatedly led to initial misunderstanding of the complex social dynamics. Most of these already motivated women have five, six, or more children. Having reached the limits of their physical, fiscal, or bother tolerances they have been using whatever methods were available to them. When local indigenous methods of contraception and taboos fail, they resort to abortions (which may be the most commonly used female method of family limitation in the world today). In many rural groups, differential care favoring boys produces a significantly higher mortality of girl babies, a highly effective population control method.

Rapid initial acceptance of a new family planning program has led to two errors of judgment among those responsible for population policy. First, forward extrapolation of the acceptance curve ignores the natural plateau when the initial 15 percent of desperate women have tried the new method. Programmers set unrealistic targets and make impossible promises that birth rates will be reduced dramatically and quickly. Failure to meet such wishful targets may cause otherwise reasonable programs and methods to be discredited and discontinued.

Second, expectations are distorted because the new acceptors are counted as being added to previous efforts to limit births. Instead, these first-stage women are merely substituting the new method for those traditionally used; reduction of the birth rate results only from whatever increased effectiveness the new method provides. Realistically, therefore, only a slight fall in birth rates should be expected as a result of these initial acceptances of family planning.

The quality of care and convenience of services provided at this stage of program development largely determines the eventual success of other efforts. In the rush of stage one, services are often swamped so that efforts to cater to patient satisfaction seem unnecessary. Precisely during this busy time, however, the quality and tone of clinical and follow-up services can set the preconditions for long-term success. The best publicity is the word of mouth endorsement of satisfied users, and they should be deliberately enlisted in health education. No one is a more effective recruiter of new patients than a previously desperate friend or neighbor. Conversely, a worried and dissatisfied woman may talk incessantly and effectively negate the favorable experience of many satisfied users.

Careful attention must be given to such apparently obvious but often ignored administrative details as convenience of time and place and sympathetic care of complications. With considerate attention, the initial plateau step may slope into a continuing rise of cumulative acceptance which will progressively reduce the birth rate. Experience with campaigns for the insertion of the intrauterine device (IUD) in India has clearly shown that, when a mass program is started without sufficient attention to quality of care, repercussions may create a backlash (34). More than a quarter of women who try presently available IUD's have some bleeding, cramping, backache, or expel the device. Many will adjust to long-term use if given assurance and supportive care during the first several months. If complications continue after a reasonable trial, the women can be encouraged to use other contraceptive methods such as oral pills.

When the official IUD program was started in India, there did not seem to be time or money for such a supportive program. In order to get as rapid mass coverage as possible, mobile teams of doctors conducted "loop camps." Auxiliary health workers rounded up candidates from rural areas. The "loop and run" visits made essentially no provision for women who bleed, cramp, or expel the device. Health personnel were not themselves sufficiently confident to instill confidence. The hazards of minor complications were magnified by gossip. Minimal or totally unrelated symptoms were publicized. Among the many rumors that spread rapidly were such imaginative gems as: The S-shaped IUD was really a worm which ate the developing embryo; a husband had gotten himself entangled in a loop and had to be surgically separated with permanent damage to both partners; and nylon in the device was said to produce static electricity and electric shocks.

Such rumors naturally led many women with no complications to have their IUD's removed. These stories probably would not have started if women had been cared for as minor complications appeared. With even minimal follow-up care by health workers who believe in the device, the community gossip network can be made to work for rather than against the family planning program.

Villagers' reactions to administrative arrangements are often unpredictable. Normally, modesty demands that getting the contraceptive not be too blatantly evident to neighbors. Family planning camps such as those used in India have in the past mainly provided good publicity for family planning administrators. They may also be effective in creating public awareness and general social support for the idea of family planning, as was shown in Ernakalum District in South India, where 63,000 vasectomies were done in July, 1971. But a village woman ordinarily prefers the anonymity of a general health center. If she then wants to publicize the family planning method as a satisfied user she will talk with her friends. If an ambivalent village woman has to wait three months for a "loop camp" or travel to a city pharmacy for supplies, she usually will not bother. Most important are consideration and kindness, understanding and patience, and conviction and assurance in the daily patient contacts of family planning and health staff.

In rural societies, initial decisions about family planning are often tentative. To eventually reach the norm of only two or three children per family, methods of contraception should be adapted to varying levels of motivation. Women may be willing to start with rhythm, a conventional contraceptive, or an oral preparation. They may then move on to an IUD or sterilization because it does not require repetitive use. Increasingly reliable and long-lasting methods will be chosen as the number of children increases. Each method has a threshold of inconvenience and cost which determines the level of motivation needed for effective use. Individual differences in motivation and physiology will obviously be met best by a varied assortment of methods. The search for any one ideal contraceptive is unrealistic.

Health Care for Mothers and Children

Decisions about phasing family planning programming require recognition of the fact that much of the initial rapid acceptance of family planning derives from the pressure of health problems. A basic dictum is that parents will not stop having children until they believe that those they already have are going to survive. In developing countries, most parents grew up in homes in which half of their brothers, sisters, and friends died. Long-term behavioral adjustments in family life were based on the cultural expectation that children had about a 50 percent chance of surviving to adulthood.

With remarkable uniformity around the world, most attitude surveys show that a completed family size of three to four children is considered ideal. If half of those born die, parents naturally feel they should start with at least six children. To have the one son demanded by many cultures, parents should start with at least two sons (35, 36). As improved living conditions and better care increase the chances of child survival, an obvious lag intervenes before the realization that mortality has improved enters subconscious recognition, especially among uneducated persons. At least one generation in which almost all children survive would normally be needed for parents spontaneously to develop sufficient confidence to limit births (37).

In many developing countries, population pressure is obviously too great to permit this spontaneous, one generation transition. Instead, each healthy child can be used as an audiovisual aid in family planning education. In a comprehensive child care program, mothers can be repeatedly reminded, "See, you don't need to have another child right away."

Growing evidence suggests that the greatest cause of death in the world may be the "weaning syndrome." This synergism between common, normally nonlethal infections and malnutrition appears to be responsible for most childhood deaths in developing countries, as it was in the more developed countries until two generations ago. Typically, death results not from an event but from a sequence. The precipitating episode is usually a common infection such as diarrhea or measles. Well-nourished children recover rapidly and completely from such infections. When nutrition is borderline because weaning consists of transferring the child directly from breast feeding to an adult diet, these common infections can precipitate overt malnutrition. A serious catabolic effect of fever is significant protein loss, while diarrheas interfere directly with nutrition. Particularly dangerous are local beliefs which restrict the food of sick children to starchy gruels. Incipient malnutrition then increases susceptibility to common infections and a spiraling deterioration follows with more infections and progressive malnutrition. Death is common. For those who survive, serious sequellae in physical and mental development are even more common (38).

This syndrome responds to better nutrition, immunization, early treatment, better home environment, the diverse benefits of enlightened mothering, and being a wanted child. Such changes follow general economic development, although they are accelerated by health education and public health programs. Prevention of the weaning syndrome appears to be one of the main immediate causes of the world's population crisis, but it also appears to be essential to population limitation among the low parity women who are most important demographically.

The health of mothers can also be effectively used in family planning education. The strain of frequent childbearing may produce complications ranging from the progressive weakness of anemia and the skeletal deformities of osteomalacia to phlebitis, the convulsions of eclampsia, and direct birth trauma. Health education should provide concrete illustrations of how ability to care for present family responsibilities will be jeopardized by additional pregnancies. The postpartum period is clearly a time of maximum susceptibility to family planning education and some of the more effective programs internationally concentrate on postpartum IUD insertions.

Economic Factors

A later stage of program development is the much discussed, but so far little used, economic approach to population control. Methods must be developed to alter a family's view of its own economic prospects and its understanding of the financial implications of more children (39). Less information is available on this motivational component than on any of the others. The more developed the society, the more economic considerations seem to influence family decisions about numbers of children. These issues are of particular concern to fathers.

One hypothesis that needs testing is that in the development process an important social transition occurs when the more labile economic motivations for change take over from relatively rigid sociocultural patterns which are historically derived and static. We must learn what the sequence of these changes is and how the balance can be manipulated before social engineering for population control can be safely tried.

Clearly, the old notion that birth rates automatically come down as economic conditions improve does not necessarily hold. With economic improvement the birth rate may go up before it starts down. The first reaction to improved financial prospects is that parents feel they can now have all the children that their traditional culture had taught them was desirable. This sequence coincides with the observation that economic improvement itself lowers child mortality. My personal observation is that when economic conditions are bad and famine threatening, village people worry about having too many children. Conversely, when crops are good and conditions stable, the same people deny that they could possibly have too many children.

Children continue to represent the major investment in social security for agrarian people. When conditions are good they naturally want to put more children in the bank. When crops are abundant they need more hands to work in the fields. The economists' dogma that village economies suffer from chronic underemployment is not supported by recent research (1). With the labor intensive methods now used, a clear correlation has been found between land productivity and the number of persons available in the family for work. Although seasonal underemployment may exist, removal of labor from villages causes a marked fall in agricultural production. A clear example was the 4 percent reduction in crop acreage planted in India after 9 percent of the labor force died in the 1918 influenza epidemic, with the decline being most marked where mortality was greatest (40). A similar reduction followed the high morbidity of the 1957 Asian influenza epidemic during rice planting time in Thailand (41). The traditional conviction that in old age one's security depends on children will diminish only as other provisions for social security are developed.

One of the greatest constraints in present village thinking about development is the idea that the progress of any individual or family can only be at the expense of others in the community. In Punjab villages the local moneylenders were considered a threat mainly because, as they foreclosed debts, they accumulated land. Since the land available was limited, they were obviously taking over more and more of what had belonged to other villagers. In a stable agrarian society, there is no obvious basis for the progressive notion that a neighbor's economic progress will promote the good of the whole village. A strong underlying motivation is to advance the family group by increasing its position in the village by sheer force of numbers.

Probably the best prospect of changing the economic motivations influencing family size will become evident only after competing economic choices become available. Village people gradually learn to balance two or three educated children against an improved plow or a share in a cooperatively owned tractor.

To get such a change in motivation spontaneously will require a total climate of change to pervade village life. Change in patterns of family size will then follow changes in education, agriculture, health, and social relationships. The process can be sharply accelerated by making such economically oriented thinking explicit in general educational programs. The whole new field of Population Education attempts to mobilize such motivational factors.

A more direct economic intervention has for many years been discussed as part of national policy in developing countries (42). Possible legal provisions would include elimination of such benefits as tax concessions based on size of family, welfare allowances, paid maternity leaves, favored housing for large families, and special educational benefits for students with dependents. Women could be encouraged to do outside work. Insufficient attention is usually paid, however, to the fact that since such provisions have never been available to rural people they could then scarcely be usefully applied to rapidly growing village populations. Most direct legal manipulations are politically hazardous and certainly must be proposed extremely cautiously by any foreign assistance group.

Modifying Sociocultural Factors and Population Education
Long range demographic change involves efforts to modify sociocultural factors in motivation. Cultural blocks can be removed or bypassed and social facilitating mechanisms strengthened. This development stage is placed last in this series because it is the most difficult to implement, although some of the problems are so evident that they have been much discussed. Many demographers have been social scientists and considerable research has been attempted on cultural orientation to family size, the value attached to children, birth practices, religious beliefs, and sexual taboos. Little is known, however, about how these complicated variables can be manipulated in organized family planning programs. Certainly learning about present beliefs and practices is an early requirement in planning a program. Family planning education must start from where the people are in their attitudes and thinking.

Although cultural beliefs and values are not usually amenable to ready change, practices change more rapidly. It is often helpful, therefore, in family planning education to interpret a desirable practice in terms of an existing belief. For instance, in India, an already established system of rhythm contraception is based on ancient Ayurvedic teachings about reproductive physiology. In an agricultural analogy, menstruation is compared with plowing a field, thus preparing the uterus for fertilization. About halfway through the intermenstrual period the uterine "soil" is considered no longer suitable and the cervix no longer open, so a safe period is thought to start. According to present evidence this is precisely the time of maximum fertility. When attempts to teach about early and late safe periods were met by incredulity, the recommendation of a few further days postponement of intercourse until the "safe period" was really safe was found to be more readily acceptable.

Some social changes are so basic and important that efforts should be started now to modify behavior patterns even though results may be delayed. In high fertility situations, postponing age at marriage has a particularly powerful effect in reducing net reproduction. In many European Catholic countries, the fact that the average age of women at marriage has risen to 25 or 30 years contributes strongly to the low birth rate (4). Promoting more education of women should delay marriages, but many developing countries are having difficulty even maintaining the status quo in education because of the rate of population increase.

Underlying village resistance to family planning is a combination of fatalism and reluctance to plan ahead. When conditions of life seem to be controlled more by outside forces, such as climate or the government, than by one's own efforts, planning seems futile. Fatalism is particularly dominant in conservative religions. A powerful force in breaking down such resistance to change is the demonstration that health is not controlled by supernatural forces. A child saved after having been diagnosed by a faith healer as being doomed by an intrusion of an evil spirit or an "evil eye" can change many associated attitudes.

In summary, the last two of the above stages of population programs are long range approaches to population control. Much wisdom and preparatory work will be needed before such economic and social variables can be readily manipulated in general programs, but study of their potential should start now. In the meantime, family planning programs can move ahead through the first two stages of program development to meet presently identified and sharply increasing demand. Success in these family planning stages will make it possible to move on to the politically more delicate population control measures.

A Diagrammatic Model for Family Planning Utilization

A simple diagrammatic model illustrates some of these relationships among program planning components (Figure 18.1A). Increments in family planning utilization over time can be shown as a series of curves, each reaching its own plateau level. For conceptual clarity the steps are separated sequentially although in actuality they must overlap. Local variation determines the strength of motivation associated with each program component, but for schematic purposes, all increments are shown as being essentially equivalent.

The first curve shows the spontaneous acceptors—parents already overwhelmed by the health, economic, or bother problems of too many children. To meet such existing demand, providing family planning services to parents regardless of race or economic status is simply a matter of social justice.

The next three curves show health service components which can most logically be combined with family planning programs. Although the curves are

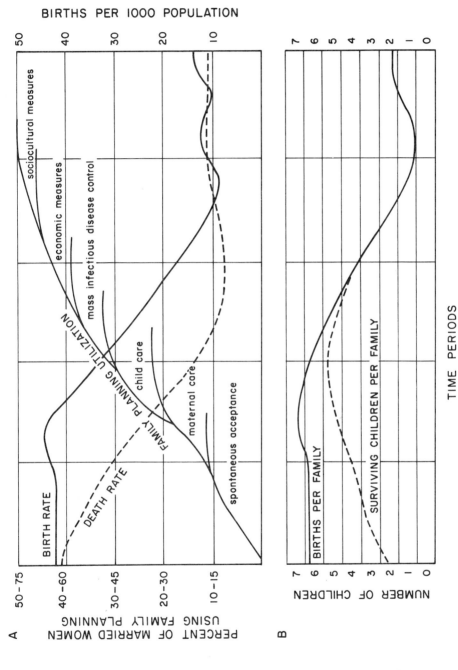

Fig. 18.1. Model of interactions between factors influencing family planning utilization, birth rate and family averages for births and surviving children.

shown separately here, the services are usually implemented in some locally determined combination having a synergistic interaction. Successive increments in family planning utilization can be expected from integration with maternal care, child care, and control programs for epidemic and endemic infections. For the greatest efficiency of personnel use, female methods of contraception can be combined with maternal and child care. Male methods can be combined with infectious disease control programs which include home visiting for surveillance; these visits can be used to provide family planning education and services to men (43).

Experience in countries such as Singapore, Korea, and Taiwan suggest that where health conditions are already fairly good, family planning acceptance may rise rapidly to a relatively high level rather than plateauing at lower levels. The cumulative effect of combined health services and family planning should bring birth rates down to about 25 per 1,000.

The next two family planning utilization curves show the effects of the economic measures and sociocultural changes which become most effective at later stages of development. Pronatalist measures should be removed and abortion legislation eased as early as possible. On the other hand, political sensitivity dictates cautious implementation of population control proposals that involve specifically antinatalist legal, social, or economic constraints or incentives.

A second set of curves (Figure 18.1B) on the same time scale shows some secondary effects during the transitional period of demographic lag. The birth rate may rise as women's health improves and they survive longer, and as cultural taboos limiting fertility are dissipated. Similarly, the number of surviving children per family rises with falling death rates until the declining number of births reduces average family size and the curves then go down together.

SPECIAL PROBLEMS IN ASSESSMENT OF NEEDS

Information Systems

Clear defintion of program objectives helps greatly in designing forms which will be most useful for such program requirements as identification of needs, quality control, establishing priorities, and evaluation. A clear distinction must be made between objectives for research purposes and for routine services.

Population programs have been strongly influenced and often dominated by demographers and social scientists with a research and survey bias. Few organized efforts in modern society have been subjected to as massive a flood of documentation. Some attempts have been made to systematize the information being collected through surveys and routine reporting, e.g., a uniform questionnaire for KAP surveys (knowledge, attitudes, and practices). An unfortunate feature of most efforts to improve data systems is that they often just add new items without cutting existing data flows. Information systems need a mechanism for raising the mortality of forms to compensate for hyperfertile production of new forms. Records and forms seem to develop lives of their own, with no one being willing to kill a form. The longer a form has persisted, the greater this protectionism becomes as administrators begin to feel that surely 30 years of files must be useful to someone. Many forms now being used originated from research interests to study causal relationships or the sources of motivation. While this is reasonable at early stages in program development, a current danger is that research data should not get built too deeply into routine forms.

Data requirements for planning fall into two categories. First are initial or periodic special surveys to identify gaps, potential program interrelations, or causal linkages relating to motivations and practice. Second is the more limited administrative information collected routinely to maintain quality control and evaluation of continuing services, with emphasis on the numbers and distribution of those served, where, by whom, for what, and with beginning information on satisfaction and outcome. A recent WHO Expert Committee listed the types of information that might be acquired through surveys to assess family planning needs (9). Publishing this extensive a list (Table 18.1) does not imply that all these data should be gathered at once, but does provide a basis for appropriate selections.

Definition of Target Groups for Family Planning Services

Planners of family planning services are increasingly developing methods of identifying target groups according to priority ranking of their need for family planning. Any definition of need will clearly be conditioned by local goals. If the dominant goals are to protect the health of mothers and children, the target groups would be those most subject to health complications from high parity. If need is defined according to human rights goals, the highest priority population groups would be minorities most subject to discrimination, but such selectivity must be applied cautiously because of the familiar stigma of genocide. Finally, for demographic goals, selection would be directed toward identifying those population groups that can be reached most efficiently to bring down birth rates.

The recurring tension between need as defined by professionals and demand as expressed by the public requires careful attention. Before making commitments on the basis of professionally defined need, the wise administrator will start by responding to existing demand in order to build a motivational base for the rest of the program. The planner's judgments about needs may be misunderstood by the public because they seem too aggressive, even on such apparently straightforward matters as deciding which contraceptives are most appropriate and safe. On the other hand, administrators and planners have also commonly made the contrary mistake of being too conservative. Surveys have

Table 18.1
Range of Information for Survey Purposes in Assessing Family Planning Needs

Population

Total population	Crude birth rate
Age and sex	Family size
Geographic (urban/rural) distribution	Distribution of birth orders
Migration patterns	Patterns of family building;
Urbanization phenomena	birth order

Cultural Considerations

Religion	Types of marital and extramarital
Languages	sexual alliances
Education and literacy	Marriage, divorce, and remarriage
Role of women	patterns
Nuclear and extended family patterns	Clan or caste groupings

Economic Aspects

Standard and cost of living	Social security and welfare
	legislation and practices

General Health Status

Crude mortality rates	Major diseases
Age or sex specific mortality rates	Nutritional status
Major causes of death	

Maternal and Child Health Status

Maternal mortality: differentials	Growth and development of
and trends; major causes	children
Infant and child mortality:	Maternal morbidities
differentials and trends;	Infant and child morbidities
major causes	Fetal, neonatal, and perinatal
Nutritional status, including	mortality
lactation status	Prematurity

Family Planning

Knowledge and attitudes	Continuation and dropout experiences
Prevalence of contraceptive	Choice of contraceptive methods
practice	and changes from one method
Consistency and quality of	to another
contraceptive practices	Substitution of one service for
Abortion practices	another
Numbers of "new" acceptors	

SOURCE: *Family Planning in Health Services.* WHO Technical Report Series No. 475. Geneva: World Health Organization, 1971, pp. 19-20.

repeatedly shown that the public is often far ahead of its leaders in its demands for family planning services (30). This is also true of specific types of family planning services such as those for unmarried women, for specific methods such as abortion, or for particular patterns of services to make them more congenial or accessible. Decisions about the balance between male and female methods have tended to focus on one partner or the other without much apparent rationale. While it seems best generally to work with the couple as a unit, the service program may usefully develop separate identification of target groups.

In many countries, efforts to identify high risk families have led to various formulas for developing community lists of eligible couples. These lists have proved most useful for organizing home visiting by either family planning staff or volunteers. Such lists usually start with identifying the married women of reproductive age (15-49 years), who usually comprise 10 to 20 percent of the population. Subcategories may be specified for priority attention on the basis of: (1) parity, (2) age, (3) health problems, (4) those who are, or are not, practicing birth control, (5) those sterilized or otherwise unable to conceive, (6) those entering the reproductive age range, (7) those currently pregnant or lactating, (8) those trying to become pregnant, (9) the infertile who want help in becoming pregnant, (10) those who reject family planning on cultural or religious grounds, (11) those who have low expectation of their children's survival and therefore fear to limit the size of their family, (12) those who have started family planning but have not returned for follow-up supplies or care, and (13) those who resort repeatedly to induced abortion for birth control. This list is offered here mainly so that an appropriate selection can be made for particular situations.

SPECIAL PROBLEMS IN ASSESSMENT OF RESOURCES

In most countries where population programs are taken seriously, services for family planning have been developed as part of the health services. Efforts to increase motivation for family planning may draw on the resources and talents of other sectors of the government or on voluntary organizations, e.g., mass media, schools, community development, professional associations, and voluntary agencies. Health planners are concerned primarily with those resources required for actual delivery of services.

As with other programs that have started as categorical activities, the general experience has been that when family planning is suddenly provided with a massive injection of resources, serious tensions and imbalance may be produced in relationships with other services. In some instances other services, especially maternal and child health, have suffered seriously when resources were diverted to family planning. This may occur indirectly when special incentives for family planning accomplishments take personnel time away from previous duties. Such experiences have clearly shown that it is best to provide for a synergistic development of family planning and maternal and child health rather than thinking in terms of either one or the other. This, of course, requires an appropriately increased allocation of funds when family planning is introduced. Dr. Cecily Williams has pointed out that more than one-half of the World Health Organization budget has been allocated to mass control of infectious disease, with 33 percent going into malaria alone (2). Maternal and child health has received less than 4 percent and until recently family planning received nothing.

Manpower

Modern services for family planning depend on health personnel. It is likely that further advances in family planning technology will only increase the involvement of health personnel because, as more specific and potent methods of modifying physiological processes or target organs are perfected, there is a greater chance that careful surveillance for complications will be needed. For instance, if prostaglandins become a recognized postconceptive birth control method, there will certainly be women who will use the method after the first month of pregnancy and thereby increase the need for facilities to care for postabortion complications. Even with such traditional contraceptive methods as condoms, the general experience has been that promotion by health workers can facilitate acceptance.

Most categories of health workers can contribute to family planning activities. Those that are most likely to be effective, however, are paramedical health workers providing care for mothers and children. The WHO Scientific Group Report (*Health Aspects of Family Planning*) lists the possible roles of various personnel (19). Greater recognition of the importance of providing routine services in homes and village subcenters has focused attention on the job description and training of auxiliary nurse midwives. Doctors and public health nurses are needed mainly for referral, support, continuing supervision, and education. In many less developed countries indigenous practitioners of medicine, and especially indigenous midwives, may be a major untapped resource for family planning.

Manpower can be increased by recruiting newly qualified personnel, by transferring workers from within the health system, or by increasing efficiency. All these approaches require careful attention to job definition and carefully structured and continuing training programs. In some countries the most important part of initiating a national family planning program has proved to be a mass training program in modern approaches to family planning for all levels of health personnel.

Efforts are being made to do special studies of family planning manpower. These range from analyses of the numbers and categories needed for specialized roles to computer models to define manpower needs (44). One example of the latter that has been effectively applied to the family planning programs of Taiwan, Korea, and Kenya is a study by Gorosh which has now been computerized for a rapid planning output (45). It is based on simplified data which are either generally available in the health system or can be approximated through expert judgment.

Facilities

An obvious general principle for good family planning care is that facilities should be as close and as convenient as possible to homes. Sometimes temporary facilities can be used for specific surgical procedures, such as the Indian-style family planning camp for vasectomies, tubectomies, and IUD insertions.The greatest weakness of such mobile activities has been the difficulty of providing follow-up. Health centers and subcenters must be strengthened to provide regular care before such intermittent mass approaches are undertaken.

Mass family planning programs face major logistic difficulties in ensuring appropriate distribution of equipment and supplies. In the delicate relationships between family planning personnel and the public, one important ingredient in maintaining confidence is that there be no break in supplies. This is most serious with certain birth control methods such as oral pills. Too much attention cannot be given to enhancing the convenience and congeniality of the environment in which services are provided, an atmosphere which does not depend necessarily on additional expenses. There are many intangibles related to whether facilities meet local standards and expectations in appearance as well as functional serviceability. Especially when auxiliary personnel are providing direct services, such as inserting IUD's, it is necessary to ensure that there is no downgrading in the provision of equipment or supplies through the sort of professional superciliousness that leads doctors to think that the best facilities must be reserved for them.

In the dramatically successful family planning camp held in Ernakulum, South India, during July, 1971, over 63,000 vasectomies were performed in one month. A surgical assembly line was set up with 50 operating tables in the town hall. A strong motivational determinant that contributed greatly to popular acceptance was confidence that good quality services were being provided. Not only was careful attention paid to good surgery and unfailing follow-up, but also the low complication rate was publicized. The physical arrangements made people conscious of the fact that cases were being carefully screened and good clinical care was provided when complications did occur.

One item that must not be slighted is the provision of transport. Functional analysis studies by the Johns Hopkins Department of International Health have shown that field workers may spend from one-quarter to one-third of their working time just walking (46). It is clearly more cost effective to invest in appropriate transportation facilities even if nothing more than bicycles can be provided or to subsidize the use of public transport. Personnel time is not only expensive but increasing personnel satisfaction and reducing their fatigue may also contribute to program accomplishments. Similarly, efficiency of services can be greatly increased by technological and educational aids. For instance, an educational and motivational process can be simplified and accelerated by an appropriate balance between audiovisual aids and personnel contact.

Finances

Sources for financing family planning need to be defined according to the goals of the program. Economic planners are sometimes so concerned about population control goals that they may say there is no limit to the funds they will make available. In some situations normal channels for distributing funds have become clogged by uncertain spurts of financing which distort other budgetary patterns at the local level. Family planning, almost more than any other service, had been a private business. Now, in a sudden shift, it has become one of the more lavishly supported public programs.

In less developed countries financing may be most severely distorted by the availability of massive financing from international agencies. Many international funding sources have placed strict limitations on how their money can be used. For justification, they sometimes express concern that health administrators will divert money to other health needs, whereas the truth is that money has more often been diverted to family planning services from other health activities. Another difficulty with international funding is that it is frequently short term and uncertain. Local officials may have to perform elaborate budgetary acrobatics to pick up activities when grants run out. Because of this, the general tendency is to use international support for short term needs such as capital construction, supplies and equipment, special training, surveys, and research.

Administrative Infrastructure

It is a truism that the effectiveness and speed of implementation of a new program will be determined largely by general administrative efficiency within the country. Even the best government services tend to have internal rigidities and constraints which may help maintain a momentum of performance once the system is established, but which almost never have the flexibility to permit the rapid development of new and innovative services. Many mass programs have started as categorical activities, partly to get out from under restrictive bureaucratic practices. If the new service can make its own rules while expanding to meet an immediate need, then once the service is established it can be integrated more readily into the rest of the health services.

Experience with other categorical programs such as malaria eradication has shown that this pattern of developing an intensive single purpose administrative structure with subsequent integration works best where there has been a longstanding gap in care for a particular disease condition or service area. Such gaps appear either because society has ignored an area of activity, as with family planning, or because a technological breakthrough provides a new method of meeting an old problem, as with malaria control. The categorical program, then, permits a period of intensive catching up in that one area.

Experience in the several categorical programs sponsored by the World Health Organization has shown that the same justifications do not apply when there are no health services. It does little good to produce a massive advance in malaria control and then have no basic services to pick up the maintenance and surveillance activities. Where all services are lacking, therefore, it is more logical to start with integrated minimum service packages which can produce maximum change.

> Many potential advantages result from providing family planning through the system of health care. Health workers have many advantages in family planning work through their opportunities to introduce the subject and services in the context of relevant activities, such as prenatal, postnatal, and post-abortal care, infant and child care and immunization, family counselling on nutrition needs, and the management of special disease problems such as tuberculosis. Health workers not only have access to people at such critical periods, but are also capable of establishing the intimate rapport that is so important in dealing with problems related to reproduction. Furthermore, many types of health worker are trained and experienced in person-to-person and group education approaches, which are essential for family planning efforts . . . .
> . . . The potential effectiveness of family planning in promoting health is further strengthened by the organizational structure established by health programmes to collect information on births, deaths, disease, the performance of health personnel, and facilities. This structure can serve as a ready means for the evaluation of the family planning components of the health services.
> There are logistic reasons also for integrating family planning with other health activities. Funds can be pooled, a stronger infrasturcture developed, supervision strengthened, and duplication of facilities avoided. Logistic problems are especially acute in the many areas of the world where women will not accept services from male workers, because of the shortages of female health personnel (9, pp. 32-33).

Program development has been greatly influenced, both favorably and unfavorably, by the personalities of individuals in authority at certain times or by the presence of influential outside consultants. A perceptive and devastating criticism of recent Indian experience is provided by Banerji, who developed the view that it was difficult for Indian administrators who rose to seniority in a colonial service where the main purpose was maintenance of law and order to adjust to post-independence programs of "social and economic uplift of the masses" (47). He was also critical of foreign consultants who were more interested in "grafting certain ideas which were developed in the Western context" than in "an experimental approach to make suitable innovations."

IMPLEMENTATION

In implementing a family planning program in the field, three chronologically definable functions need to be planned for.

First, establishing contact between the services and eligible couples may occur with the initiative coming either from the family or from health personnel. The case finding process starts with informational and educational activities to create awareness and develop knowledge and proceeds to more personalized efforts to change attitudes. Once the individual is contacted, specific identification data, a clinical history, and some sort of physical examination provide the start for a systematic record.

In the second stage, family planning practice is started. Opportunities for discussion between the couple and those providing the services are needed to get appropriate selection of suitable methods. An actual trial of different methods may be indicated with opportunity for shifting from one method to another as the couple's needs change. A dogma that has become accepted in family planning literature is that parents in less developed countries prefer to have all their children and then stop childbearing with a permanent method of contraception. This notion started from survey results in Taiwan. In other countries, however, parents seem to prefer spacing to stopping childbearing (48). In discussions about selection of contraceptive methods, it is important to be absolutely frank and open about the possibility of complications, without exaggerating the dangers.

The third stage is continuing care. Follow-up is essential with all clinical methods. It also enhances continuation rates for conventional methods. Follow-up visits must be routinely scheduled otherwise individuals most in need often end up being those who cannot or will not come spontaneously for help. Particular efforts should be made to maintain contact with dropouts.

A complicated problem in most family planning programs is to provide for an appropriate balance between central, regional, and local activities. Clearly, a strong regionalized framework is necessary in order to get rapid implementation at the periphery. Since the ultimate success of combined family planning/MCH programs will be determined largely by the performance of auxiliaries in peripheral units, primary emphasis should be placed on supportive supervision and education. It often takes time and careful guidance for health workers to get over showing that they are ill at ease when discussing family planning. When clients sense such attitudes they, too, feel uncomfortable, with deleterious effects on rapport and continuing utilization. Supervisory personnel must be supportive rather than critical in educating an auxiliary worker to communicate through the silent language of behavior a calm reassurance to parents who may be approaching the subject of family planning with considerable ambivalence. The age, sex, and marital status of health workers may influence clients receptivity in obvious ways.

Targets and Incentives

The right use of targets and incentives is an essential part of good program administration. The efficiency of personnel will be improved if they are challenged with appropriate targets and feel that good work is being recognized through reasonable rewards. In the rapid implementation of family planning programs, however, targets and incentives have often been severely abused.

Targets must be realistic rather than being so impossibly high that health workers may be left with only two alternatives, both of them bad: either to apply coercion to eligible couples or to falsify their reports of accomplishments. Such inflated targets have been set not according to what is possible but rather because of assumed demographic requirements for population control goals.

The use of monetary incentives for family planning is much argued. The massive influx of money into family planning programs has produced an almost commercial approach. More than with any other health services there has been a tendency to "buy" participation. Two patterns have emerged. In some situations health and family planning personnel receive monetary rewards usually as direct payments for each case served. A second pattern has been to make the incentive payment to the client who accepts family planning or to a "motivator" who brings in the new client. Such immediate payment arrangements work only with permanent methods of contraception. Several proposals for deferred payment through bonds or social security according to the number of years a woman is nonpregnant have also been made. These incentive programs have potential negative features and require considerable machinery in order to maintain financial control. They require carefully designed safeguards to prevent a backlash of resentment from the public and to ensure that they do not interfere with the long term motivation of personnel.

Population Education

A new emphasis in population programs is the organization of educational activities to build awareness and support for family planning into general public understanding. Included are efforts to promote understanding of demographic trends and ecological change and to develop a small family norm. Such themes are increasingly being built into educational programs in schools.

EVALUATION

The intensive involvement of multiple academic disciplines in family planning programs has led to considerable emphasis on evaluation. Because of the urgent need for research in this new field, certain evaluation activities have been somewhat esoteric. Then, too, because of the international flow of funds, evaluations have frequently been done by individuals with little understanding of local culture or program potential. Judgments have been based on comparisons between national programs rather than on understanding of local constraints. Some notable examples of such outside evaluation are the prestigious United Nations evaluation teams which have periodically reviewed the programs of countries such as India and Pakistan (49). Such major periodic exercises are most useful when they provide some objectivity in putting together ideas supplied by those running the local programs. More important, perhaps, is better continuing evaluation by those administering the programs in order to get improvement in services and to prevent early development of bureaucratic rigidities.

A variety of parameters may be used for either periodic or continuing approaches to family planning evaluation (42). The most straightforward measurement parameters are simple statistical indices of reduced numbers of births. The crude birth rate is so influenced by demographic factors such as the age distribution of the population that it is usually better to use fertility rates if data of appropriate precision can be gathered. More sophisticated analyses proceed to various measures of births prevented. Such formulations are most useful when attempting to quantify the effects of specific family planning approaches. More straightforward program-oriented evaluations depend on estimates derived from service statistics of couples accepting particular contraceptives, and some indication of current use is desirable. Time trends permit correlations with other program variables including costs. Even simpler evaluations can be made on the basis of actual program inputs, such as patients seen, personnel involved, training programs, facilities, and so forth. Again, as in so much of program planning, final decisions about evaluation methods will have to be determined by clear definition of objectives.

CONCLUDING COMMENTS

The planning of family planning programs is a new and exciting endeavor. General recognition that rapid population growth has become a worldwide crisis has led to a surge of interest and involvement by many different administrative sectors and academic disciplines. Health planners involved in family planning have a unique opportunity to establish effective collaborative relationships on a broad interdisciplinary front. In most countries, health services have been given the responsibility for organizing the expanding family planning programs. In order to justify this responsibility, we need more than intuitive evidence that integration of health and family planning works.

Since this is a new field there are more questions than answers. Program development cannot wait for the needed research findings; rather, research and services must be developed concurrently. This means that planning must be flexible and innovative. Much can be done to implement what we know now, especially the long hard process of building good local services. Some international experts recommend that money and efforts be concentrated on stimulating motivation with the expectation that more people will generate their own services. Among the poor, however, a more logical sequence seems to be to satisfy present unmet demand for combined health and family planning services so that later measures for strengthening population motivation can be more productive.

Finally, in family planning more than in most problem areas, ethical issues and values are crucial in policy decisions. The planner must develop an intuitive sensitivity to the long range implications of demographic decisions that are necessarily subject to moral judgments about right and wrong.

REFERENCES

1. Taylor, C. E. and Hall, M.-F. "Health, Population, and Economic Development." *Science* 157:651-657, 1967.
2. Williams, Cecily and Jelliffe, D. *Mother and Child Health –Delivering the Services.* New York: Oxford Medical Publishers, 1971.
3. McKeown, T. and Brown, R. G. "Medical Evidence Related to English Population Changes in the Eighteenth Century." *Population Studies* 9:119-141, 1955.
4. Coale, A. J. "The Decline of Fertility in Europe from the French Revolution to World War II." In: Behrman, S. J., Corsa, L., and Freedman, R., editors. *Fertility and Family Planning: A World View.* Ann Arbor: University of Michigan Press, 1969.
5. Frederiksen, H. "Economic and Demographic Consequences of Malaria Control in Ceylon." *Indian Journal of Malariology* 16:379-391, 1962.
6. Omran, A. R. "The Epidemiologic Transition: A Theory of the Epidemiology of Population Change." *Milbank Memorial Fund Quarterly* 49:509-538, No. 4, Part 1, October, 1971.
7. Rulison, M. *Report on Topical Investigation and Analysis of Nutritional Supplements in Family Planning Programs in India and Pakistan.* Research Triangle Park, North Carolina: Research Triangle Institute, 1970.
8. Heer, D. "Economic Development and Fertility." *Demography* 3:423-444, 1966.
9. *Family Planning in Health Services.* WHO Technical Report Series No. 476. Geneva: World Health Organization, 1971.
10. Tatochenko, V. "The Provision of Services for Regulation of Childbirth by Health Institutions in the USSR." Unpublished report of the Expert

Committee on Family Planning in Health Services, Geneva, 24-30 November 1970 (WHO HR/EC/70.3).

11. Brackett, J. W. "The Evolution of Marxist Theories of Population: Marxism Recognizes the Population Problem." *Demography* 5:158-173, 1968.

12. Davis, K. "Population Policy: Will Current Programs Succeed?" *Science* 158:730-739, 1967.

13. Hardin, G. "The Tragedy of the Commons." *Science* 162:1243-1248, 1968.

14. Blake, J. "Population Policy for Americans: Is the Government Being Misled?" *Science* 164:522-529, 1969.

15. Harkavy, O., Jaffe, F., and Wishik, S. "Family Planning and Public Policy: Who Is Misleading Whom?" *Science* 163:367-373, 1969.

16. Berelson, B. "Beyond Family Planning." *Science* 163:533-542, 1969.

17. Kangas, L. "Integrated Incentives for Fertility Control." *Science* 169:1278-1283, 1970.

18. Reinke, W., Taylor, C., and Immerwahr, G. "Nomograms for Simplified Demographic Calculations." *Public Health Reports* 84:431-444, 1969.

19. *Health Aspects of Family Planning.* WHO Technical Report Series No. 442. Geneva: World Health Organization, 1970.

20. Wyon, J. and Gordon, J. "A Long Term Prospective-Type Field Study of Population Dynamics in the Punjab, India." In: Kiser, C., editor. *Research in Family Planning.* Princeton: Princeton University Press, 1962.

21. Wray, J. D. "Population Pressure on Families: Family Size and Child Spacing." *Reports on Population/Family Planning (Population Council)*: Number Nine, August, 1971.

22. Kessler, A. "Health Aspects of Family Planning." Paper presented at the Fifteenth Nobel Symposium, Stockholm, 27-29 May 1970 (in press).

23. Taylor, C. E. "An Epidemiologic Approach to Family Planning Research." *Proceedings of Second All India Conference on Family Planning.* Delhi: Indian Family Planning Association, 1955.

24. Rosa, R. and Gulick, F. "A Quantification of the Impact of Maternity Care, Including Family Planning, on Infant-Childhood Mortality." Unpublished report of WHO Meeting on Maternity-Centered Approach to Family Planning, New Delhi, 26-28 July 1971 (WHO/MCH/71.6).

25. Taylor, C. E. "Health and Population." *Foreign Affairs* 43:475-486, 1965.

26. Taylor, C. E. "Population Trends in an Indian Village." *Scientific American* 223:106-114, 1970.

27. Taylor, C. E. "Five Stages in a Practical Population Policy." *International Development Review* 10:2-7, 1968.

28. Taylor, C. E. "Nutrition and Population." Paper presented at the International Conference on Nutrition, Massachusetts Institute of Technology, Cambridge, Massachusetts, 19-21 October 1971 (to be published).

29. Wyon, J. and Gordon, J. *The Khanna Study: Population Problems in the Rural Punjab.* Cambridge: Harvard University Press, 1971.

30. Berelson, Bernard, editor. *Family-Planning Programs: An International Survey.* New York: Basic Books, 1970.

31. Dow, T. E., Jr. "Fertility and Family Planning in Africa." *Journal of Modern African Studies* 8:445-457, 1970.

32. Pradervand, P. "Family Planning Programmes in Africa." Paper presented at

an Expert Group Meeting, OECD Development Centre, Paris, 6-8 April 1970.

33. Jaffe, F. S. "Estimating the Need for Subsidized Family Planning Services." *Family Planning Perspectives* 3:51-55, 1971.

34. *Family Planning Programme in India: An Evaluation.* P.E.O. Publication No. 71. New Delhi: Planning Commission, Program Evaluation Organization, 1970.

35. Heer, D. and Smith, D. O. "Mortality Level, Desired Family Size, and Population Increase." *Demography* 5:104-121, 1968.

36. Immerwahr, G. "Survivorship of Sons under Conditions of Improving Mortality." *Demography* 4:710-720, 1967.

37. David, A. F., editor. *Infant and Child Mortality and Fertility Behavior.* Report of a Conference held on February 17, 1971. Research Triangle Park, North Carolina: Research Triangle Institute, 1971.

38. Scrimshaw, N., Taylor, C., and Gordon, J. *The Interactions of Nutrition and Infection.* WHO Monograph Series No. 57. Geneva: World Health Organization, 1968.

39. Myrdal, Gunnar. *Asian Drama: An Inquiry into the Poverty of Nations.* pp. 1463-1531. New York: The Twentieth Century Fund, 1968.

40. Schultz, T. *Transforming Traditional Agriculture.* New Haven: Yale University Press, 1964.

41. Griffith, D., Ramana, D., and Mashaal, H. "Contribution of Health to Development." *International Journal of Health Services* 1:253-270, 1971.

42. Ruprecht, T. and Wahren, C. *Population Programmes and Economic and Social Development.* Paris: Development Centre of the Organization for Economic Co-operation and Development, 1970.

43. Frederiksen, H. *Epidemiographic Surveillance: A Symposium.* Monograph 13. Chapel Hill: Carolina Population Center, University of North Carolina, 1971.

44. Bean, L., Anderson, R., and Tatum, H. "Population and Family Planning in the United States: Manpower Development and Training." Unpublished paper of The Population Council, New York, March 19, 1970.

45. Gorosh, M. "A Systems Model for Determining the Manpower and Related Organizational and Administrative Dimensions of Family Planning/Population Control Programs." Projected Doctoral Thesis, The Johns Hopkins University, School of Hygiene and Public Health, n.d.

46. Reinke, W., Taylor, C., and Parker, R. "Functional Analysis of Health Needs and Services." In: *Proceedings of the Sixth International Scientific Meeting of the International Epidemiological Association*, Primosten, Yugoslavia, September, 1971 (in press).

47. Banerji, D. *Family Planning in India: A Critique and Perspective.* New Delhi: People's Publishing House, 1971.

48. *Integration of Health and Family Planning in Village Subcentres.* Report of the Fifth Narangwal Conference, November, 1970. Narangwal (Punjab), India: Johns Hopkins Rural Health Research Centre, 1971.

49. United Nations Advisory Mission. *An Evaluation of the Family Planning Programme of the Government of India.* United Nations Report TAO/IND/50. New York: United Nations, 1969.

ADDITIONAL READINGS

Primary

Berelson, Bernard, editor. *Family-Planning Programs: An International Survey.* New York: Basic Books, 1969.

A detailed review of the national programs for family planning in 13 countries comprises the first half of this book. Another long section deals with special topics relating to fertility control, including postpartum programs, population surveys, modern methods and new developments in birth control, and population and medical education. Several chapters describe various international advisory services.

Calderone, Mary S., editor. *Manual of Family Planning and Contraceptive Practice.* Second edition. Baltimore: The Williams & Wilkins Co., 1970.

A comprehensive survey of the medical, psychological, social, and legal aspects of contraception, with an extensive section on family planning. This volume is a significant textbook on family planning and contraceptive practice.

Family Planning in Health Services. WHO Technical Research Series No. 476. Geneva: World Health Organization, 1971.

Report of an Expert Committee dealing with the planning, administration, organization, operation, and evaluation of family planning programs within the over-all health care system. In regard to planning, consideration is given to the assessment of needs and resources and to the establishment of objectives, priorities, strategies, and phasing. In regard to implementation, the monograph deals with such topics as integration of family planning activities into health services, special aspects of manpower, facilities, finances, and utilization. Evaluation structures and methodology are also discussed.

Health Aspects of Family Planning. WHO Technical Report Series, No. 442. Geneva: World Health Organization, 1970.

A report of a WHO Scientific Group which discusses the impact of family planning on health through avoidance of unwanted pregnancies and through changes in the number of pregnancies and births and in the times at which births (particularly the first and last) occur in relation to the age of the parents. Another section considers how family planning services can be provided within the context of other health activities. The methodology of assessing health aspects of family planning is also covered.

Peel, John and Potts, Malcolm. *Textbook of Contraceptive Practice.* Cambridge: Cambridge University Press, 1969.

A comprehensive and authoritative text on the medical and sociological aspects of contraception, sterilization, and abortion. Fertility control methods are described in some detail, and one chapter is devoted to the legal and administrative aspects of birth control.

Program Area Committee on Population and Public Health. *Family Planning. A Guide for State and Local Agencies.* New York: American Public Health Association, 1968.

A compilation of the medical, social, and administrative information needed by state or local agency personnel in setting up family planning programs in the United States.

Zatuchni, Gerald I., editor. *Post-Partum Family Planning.* New York: McGraw-Hill Book Company, 1970.

Detailed report of the first two years of a study of postpartum programs in 26 hospitals in 15 countries (including Chile, India, Japan, Thailand, Mexico, Turkey, the United Arab Republic, and the United States). Sections of the book are devoted to an overview of postpartum services, education and training, achievements and problems of hospital programs, contraceptive methods, and other aspects of family planning.

Secondary

Hall, M.-F. "Birth Control in Lima, Peru: Attitudes and Practices." *Milbank Memorial Fund Quarterly* 43:409-438, No. 4, Part 1, October, 1965.

Hall, M.-F. "Male Use of Contraception and Attitudes toward Abortion, Santiago, Chile, 1968." *Milbank Memorial Fund Quarterly* 48:145-166, No. 2, Part 1, April, 1970.

Hall, M.-F. "Male Attitudes toward Family Planning Education in Santiago, Chile." *Journal of Biosocial Science* 3:403-416, 1971.

Hall, M.-F. "Male Sexual Behavior and Use of Contraception in Santiago, Chile." *American Journal of Public Health* 62: June, 1972 (in press).

Muramatsu, M. and Harper, P. A., editors. *Population Dynamics.* Baltimore: Johns Hopkins Press, 1965.

Planned Parenthood-World Population. Department of Program Planning and Development. *Family Planning Programs in the War against Poverty: A Guide for Community Action Programs.* Program Development Series No. 1. New York: Planned Parenthood, 1966.

Planned Parenthood-World Population. Department of Program Planning and Development. *Family Planning Services in Public Health Programs.* Program Development Series No. 2. New York: Planned Parenthood, 1966.

Sheps, M. C. and Ridley, J. C., editors. *Public Health and Population Change.* Pittsburgh: University of Pittsburgh Press, 1965.

United Nations. *Proceedings of the World Population Conference, Belgrade, 1965.* Three volumes. New York: United Nations, 1966.

Bibliographies of Topics in Health Planning

Aldous, J. and Hill, R. *International Bibliography of Research in Marriage and the Family, 1900-1964.* Minneapolis: University of Minnesota Press, 1969.

Altman, I., Anderson, A. J., and Barker, K. *Methodology in Evaluating the Quality of Medical Care: An Annotated Selected Bibliography, 1955-68.* Pittsburgh: University of Pittsburgh Press, 1969.

Barr, C. W. *Housing-Health Relationships: An Annotated Bibliography.* Exchange Bibliography No. 82. Monticello, Illinois: Council of Planning Librarians, 1969.

Battistella, Roger M. and Weil, Thomas P. *Health Care Organization. Bibliography and Guide Book.* Washington, D.C.: Association of University Programs in Hospital Administration, April, 1971.

Bibliography for Regional Health Planning. Baltimore: Regional Planning Council, May, 1969.

Blackman, Allan. *A Bibliography of Bibliographies on Comprehensive Planning for Health and Related Topics.* Ann Arbor: Association of University Programs in Hospital Administration, July, 1970.

Bolton, C. K. and Corey, K. E. *A Selected Bibliography for the Training of Citizen-Agents of Planned Community Change.* Exchange Bibliography No. 206. Monticello, Illinois: Council of Planning Librarians, 1971.

Bolton, C. K. and Lenz, D. W. *A Selected Bibliography on Planned Change and Community Planning Practice: Making Things Happen.* Exchange Bibliography No. 224. Monticello, Illinois: Council of Planning Librarians, 1971.

Booth, W., Beetham, M. A., and Strauss, M. *Consumer Participation in Comprehensive Health Planning.* Exchange Bibliography No. 72. Monticello, Illinois: Council of Planning Librarians, 1969.

Brennan, Maribeth. *PERT and CPM. A Selected Bibliography.* Exchange Bibliography No. 53. Monticello, Illinois: Council of Planning Librarians, 1968.

Brown, M. V. and Harten, C. J. *Health Manpower Planning.* Exchange Bibliography No. 134. Monticello, Illinois: Council of Planning Librarians, 1970.

Clark, V. V. and Davidson, L. P. *Ambulatory Nursing Care: An Annotated Bibliography.* New York: Health and Hospital Planning Council of Southern New York, May, 1969.

Community Health Service. *Utilization Review. A Selected Bibliography, 1933-1969.* Washington, D.C.: United States Public Health Service, Health Services and Mental Health Administration, 1969.

Corey, K. E. and Stafford, H. A. *Planning for Locational Change in the Delivery of Medical Care: A Selected Bibliography.* Exchange Bibliography No. 100. Monticello, Illinois: Council of Planning Librarians, 1969.

Cross, R. E. and Jordan, L. R. *Comprehensive Health Planning. A Selected Bibliography, 1960-1969.* Birmingham, Alabama: Baptist Hospitals Foundation of Birmingham, Inc., April, 1970.

Denison, R. S., Wild, R., and Martin, M. J. C. *A Bibliography of Operations Research in Hospitals and the Health Services.* Ann Arbor: University Microfilms, n.d.

Department of Health, Education, and Welfare. *Comprehensive Health Planning: A Selected Annotated Bibliography.* U.S.P.H.S. Publication No. 1753. Washington, D.C.: Government Printing Office, 1968.

Division of Regional Medical Programs. *Selected Bibliography of Regional Medical Programs.* Washington, D.C.: United States Public Health Service, Health Services and Mental Health Administration, January, 1970.

Dunaye, T. M. *Health Planning: A Bibliography of Basic Readings.* Exchange Bibliography No. 168. Monticello, Illinois: Council of Planning Librarians, 1971.

Edwards, S. A. and Hurst, O. R. *Health Care System Variables. An Annotated Bibliography, 1969.* San Antonio, Texas: Health Resources Planning Unit, Texas Hospital Association, Trinity University, 1969; Supplement 1, 1970; Supplement 2, 1971.

Federal Health Programs Service. *Automated Multiphasic Health Testing Bibliography.* U.S.P.H.S. Publication No. 2077. Washington, D.C.: Government Printing Office, May, 1970.

Golay, G. *Regional Planning and Development in Developing Countries.* Exchange Bibliography No. 43. Monticello, Illinois: Council of Planning Librarians, 1968.

Goodman, W. *Planning Legislation and Administration: An Annotated Bibliography.* Exchange Bibliography No. 57. Monticello, Illinois: Council of Planning Librarians, 1968.

Hastings, P. K., editor. *Population Control: A Bibliography of Survey Data, 1938-1970.* Williamstown, Massachusetts: Roper Public Opinion Research Center, 1970.

Hebert, B. H. and Murphy, E. *Network Analysis: A Selected Bibliography.* Exchange Bibliography No. 165. Monticello, Illinois: Council of Planning Librarians, 1970.

Hilleboe, H. E. and Schaefer, M. *Papers and Bibliography on Community Health Planning*. Albany: State University of New York, Graduate School of Public Affairs, 1967.

Kasdon, D. L., editor. *International Family Planning, 1966-1968: A Bibliography*. U.S.P.H.S. Publication No. 1917. Washington, D.C.: Government Printing Office, 1969.

Leo, Patricia A. "A Bookshelf on Poverty and Health." *American Journal of Public Health* 59:591–607, 1969.

LeRocco, A. *Planning for Hospital Discharge: A Bibliography with Abstracts and Research Reviews*. HSRD-70-17. Rockville, Maryland: National Center for Health Services Research and Development, August, 1970.

May, J. V. *Citizen Participation: A Review of the Literature*. Exchange Bibliography Nos. 210-211. Monticello, Illinois: Council of Planning Librarians, 1971.

McVeigh, T. *Social Indicators: A Bibliography*. Exchange Bibliography No. 215. Monticello, Illinois: Council of Planning Librarians, 1971.

National Center for Health Statistics. *Annotated Bibliography on Vital and Health Statistics*. U.S.P.H.S. Publication No. 2094. Washington, D.C.: Government Printing Office, 1970.

Office of Health Affairs, Comprehensive Health Service, Department of Health, Education, and Welfare. *Bibliography on Comprehensive Health Service Program*. Washington, D.C.: Government Printing Office, January, 1970.

Population Reference Bureau. "A Sourcebook on Population." *Population Bulletin* 25:1–51, 1969.

Schneidermeyer, J. *The Metropolitan Social Inventory: Procedure for Measuring Human Well-Being in Urban Areas*. Exchange Bibliography No. 39. Monticello, Illinois: Council of Planning Librarians, 1968.

Starkweather, D. B. and Taylor, S. J. *Health Facility Combinations and Mergers: An Annotated Bibliography*. Chicago: American College of Hospital Administrators, 1970.

Stoots, C. F. *Regional Planning: An Introductory Bibliography*. Exchange Bibliography No. 51. Monticello, Illinois: Council of Planning Librarians, 1968.

Strauss, M. D. "A Bookshelf on Community Planning for Health." *American Journal of Public Health* 61:656–679, 1971.

Strauss, M. *Policy Formulation in Comprehensive Health Planning*. Exchange Bibliography No. 95. Monticello, Illinois: Council of Planning Librarians, 1969.

Strauss, M. and Aronoff, L. *Bibliography of Periodicals for the Health Planner*. Exchange Bibliography No. 102. Monticello, Illinois: Council of Planning Librarians, 1969.

Tudor, D. *Planning-Programming-Budgeting Systems*. Exchange Bibliography No. 121. Monticello, Illinois: Council of Planning Librarians, 1970.

Weaver, C. *The Development of a Simulation Model of a Community Health Service System. Vol. 4. General and Annotated Bibliography.* Research Triangle Park, North Carolina: Research Triangle Institute, 1968.

Williams, H. E. *General Systems Theory, Systems Analysis and Regional Planning: An Introductory Bibliography.* Exchange Bibliography No. 164. Monticello, Illinois: Council of Planning Librarians, 1970.

Index